STUDIES IN ELOCUTION

ADAPTED AND ARRANGED

BY

T. HARROWER, F.S.Sc., LOND.,

ONE OF THE TEACHERS OF ELOCUTION TO GLASGOW UNIVERSITY,
LECTURER ON ELOCUTION IN THE UNITED FREE CHURCH COLLEGE, GLASGOW.

ENLARGED EDITION

CONTENTS.

Introduction to the Study of Elocution, ... 11

SELECTIONS IN PROSE.

The Art of Reading, ...	Mrs. Ellis, ...	21
On Reading Aloud, ...	Robert Chambers, ...	22
The Vision of Mirza, ...	Joseph Addison, ...	24
The Three Cherry-Stones, ...	Anon., ...	29
The Voyage, ...	Washington Irving,	31
The St. George, ...	Scottish Annual, ...	34
The Boat Race, ...	O. W. Holmes, ...	37
The Death of Paul Dombey, ...	Dickens, ...	39
Caleb Plummer and his Blind Daughter,	Dickens, ...	43
On the Death of President Garfield, ...	James G. Blaine, ...	49
The Story of Le Fevre, ...	Rev. L. Sterne, ...	51
Escape of Sir Arthur and Miss Wardour,	Sir Walter Scott, ...	56
A Wild Night at Sea, ...	Dickens, ...	60
Old Scrooge, ...	Dickens, ...	62
Marley's Ghost, ...	Dickens, ...	65
An Irishman's Love for his Children, ...	Anon., ...	68
A City by Night, ...	Carlyle, ...	71
Old Parson Rayne, ...	George R. Sims, ...	72
Christmas Eve in a Belfry, ...	L. Mosley, ...	82

CONTENTS.

HOUP-LA,	John S. Winter,	86
ONE NICHE THE HIGHEST,	Elihu Burritt,	93
THE MOTHER AND HER DEAD CHILD,	Hans C. Andersen,	96
A NOBLE REVENGE,	Thomas de Quincey,	102

SELECTIONS IN POETRY.

THE GAIN OF GIVING,	The Young Pilgrim,	104
THE KING'S TEMPLE,	Anon.,	105
THE GIFT OF TRITEMIUS,	J. G. Whittier,	107
A LITTLE HELP WORTH A GREAT DEAL OF PITY,	A. H. Miles,	108
KING JOHN AND THE ABBOT OF CANTERBURY,	Old Ballad,	109
ROBERT OF LINCOLN,	W. C. Bryant,	112
THE CHARCOAL MAN,	J. T. Trowbridge,	113
THE NIGHT BEFORE CHRISTMAS,	C. S. Moore,	114
MARJORIE'S ALMANAC,	J. B. Aldrich,	116
A CATASTROPHE,	P. Arkwright,	118
A MODEST WIT,	Anon.,	118
THE GLOVE AND THE LIONS,	Leigh Hunt,	119
LOCHINVAR,	Sir Walter Scott,	120
THE RIDE OF JENNIE MACNEAL,	Will Carleton,	122
THE BATTLE OF BLENHEIM,	Robert Southey,	124
PAPA'S LETTER,	Anon.,	125
THE CAPTAIN'S CHILD,	Mrs. Leeson,	127
THE DRUM,	D. Jerrold's Magazine,	129
THE NEWS-BOY'S DEBT,	Harper's Magazine,	131
A LAPSUS LINGUÆ,	Anon.,	133
EXCELSIOR,	Longfellow,	134
MEASURING THE BABY,	E. A. Brown,	135
BARBARA FRIETCHIE,	J. G. Whittier,	136
A MOTHER'S ANSWER,	L. E. Barr,	137
THE PIED PIPER OF HAMELIN,	Robert Browning,	138

CONTENTS.

DIMES AND DOLLARS, ...	Henry Mills,	... 142
ELKANO AND THE WIDOW, ...	J. T. Trowbridge,	... 148
MAUD MÜLLER, ...	J. G. Whittier,	... 151
CURFEW MUST NOT RING TO-NIGHT, ...	Rose H. Thorpe,	... 153
JANE CONQUEST, ...	J. Milne, ...	... 156
BECALMED, ...	Samuel K. Cowan,	... 160
THE LADY OF PROVENCE, ...	Mrs. Hemans,	... 162
FITZ-JAMES AND RODERICK DHU, ...	Sir Walter Scott,	... 164
THE RUINED COTTAGE, ...	Mrs. Maclean,	... 172
MARY, QUEEN OF SCOTS, ...	H. G. Bell, ...	... 174
THE BURIAL OF MOSES, ...	Mrs. C. F. Alexander,	179
THE LEPER, ...	N. P. Willis,	... 180
THE FALCON OF SER FEDERIGO, ...	H. W. Longfellow,	... 183
KING ROBERT OF SICILY, ...	H. W. Longfellow,	... 188
THE DEATH OF MARMION, ...	Sir Walter Scott,	... 192
WILLIAM TELL TO HIS NATIVE MOUNTAINS,	Knowles, ...	... 196
THE SEVEN AGES, ...	Shakespeare,	... 198
CATO ON THE IMMORTALITY OF THE SOUL, ...	Addison, ...	... 199
THE WATER-MILL, ...	D. C. M'Callum,	... 200
TO-MORROW, ...	Nath. Cotton,	... 202
THE OLD CLOCK ON THE STAIRS, ...	H. W. Longfellow,	... 203
ELEGY WRITTEN IN A COUNTRY CHURCHYARD,	Thomas Gray,	... 204
THE BELLS, ...	Edgar Allan Poe,	... 207
COMING, ...	B. M., ...	... 208

DIALOGUES AND SCENES FROM

CANUTE AND HIS COURTIERS, ...	Barbauld, ...	... 213
THE TWO ROBBERS, ...	Barbauld, ...	... 214
WILLIAM TELL, ...	Knowles, ...	... 216
A GAOL MOUSE, ...	John Cox, ...	... 219
THE HEART OF MIDLOTHIAN, ...	Sir Walter Scott,	... 221

CONTENTS.

THE FORTUNES OF NIGEL,	Sir Walter Scott,	226
THE OLD LIEUTENANT AND HIS SON,	Dr. Norman Macleod,	230
THE SCHOOL FOR SCANDAL,	Sheridan,	234
THE SCHOOL FOR SCANDAL,	Sheridan,	239
THE RIVALS,	Sheridan,	243
KING JOHN,	Shakespeare,	246
ROMEO AND JULIET,	Shakespeare,	250
HENRY V.,	Shakespeare,	253
RICHARD III.,	Shakespeare,	255
HENRY VIII.,	Shakespeare,	257
HAMLET,	Shakespeare,	261
THE MERCHANT OF VENICE,	Shakespeare,	265
THE MERCHANT OF VENICE,	Shakespeare,	269
AS YOU LIKE IT,	Shakespeare,	277
PYGMALION AND GALATEA,	W. S. Gilbert,	305

SACRED READINGS.

O GOD OF BETHEL,	312
PSALM C.,	313
PSALM XXIII.,	314
ECCLESIASTES XII. 1-7,	314
PART OF ISAIAH XL.,	315
LUKE XV. 11-32,	317
1 CORINTHIANS XIII.,	318

ADDITIONAL STUDIES.

POETRY.

THE MOUSE, ...	Anon., ...	322
THE DEAD DOLL, ...	American Magazine,	323
SOMEBODY'S MOTHER, ...	Anon., ...	324
GUILTY, OR NOT GUILTY?	Anon., ...	326
"NAY; I'LL STAY WITH THE LAD,"	L. E. Barr, ...	327
NOTTMAN, ...	Alex. Anderson, ...	329
JACK CHIDDY, ...	Alex. Anderson, ...	332
THE FIREMAN'S WEDDING, ...	W. E. Eaton, ...	334
KARL THE MARTYR, ...	Anon., ...	338
THE BRIDGE OF SIGHS, ...	Hood, ...	342
THE EXECUTION OF MONTROSE, ...	Aytoun, ...	344
THE FIELD OF WATERLOO, ...	Byron, ...	347
HORATIUS, ...	Macaulay, ...	349
VIRGINIA, ...	Macaulay, ...	353
THE RAVEN, ...	E. A. Poe, ...	357
THE MAISTER AND THE BAIRNS, ...	W. Thomson, ...	413
THE COTTER'S SATURDAY NIGHT, ...	Robert Burns, ...	414
SCOTS WHA HAE, ...	Robert Burns, ...	419
THE DOWIE DENS O' YARROW, ...	Old Scottish Ballad,	420
CHARLES EDWARD ON THE ANNIVERSARY OF CULLODEN, ...	Aytoun, ...	422
A PSALM OF LIFE, ...	H. W. Longfellow, ...	424
GIRLS THAT ARE IN DEMAND, ...	Anon., ...	425
HOW HE SAVED ST. MICHAEL'S, ...	M. A. P. Stansbury,	426
OUR FOLKS, ...	Ethel Lynn, ...	430
THE UNCLE, ...	H. G. Bell, ...	432
THE OLD MAN DREAMS, ...	O. W. Holmes, ...	437
THE BOYS, ...	O. W. Holmes, ...	438
LITTLE ORPHANT ANNIE, ...	J. W. Riley, ...	439
THE KITCHEN CLOCK, ...	J. V. Cheney, ...	441
THE OWL CRITIC, ...	Harper's Magazine,	442
JAMIE DOUGLAS, ...	Scotch Ballad, ...	529

CONTENTS.

ME AND HIM,	Anon.,	524
THE MINUET,	Anon.,	525
A FEAST OF ALL NATIONS,	Anon.,	526
IF I COULD KEEP HER SO,	Anon.,	529
THE STORY OF A FAITHFUL SOUL,	Adelaide Procter,	530
THE DOG AND THE TRAMP,	Eva Best,	532
ABOU BEN ADHEM AND THE ANGEL,	Leigh Hunt,	533
DAINTY LITTLE LADY,	Anon.,	533
CAN I GO HOME?	Anon.,	534
BABY IN CHURCH,	Anon.,	535
A PERFECT FAITH,	Anon.,	537
THE AUCTIONEER'S GIFT,	Anon.,	538
THE CHILD'S MIRROR,	Anon.,	539
THE CHILD CHRIST,	J. W. Riley,	540
TWO SURPRISES,	R. W. M'Alpine,	541
THE THREE KINGDOMS,	J. E. Bendall,	542
AN ORDER FOR A PICTURE,	A. M. Carey,	544
HER HERO,	Anon.,	546

PROSE.

JUD. BROWNIN' ON RUBENSTEIN'S PLAYING,	Adams,	362
THE BABIES,	Mark Twain,	365
THE RAPIDS,	J. B. Gough,	368
EUROPEAN GUIDES,	Mark Twain,	370
LITTLE "LORD FAUNTLEROY,"	F. H. Burnett,	445
EDITHA'S BURGLAR,	F. H. Burnett,	453
THE MORMONS,	Artemus Ward,	457
THE CELEBRATED JUMPING FROG,	Mark Twain,	459
THE THREE PARSONS,	Robert Overton,	463
DEATH OF GENERAL WAUCHOPE,	Letter,	520
THE LITTLE SCOTTISH MARTYRS,	Anon.,	551

DIALOGUES AND SCENES.

EXAMINATION OF MR. WINKLE AND SAM WELLER,	Dickens,	372
"SAM WELLER'S VALENTINE,"	Dickens,	376
FROM "HAMLET,"	Shakespeare,	379
FROM "MACBETH,"	Shakespeare,	384

CONTENTS.

From "Julius Cæsar,"	Shakespeare,	387
From "The Merchant of Venice,"	Shakespeare,	391
The Two Grave-Diggers in "Hamlet,"	Shakespeare,	393
From "The Rivals,"	Sheridan,	396
From "Rob Roy,"	Scott,	402
Mr. Pickwick and the Wellers,	Dickens,	466
Helen and Modus,	Sheridan Knowles,	471
Dialogue from "She Stoops to Conquer,"	Goldsmith,	476
Cardinal Richelieu,	Lord Lytton,	481
Scenes from "King Louis the Eleventh,"	Delavigne,	488
From "Much Ado about Nothing,"	Shakespeare,	494
Scenes from "Love's Labour's Lost,"	Shakespeare,	499
Sleep-Walking Scene from "Macbeth,"	Shakespeare,	508
Hamlet's Advice to the Players,	Shakespeare,	508
Polonius's Advice to Laertes,	Shakespeare,	509
Hamlet on a Future State,	Shakespeare,	510
Cassius instigating Brutus,	Shakespeare,	511
Brutus on the Death of Cæsar,	Shakespeare,	512
Britannia and her Colonies,	Anon.,	548

PULPIT ORATORY.

The Consequences of Sin,	Archdeacon Farrar,	406
God is Love,	Watson,	409
Love one Another,	F. W. Robertson,	410
The Field is the World,	Archdeacon Farrar,	410
Extracts from "Eternal Hope,"	Archdeacon Farrar,	513
The Loneliness of Christ,	F. W. Robertson,	516

INTRODUCTION
TO THE STUDY OF ELOCUTION.

1. **Breathing.**—Some years ago a teacher of elocution imparted "a great secret" to his pupils, for which they had to pay an extra fee, and give their word of honour not to reveal it. Like some other great secrets, this one leaked out: it was simply this—"*Breathe through the nostrils.*"

By all means practise this method of breathing, not only when reading, but at all times. Breathing habitually thus, and combining with it the constant practice of taking long, deep inspirations, you will not only acquire the first requisite for reading—namely, the full inflation of the lungs—but will also possess an invaluable means of strengthening these organs.

Again: this method of breathing imparts a strength of expression to the face which, you will observe, is altogether lacking in the weak and vacant expression of those who breathe through the open mouth.

Breathe silently. Breathing audibly gives one the idea that the speaker is straining after effect, or causes the equally unpleasant feeling that the reading is laboured, and that the reader is not at ease.

2. **Formation of Mouth.**—As in singing, so in speaking: don't speak or read in any *other* way than by forming the mouth into an *oval* shape. In the first place, that shape gives a clear channel for the emission of sound; and, in the second place, it prevents the possibility of that distortion of face which ensues

when a person reads or speaks with the mouth distended from "ear to ear."

3. Voice Production.—There are two ways in which voice sounds are produced—the one from the throat, the other from the chest.

To speak from the *throat* is utterly wrong. True, all voice sounds must come *through* the throat; but whoever throws the strain of speaking *on* the throat is violating a natural law. That habit can only result, in the case of any who speak in public, in serious injury. It is the cause, for one thing, of that disease known as "clerical sore throat." Further, in speaking from the throat you cannot produce either a mellow or a natural sound, nor can you read with ease to yourself or with pleasure to your hearers.

Produce the voice from the *chest*.

The constant practice of this method of voice production will result in the strengthening and deepening of the voice, in imparting to it quality of tone, and in affording ease and pleasure to the speaker.

Let me enforce this with all the emphasis I can use—*Speak from the chest*. As a test, place the open palm firmly on the breast: if you feel a distinct vibration, the voice production is from the chest; if there is little or no vibration, you are straining the throat, for which violation of nature you must pay the penalty of acquiring a weak, false voice. If the habit is persevered in, "worse remains behind." *Speak from the chest.*

4. Pronunciation.—Mispronunciation must ever be a fatal stumbling-block in the way of forming a refined and cultured manner in either speaking or reading.

It has been well said: "Slovenly speaking may pass in common conversation, but when speakers are required to pronounce with emphasis, and for that purpose to be more distinct and definite in their utterance, they have been so accustomed to loose, indistinct articulation that here they utterly fail. A thousand faults lie concealed in a miniature, which a microscope

INTRODUCTION TO THE STUDY OF ELOCUTION. 13

brings to view; so it is chiefly by pronouncing on a large scale, as public speaking may be called, that we prove the propriety of elocution."

While agreeing with the above, I shall be surprised indeed if pupils, *young* pupils especially, do not find, after a course of training, that they are able to *speak* more correctly than before. The study of elocution misses its mark if it does not improve *speaking* as well as *reading*.

First of all, let me impress upon learners the absolute necessity of speaking distinctly and with deliberation. Let them give to each word and to every syllable its true balance.

The following examples of the opposite practice are neither fictions nor exaggerations: they have assailed my ears for many a long day. I have heard them over and over again in the ordinary course of teaching, and I am within the mark when I affirm that ten out of every twelve pupils, at the beginning of their elocutionary studies, commit these very serious faults. The words and syllables in italics indicate the mispronunciations.

At this the mayor *an* corpora*shin*
Quaked with a mighty consterna*shin*.
Eng*lan's* sun was slowly setting.
And the royal *beas's* below.
Only by *pries's* and in the Latin tongue.
His-*kin* grew dry *an* blood*liss*.
For far the day was *pent*.
A mo*mint* speech*liss*, mo*shnliss*, amazed.
The throne*liss* monarch on *th' ange'l* gazed.
The roaring tor*rint* is deep *an* wide.
His *axe* being seven ag*is*.
The *sixt* age *shif's* into the lean *an* slippered pantaloon.
Her tall ma*s*-trembling, and her timbers *t*arting on the strain.
The close of the *las'* century.
All the pit with sand and mane
Was in a thunderous *m*other.
Th' ocazhin is divine.
Mo*s t*rangely sweet.

14   INTRODUCTION TO THE STUDY OF ELOCUTION.

Leprous 'cales.
His 'tature mod*dled* with a per*fec*' grace.
And piti*liss* manhood.
And with no *strenth* to flee.
Opening inno*cince* of a child.
With *th'* as*his* on his brow.
The *forrms* of ag*is* passed away.
The *nex'* great event was the *firs'* meeting of this board.
An ho*nist* man's the nob*list* work of God.
Jus' two days after.
Made nes'*s* inside men's Sunday hats.
Al*mos'* five hund*rid* years ago.
A*n* no*buddy* could enough admire.
All the little boys *an gurrls*,
With rosy cheeks *an* flaxen *currls*,
A*n* spar*r*kling eyes, *an* teeth like *pearrls*.
Crom*wull* will not come till sunset.
The bell *ceas's* swaying.

And now turn back and read each of these quotations *correctly*—say twice a day for a week, or *till you have mastered them*. This exercise will amply repay you.

Terminations.—The correct pronunciation of terminations seems to be almost "a lost art." Let me endeavour to show how the art may be recovered; for, without it, you can never read but in a slovenly, uncultured manner.

The termination *ed* should be pronounced *ĕd*, not *id*—*boundĕd, ĕxpandĕd, repeatĕd*.

The termination *el* should be pronounced *ĕl*, not *il*—*angĕl, gospĕl, modĕl, cruĕl, rebĕl, apparĕl, minstrĕl*. To this termination there are a few exceptions—*hazel, weasel, snivel, ravel;* pronounced as if written *hazle, weasle*, etc.

The terminations *em* and *emn* should be pronounced *ĕm*, not *um*—*emblĕm, solĕmn*.

In the termination *en*, the *e* is, as a rule, suppressed—*heaven, given, open, maiden, sudden, garden, heathen, dozen;* pronounced *heav'n, giv'n,* etc.

The termination *ence* should be pronounced *ĕnce*, not *ince*

—*consciĕnce, impatiĕnce, eminĕnce, providĕnce, silĕnce, turbulĕnce.*

The termination *est* should be pronounced *ĕst*, not *ist*—*mightiĕst, weightiĕst, heaviĕst, tenderĕst, cruellĕst, hardiĕst.*

The termination *eth* should be pronounced *eth*, not *ith*—*failĕth, enviĕth, suffĕrĕth, vauntĕth, thinkĕth, rejoicĕth, hopĕth, believĕth, endurĕth.*

The termination *ent* should be pronounced *ĕnt*, not *int*—*evidĕnt, providĕnt, eminĕnt, silĕnt.*

The termination *less* should be pronounced *lĕss*, not *liss*—*motionlĕss, restlĕss, recklĕss, resistlĕss.*

The termination *ment* should be pronounced *mĕnt*, not *mint*—*battlemĕnt, contentmĕnt, judgmĕnt, treatmĕnt, parliamĕnt, regimĕnt, momĕnt.*

The termination *ness* should be pronounced *nĕss*, not *niss*—*goodnĕss, wickednĕss, righteousnĕss, wildernĕss, darknĕss.*

The terminations *il* and *in* should be pronounced as in *pencĭl, pupĭl, vigĭl, Latĭn, urchĭn.* Exceptions—*evil, devil, raisin, cousin;* pronounced as *ev'l, dev'l, rais'n, cous'n.*

The termination *es* should be pronounced as *ĕz*, not *iz*—*agĕs, wishĕs, crossĕs, lossĕs.*

The termination *let* should be pronounced *lĕt*, not *lit*—as in *goblĕt, ringlĕt.*

The terminations *tion* and *sion.* The vicious habit is almost universal, of pronouncing these terminations as if *nation, motion, occasion, profession,* etc., were written *nashn, moshn, ocazhn, professhn.* These terminations should be pronounced as distinctly as if written *nashun, moshun, ŏccazhun, professhun,* the *tion* in every word receiving the sound of *shun.*

The sound of *ts* is often crushed out altogether; *beasts, bursts, nests, priests, hosts, requests, lost sheep, Christ's sake* receiving only the mutilated sound of *beass, ness, priess, loss sheep, Chris' sake.* In every case sound the termination before going on to the next word.

The termination *on.* The *o* is suppressed in *bacon, beacon, deacon, beckon, reckon, pardon, capon, prison, reason, treason, poison, crimson, person, lesson, cotton, blazon,* etc.; pronounced *bac'n, beac'n,* etc. To sound the *o* in these and other words would be pedantic. The *o* is sounded as *u* in *Milton, sexton, Stilton, wanton;* pronounced as *Miltun, sextun,* etc.

My—when not accented, the *y* is pronounced as in *ably, lady.*

The letter *r* has two sounds, the one rough and trilled, the other smooth and soft. When *r* begins a word, as in *rough, rugged, rain, ring, robber,* or is the second letter, as in *broad, drown, dreadful,* the rough or trilled sound should be given; but when the *r* is far on in a word, or is the last letter of a syllable, the smooth or soft sound should be used, as in *dark, storm, curse, father, curfew, murmur, leper, murder.* The soft *r* is also used in *arm, ark, art.*

The definite article. When it precedes a word beginning with a vowel, the *e* is sounded long, as, *thē acorn, thē eye, thē innocent, thē oak, thē occasion.* Before a word beginning with a consonant, the *e* is elided, as, *th' bird, th' desk, th' man, th' school.*

The prefix *ex* should be pronounced *ĕx,* not *ix—ĕxclaim, ĕxplain, ĕxperience; ex* pronounced *egz—example, examine, exalt, exaggerate, exemplary; ex* pronounced *ek—except, excess, excelsior.*

5. **Modulation.**—Both in prose and in poetry, when the sense is incomplete, keep the voice sustained; but when the meaning is clearly defined, although you have not reached the end of a sentence, or of a stanza, the voice should take the falling inflection: for instance :—

And he said, A certain man had two sons : and the younger of them said to his father, Father, give me the portion of goods that falleth to me; and he divided unto them his living.

        All people that on earth do dwell,
        Sing to the Lord with cheerful voice.

INTRODUCTION TO THE STUDY OF ELOCUTION. 17

Him serve with mirth, his praise forth tell,
Come ye before him and rejoice.

I go into my library, and all history unrolls before me. I am a sovereign in my library; but it is the dead, not the living, that attend my levees.

Hamelin town's in Brunswick,
By famous Hanover city;
The River Weser, deep and wide,
Washes its walls on the southern side:
A pleasanter spot you never spied.
Rats!
They fought the dogs, and killed the cats,
And bit the babies in the cradles;
Made nests inside men's Sunday hats;
And even spoiled the women's chats,
By drowning their speaking
With shrieking and squeaking
In fifty different sharps and flats.

6. **Pauses.**—It is a common and stupid mistake to pause at the end of a line of poetry, when the sense is not completed; as in the following :—

To see the townsfolk suffer so /
From vermin was a pity.

Instead of—

To see the townsfolk suffer so
From vermin / was a pity.

Just as he said this what should hap /
At the chamber door but a gentle tap.

Instead of—

Just as he said this / what should hap
At the chamber door / but a gentle tap.

Tripping and skipping ran merrily after/
The wonderful music with shouting and laughter.

Instead of—

Tripping and skipping / ran merrily after
The wonderful music / with shouting and laughter.

O'er the distant hills came Cromwell ;
Bessie saw him and her brow/
Lately white with sickening horror
Glows with sudden beauty now.

Instead of—

O'er the distant hills came Cromwell ;
Bessie saw him / and her brow
Lately white with sickening horror/
Glows with sudden beauty now.

And summoned Rizzio with his lute, and bade the minstrel play/
The songs she loved in early years.

Instead of—

And summoned Rizzio with his lute, and bade the minstrel play
The songs she loved in early years.

A very striking example of the error of pausing at the end of a line is seen in the following :—

Our blest Redeemer, ere he breathed/
His tender, last farewell,
A Guide, a Comforter bequeathed/
With us to dwell.

Instead of—

Our blest Redeemer, ere he breathed
His tender, last farewell,
A Guide, a Comforter / bequeathed
With us / to dwell.

Interrogative sentences, which admit of a simple affirmative or negative answer, should end with the rising inflection; as—

Who art thou? and why comest thou here?

INTRODUCTION TO THE STUDY OF ELOCUTION.

Open ! 'tis I, the kìng ! Art thou afraíd ?

Do you see yonder cloud that's almost in shape of a camél ?

Will you go and gossip with your stable-boy / when you may talk with kings and queéns ?

Awaked you not in this sore agóny ?

Had you such leisure in the time of death / to gaze upon these secrets of the deép ?

Interrogative sentences, which do not admit of a simple affirmative or negative answer, take the falling inflection; as—

    What ! my young màster !
    Why, what make you hère ?
    Why are you vìrtuous ?
    Why do people lòve you ?
  And wherefore are you gèntle, stròng, and vàliant ?

Who is it that causes this river to rise in the high mountains, and to empty itself in the òcean ? Who is it that causes to blow the loud winds of winter, and that calms them again in the sùmmer ? Who is it that rears up the shade of these lofty forests, and blasts them with the quick lightning of his plèasure ? The same Great Spirit who gàve to you a country on the other side of the wàters, and gave ours to ùs.

In issuing this new Text-book, I have again to thank, very sincerely, those authors and publishers who have kindly granted me permission to insert extracts from copyright works.

                T. HARROWER.

SELECTIONS IN PROSE.

THE ART OF READING.

IF, in our ideas of the *fine arts* / we include all those embellishments of civilized life / which combine, in a high degree, the gratification of a refined taste / with the exercise of an enlightened intellect, then / must reading aloud / hold a prominent place amongst those arts / which impart a charm to social intercourse, and purify the associations of ordinary life. But it must be *good* reading, or the enjoyment is exchanged for unspeakable annoyance: not pompous or theatrical reading, but easy, familiar, and judicious reading; such reading as best conveys to the hearers / the true meaning of the writer.

It certainly does appear strange / that those who speak every day / with the tone of right reason / and the emphasis of truth, should so pervert that beautiful instrument of music, the human voice, as to read aloud with any tone and emphasis / but those which are right and true. Yet, so it is; and many a youth / now sent home from school or college, after a costly, and what is called a *finished*, education, is wholly incapable of reading / so as not at the same time / to disgrace himself / and offend his hearers.

It is sometimes said / that nothing can be easier / than to read well, if persons understand what they are reading. But where, then, *are* the good readers / who find it so easy? or where, in other words, are the people of understanding? for certainly many of our readers / would be utterly unable to understand *themselves*, were not the sense of what they utter / conveyed to their minds / through the medium of sight.

When all the necessary requisites for a good reader / are taken into account, we wonder / not so much that this accomplishment is neglected, as that it does not constitute, with all who look upon education / in its true light, an important means of refining / and elevating the mind, of cultivating the sympathies, and of improving those habits of perception and adaptation / which are so valuable to all.

Reading aloud, and reading well, ought not to be considered / as mere amusement. A good book / well read / is like the conversation of an intelligent friend, and ought to be treated / with the same respect. It forms, in fact, a rallying point, around which different tempers, feelings, and constitutions can meet / without discord; it tends to draw each mind / out of its petty cares / and perplexities, to meet with other minds / on common ground, where a wider extent of interest, and often a nobler range of thought, have the effect of showing, by contrast, how trivial and unimportant / are the things of self, when compared with the great aggregate / of human happiness / and misery.

Mrs. Ellis.

ON READING ALOUD.

Charles Kemble / has been reading Shakespeare / to London audiences; and it would be well if, from among the thousands who listened to him, a few could be induced / to carry the practice / into private life. We know of no accomplishment so valuable / as that of reading "with good emphasis and discretion," of catching the meaning and spirit of an author, and conveying them to others / with a distinct and intelligible utterance; and yet, strange to say, there is no department of modern education / so much neglected. Indeed, so general is this neglect, that scarcely one young lady or gentleman in a dozen / who boast of having "finished" their education can, on being requested, read aloud to a private company / with that ease / and graceful modulation / which is necessary to the perfect appreciation of the author. There is either a forced and unnatural mouthing, a hesitating and imperfect articulation, or a monotony of tone / so thoroughly painful that one listens with impatience, and is glad when some excuse presents itself / for his absence. Whatever may be the imperfections of our school tuition, the main evil / arises from the unequal value / which seems to be attached to good reading / as compared with music, dancing, painting, and other fashionable acquirements. Why it should be so, we can discover no good cause, but, on the contrary, see many substantial reasons / why reading aloud should be cultivated / as one of the most useful / and attractive / of domestic accomplishments.

To young ladies / the habit of reading aloud / has much to recommend it. The mental pleasure to be derived therefrom / is one of the most delightful / that can adorn the family circle. Gathered round the winter's fire, what could be more cheerful / for the aged and infirm, what more instructive to the younger branches or more exemplary to the careless, than the reading aloud / of some entertaining author?

Another advantage / which it would confer on the readers themselves / would be the improved utterance and intonation / which correct reading would produce, instead of that simpering and lisping / which are so often to be met with / even among ladies of the higher classes.

To young men preparing for professional labours / the art of reading aloud / is indispensable; and though not equally necessary / for what are called business men, still to such / it is a becoming / and valuable acquirement. Ask your son, who has lately gone to business, to read you the last debate in Parliament, and ten to one / he will rattle through it / with such a jumbling indistinctness of utterance, that you are glad when his hour calls him away, and leaves you / to the quiet enjoyment / of self-perusal. And why is this? Simply because he has never been taught / to regard reading aloud / in the light of a graceful accomplishment. At school / he learned to know his words, and that was so far useful ; but to read in the spirit and meaning of the author—this is what he has yet to acquire.

Music is cried up on all hands ; why not reading ? We have in almost every family / evidence of what practice has done for vocal music; why not the same for reading aloud ? The one art / is chiefly valued as an amusement / and refining accomplishment; the other / is equally entertaining, quite as necessary for the adornment of public or private life, and certainly more directly productive / of utility and knowledge.   CHAMBERS.

THE VISION OF MIRZA.

On the fifth day of the moon, which, according to the custom of my forefathers, I always keep holy, after having offered up my morning devotions, I ascended the high hills of Bagdat, in order to pass the rest of the day / in meditation and prayer. As I was here airing myself on the tops of the mountains, I fell into a profound contemplation / on the vanity of human life; and passing from one thought to another, "Surely," said I, "man is but a shadow, and life a dream." Whilst I was thus musing, I cast mine eyes towards the summit of a rock / that was not far from me, where I discovered one in the habit of a shepherd, with a little musical instrument in his hand. As I looked upon him, he applied it to his lips, and began to play upon it. The sound of it was exceeding sweet, and wrought into a variety of tunes / that were inexpressibly melodious, and altogether different / from anything I had ever heard. They put me in mind of those heavenly airs / that are played to the departed souls of good men / upon their first arrival in paradise, to wear out the impressions of their last agonies, and qualify them for the pleasures of that happy place. My heart melted away in secret raptures.

I had been often told / that the rock before me / was the haunt of a Genius, and that several had been entertained with music / who had passed by it; but never heard that the musician had before made himself visible. When he had raised my thoughts, by those transporting airs which he played, to taste the pleasures of his conversation, as I looked upon him like one astonished, he beckoned to me, and by the waving of his hand / directed me to approach the place where he sat. I drew near with that reverence / which is due to a superior nature; and as my heart was entirely subdued by the captivating strains I had heard, I fell down at his feet and wept. The Genius smiled upon me / with a look of compassion and affability / that familiarized him to my imagination, and at once dispelled all the fears and apprehensions / with which I approached him. He lifted me from the ground, and taking me by the hand, "Mirza," said he, "I have heard thee in thy soliloquies; follow me."

He then led me to the highest pinnacle of the rock, and placing me on the top of it, "Cast thy eyes eastward," said he, "and tell me what thou seest." "I see," said I, "a huge valley, and a prodigious tide of water rolling through it." "The valley that thou seest," said he, "is the Vale of Misery; and the tide of water that thou seest / is part of the great tide of Eternity." "What is the reason," said I, "that the tide I see / rises out of a thick mist at one end, and again loses itself / in a thick mist at the other?" "What thou seest," said he, "is that portion of Eternity which is called Time, measured out by the sun, and reaching from the beginning of the world to its consummation. Examine now," said he, "this sea that is bounded with darkness at both ends, and tell me what thou discoverest in it." "I see a bridge," said I, "standing in the midst of the tide." "The bridge thou seest," said he, "is Human Life; consider it attentively." Upon a more leisurely survey of it, I found that it consisted of threescore and ten entire arches, with several broken arches, which, added to those that were entire, made up the number to about an hundred.

As I was counting the arches, the Genius told me / that this bridge consisted at first / of a thousand arches, but that a great flood / swept away the rest, and left the bridge / in the ruinous condition / I now beheld it. "But tell me further," said he, "what thou discoverest on it?" "I see multitudes of people / passing over it," said I, "and a black cloud / hanging on each end of it." As I looked more attentively, I saw several of the passengers / dropping through the bridge / into the great tide / that flowed underneath it; and, upon further examination, perceived there were innumerable trap-doors / that lay concealed in the bridge, which the passengers no sooner trod upon / but they fell through them / into the tide, and immediately disappeared. These hidden pit-falls / were set very thick at the entrance of the bridge, so that throngs of people / no sooner broke through the cloud / but many of them fell into them. They grew thinner / towards the middle, but multiplied and lay closer together / towards the end of the arches that were entire.

There were, indeed, some persons, but their number was very small, that continued a kind of hobbling march / on the broken arches, but fell through one after another, being quite tired and spent / with so long a walk.

I passed some time in the contemplation of this wonderful structure / and the great variety of objects which it presented. My heart was filled with a deep melancholy / to see several dropping / unexpectedly / in the midst of mirth and jollity, and catching at everything that stood by them / to save themselves. Some were looking up towards the heavens / in a thoughtful posture, and in the midst of a speculation / stumbled and fell out of sight. Multitudes were very busy in the pursuit of bubbles / that glittered in their eyes / and danced before them; but often when they thought themselves within the reach of them, their footing failed, and down they sank. In this confusion of objects, I observed many with scimitars in their hands, who ran to and fro upon the bridge, thrusting several persons on trap-doors / which did not seem to lie in their way, and which they might have escaped / had they not been thus forced upon them.

The Genius, seeing me indulge myself on this melancholy prospect, told me I had dwelt long enough upon it. "Take thine eyes off the bridge," said he, "and tell me if thou yet seest anything thou dost not comprehend." Upon looking up, "What mean," said I, "those great flights of birds / that are perpetually hovering about the bridge, and settling upon it from time to time? I see vultures, harpies, ravens, cormorants, and, among many other feathered creatures, several little winged boys, that perch in great numbers upon the middle arches." "These," said the Genius, "are Envy, Avarice, Superstition, Despair, Love, with the like cares and passions / that infest human life."

I here fetched a deep sigh. "Alas!" said I, "man was made in vain! How is he given away to misery and mortality, tortured in life / and swallowed up in death!" The Genius, being moved with compassion towards me, bade me quit so uncomfortable a prospect. "Look no more," said he, "on man in the first stage of his existence, in his setting out for Eternity; but cast thine eye / on that thick mist into which the tide bears the several generations of mortals / that fall into it." I directed my sight as I was ordered, and (whether or no the good Genius strengthened it / with any supernatural force, or dissipated part of the mist / that was before too thick for the eye to penetrate) I saw the valley / opening at the farther end, and spreading forth / into an immense ocean, that had a huge rock of adamant / running through the midst of it, and dividing it into two equal parts. The clouds still rested on one half of it, insomuch that I could discover nothing in it; but the other appeared to me a vast ocean / planted with innumerable islands, that were covered with fruits and flowers, and interwoven with a thousand little shining seas / that ran among them. I could see persons dressed in glorious habits, with garlands upon their heads, passing among the trees, lying down by the sides of fountains, or resting on beds of flowers; and could hear a confused harmony of singing birds, falling waters, human voices, and musical instruments. Gladness grew in me / upon the discovery of so delightful a scene. I wished for the wings of an eagle / that I might fly away to those happy seats; but the Genius told me / there was no passage to them / except through the gates of death / that I saw opening every moment upon the bridge. "The islands," said he, "that lie so fresh and green before thee, and with which the whole face of the ocean / appears spotted as far as thou canst see, are more in number than the sands on the sea-shore. There are myriads of islands behind those which thou here discoverest, reaching further than thine eye, or even thine imagination, can extend itself. These are the mansions of good men / after death, who, according to the degree and kinds of virtue / in which they excelled, are distributed among these several islands, which abound with pleasures of different kinds and degrees, suitable to the relishes and perfections / of those who are settled in them. Every island is a paradise / accommodated to its respective inhabitants. Are not these, O Mirza! habitations worth contending for? Does life appear miserable, that gives thee opportunities / of earning such a reward? Is death to be feared, that will convey thee / to so happy an existence? Think not / man was made in vain, who has such an eternity / reserved for him." I gazed with inexpressible pleasure on these happy islands. "At length," said I, "show me now, I beseech thee, the secrets that lie hid / under those dark clouds / which cover the ocean on the other side / of the rock of adamant." The Genius making me no answer, I turned about to address myself to him a second time; but I found that he had left me. I then turned again to the vision / which I had been so long contemplating; but instead of the rolling tide, the arched bridge, and the happy islands, I saw nothing but the long, hollow valley of Bagdat, with oxen, sheep, and camels grazing upon the sides of it.

JOSEPH ADDISON.

THE THREE CHERRY-STONES.

Three young gentlemen, who had finished the most substantial part of their repast, were lingering over their fruit and wine at a tavern in London, when a man of middle age entered the public room where they were sitting. He sat down at one end of a small, unoccupied table, and calling the waiter, ordered a mutton chop and a glass of ale. His appearance, at first view, was not likely to arrest the attention of any one. His hair was beginning to be thin and gray; the expression of his countenance was sedate, with a slight touch perhaps of melancholy; and he wore a gray surtout with a standing collar, which manifestly had seen service, if the wearer had not. He might have been taken for a country magistrate, an attorney of limited practice, or a schoolmaster.

He continued to masticate his chop and sip his ale in silence, without lifting his eyes from the table, until a cherry-stone, sportively snapped from the thumb and finger of one of the gentlemen at the opposite table, hit him upon his right ear. His eye was instantly upon the aggressor, and his ready intelligence gathered from the ill-suppressed merriment of the party that this petty impertinence was intentional.

The stranger stooped, and picked up the cherry-stone. A scarcely preceptible smile passed over his features as he carefully wrapped it up in a piece of paper and put it in his pocket. This singular procedure, with their preconceived impressions of the stranger, somewhat elevated, as the young gentlemen were, by the wine they had partaken of, upset their gravity entirely, and a burst of laughter broke from the group.

Unmoved by this rudeness, the stranger continued to finish his frugal repast in quiet, until another cherry-stone, from the same hand, hit him upon his right elbow. This also, to the infinite amusement of the other party, he picked from the floor, and carefully placed with the first stone.

Amidst shouts of laughter, a third cherry-stone was soon

after discharged, which hit him upon his left breast. This also he very deliberately lifted, and placed beside the other two.

As he rose, and was paying for his repast, the gaiety of these sporting gentlemen became slightly subdued. It was not easy to account for this. There was not the slightest evidence of irritation or resentment upon the features of the stranger. He walked to the table at which they were sitting, and with that air of dignified calmness which is a thousand times more terrible than wrath, drew a card from his pocket, and presented it with perfect civility to the offender, who could do no less than offer his own in return. While the stranger unbuttoned his surtout to take the card from his pocket, they saw he wore the undress coat of a military officer. The card disclosed his rank, and a brief inquiry at the bar was sufficient for the rest. He was a captain whom ill-health and long service had entitled to half-pay. In earlier life he had been engaged in several affairs of honour, and, in the dialect of the day, was "a dead shot."

The next morning a note arrived at the aggressor's residence, containing a challenge, and *one* of the cherry-stones. The truth then flashed before the challenged party—it was the challenger's intention to make three separate affairs out of this unwarrantable frolic! The challenge was accepted, and the challenged party, in deference to the challenger's reputed skill with the pistol, had half decided upon the small sword; but his friends, who were on the alert, soon discovered that the captain, who had risen by his merit, had been in his earlier days an accomplished instructor in the use of that weapon.

They met, and fired alternately, by lot. The young man had selected this mode, thinking he might win the first fire: he did —fired, and missed his opponent. The captain levelled his pistol and fired: the ball passed through the flap of the right ear, and grazed the bone; and, as the wounded man involuntarily put his hand to the place, he remembered it was the right ear of his antagonist on which the cherry-stone had fallen.

Here ended the first lesson. A month passed. His friends cherished the hope that he would hear nothing more from the captain, when one day another challenge and another of those ominous cherry-stones arrived, with the captain's apology, on the score of ill-health, for not sending it before.

Again they met, fired simultaneously, and the captain, who was unhurt, shattered the right elbow of his antagonist—the very point upon which he had been struck with the cherry-stone. Here ended the second lesson. There was something awfully impressive in the *modus operandi*, and exquisite skill, of his antagonist. The third cherry-stone was still in his possession, and the aggressor had not forgotten that it had struck the unoffending gentleman upon the left breast. A month passed—another—and another, of terrible suspense; but nothing was heard from the captain.

One day the gentleman who had been his second in the former duels called, and tendered another note. The address was written in the captain's well-known hand, but it was the writing of one who wrote feebly. There was an unusual solemnity also in the manner of him who delivered it. The seal was broken, and there was the cherry-stone in a blank envelope.

"And what, sir, am I to understand by this?" inquired the aggressor.

"You are to understand, sir, that my friend forgives you—he is dead!" ANONYMOUS.

THE VOYAGE.

I said that at sea all is vacancy: I should correct the expression. To one given to day-dreaming, and fond of losing himself in reveries, a sea voyage is full of subjects for meditation; but then they are the wonders of the deep, and of the air, and rather tend to abstract the mind from worldly themes. I delighted to loll over the quarter railing, or climb to the main-top on a calm day, and muse for hours together on the tranquil bosom of a summer's sea; to gaze upon the piles of golden clouds just peering above the horizon, fancy them some fairy realms, and people them with a creation of my own; to watch the gentle, undulating billows rolling their silver volumes, as if to die away on those happy shores.

There was a delicious sensation of mingled security and awe, with which I looked down from my giddy height on the monsters of the deep at their uncouth gambols—shoals of porpoises tumbling about the bow of the ship, the grampus slowly heaving his huge form above the surface, or the ravenous shark darting like a spectre through the blue waters. My imagination would conjure up all that I had heard or read of the watery world beneath me—of the finny herds that roam its fathomless valleys, of the shapeless monsters that lurk among the very foundations of the earth, and of those wild phantasms that swell the tales of fishermen and sailors.

Sometimes a distant sail, gliding along the edge of the ocean, would be another theme of idle speculation. How interesting this fragment of a world, hastening to rejoin the great mass of existence! What a glorious monument of human invention, that has triumphed over wind and wave; has brought the ends of the world into communion; has established an interchange of blessings, pouring into the sterile regions of the north all the luxuries of the south; has diffused the light of knowledge and the charities of cultivated life; and has thus bound together those scattered portions of the human race between which nature seemed to have thrown an insurmountable barrier!

We one day descried some shapeless object drifting at a distance. It proved to be the mast of a ship that must have been completely wrecked; for there were the remains of handkerchiefs, by which some of the crew had fastened themselves to this spar, to prevent their being washed off by the waves. There was no trace by which the name of the ship could be ascertained. The wreck had evidently drifted about for many months; clusters of shell-fish had fastened about it, and long sea-weeds flaunted at its sides. But where, thought I, is the crew? Their struggle has long been over; they have gone down amidst the roar of the tempest; their bones lie whitening among the caverns of the deep! Silence, oblivion, like the waves, have closed over them, and no one can tell the story of their end. What sighs have been wafted after that ship! what prayers offered up at the deserted fireside of home! How often has the wife, the mother, pored over the daily news, to catch some casual intelligence of this rover of the deep! How has expectation darkened into anxiety, anxiety into dread, and dread into despair! Alas! not one memento shall ever return for love to cherish. All that shall ever be known is, that she sailed from her port, "and was never heard of more!"

In the evening, the weather, which had hitherto been fair, began to look wild and threatening, and gave indications of one of those sudden storms that will sometimes break in upon the serenity of a summer voyage. The storm increased with the night. The sea was lashed into tremendous confusion. There was a fearful, sullen sound of rushing waves and broken surges. Deep called unto deep. At times the black volume of clouds overhead seemed rent asunder by flashes of lightning that quivered along the foaming billows, and made the succeeding darkness doubly terrible. The thunders bellowed over the wild waste of waters, and were echoed and prolonged by the mountain waves. As I saw the ship staggering and plunging among these roaring caverns, it seemed miraculous that she regained her balance or preserved her buoyancy. Her yards would dip into the water; her bow was almost buried beneath the waves. Sometimes an impending surge appeared ready to overwhelm her, and nothing but a dexterous movement of the helm preserved her from the shock.

When I retired to my cabin the awful scene still followed me. The whistling of the wind through the rigging sounded like funereal wailings. The creaking of the masts, the straining and groaning of bulkheads, as the ship laboured in the weltering sea, were frightful. As I heard the waves rushing along the side of the ship, and roaring in my very ear, it seemed as if Death were raging round this floating prison, seeking for his prey; the mere starting of a nail, the yawning of a seam, might give him entrance.

A fine day, however, with a tranquil sea and favouring breeze, soon put all these dismal reflections to flight. It is impossible to resist the gladdening influence of fine weather and fair winds at sea. When the ship is decked out in all her canvas, every sail swelled, and careering gaily over the curling waves, how lofty, how gallant she appears—how she seems to lord it over the deep! I might fill a volume with the reveries of a sea voyage, for with me it is almost a continual reverie.

WASHINGTON IRVING.

THE ST. GEORGE.

It stood in the artist's studio: all Florence came to look at it; all examined it with curiosity; all admired it with eagerness. The whole town was in raptures, and ladies, as they bent from their carriages to answer the salutes of princes and dukes, instead of the commonplace frivolities of fashion, said, "Have you seen the new statue by Donatello?"

Is there an art like that of sculpture? Painting is a brilliant illusion—a lovely cheat; but the chisel works in eternal marble—strikes out a creation immortal as the globe.

"I told thee, Donatello," said Lorenzo, "thou wouldst excel all thy rivals!"

"Fling by thy chisel now," cried another, "thou canst add nothing to that!"

"I shall cease, hereafter, my devotion to the antique!" cried a third.

"The power of Phidias!" exclaimed one.

"The execution of Praxiteles!" said another.

"You will draw votaries from Venus," whispered a soft Italian girl, as she turned her melting eyes on the old man.

"The Apollo will hereafter draw his bow unheeded!" cried an artist, whom many thought the best of his day.

Among the crowds who flocked to the studio of Donatello, there was a youth who had given some promise of excellence. Many said that, with intense-study, he might one day make his name heard beyond the Alps; and some went so far as to hint that, in time, he might tread close on the heels even of Donatello himself. But these were sanguine men, and great friends of the young man; besides, they spoke at random. They called this student Michael Angelo.

He had stood a long time regarding it with fixed eyes and folded arms. He walked from one position to another, measured it with his keen glance from head to foot, regarded it before, behind, and studied its profiles from various points. The venerable Donatello saw him, and awaited his long and absorbed examination with the flattered pride of an artist and the affectionate indulgence of a father. At length Michael Angelo stopped once before it, inhaled a long breath, and broke the profound silence. "It wants only one thing," muttered the gifted boy.

"Tell me," cried the successful artist, "*what* it wants. This is the first censure which my St. George has elicited. Can I improve? Can I alter? Is it in the clay or the marble? Tell me!"

But the critic had disappeared.

Donatello knew the mighty genius of Michael Angelo. He had beheld the flashes of the sacred fire, and watched the development of the spirit within him.

"What!" cried the old man, "Michael Angelo gone to Rome, and not a word of advice about my statue! The scapegrace! but I shall see him again, or, by the mass, I will follow him to the eternal city. His opinion is worth that of all the world!— 'But one thing!'" He looked at it again—he listened to the murmurs of applause which it drew from all who beheld it—a placid smile settled on his face. "But one thing!—what can it be?"

Years rolled by. Michael Angelo remained at Rome, or made excursions to other places, but had not yet returned to Florence. Wherever he had been, men regarded him as a comet—something fiery, terrible, tremendous, sublime. His fame spread over the globe; what his chisel touched, it hallowed. He spurned the dull clay, and struck his vast and intensely brilliant conceptions at once from the marble. Michael Angelo was a name to worship; an honour to Italy—to the world. What he praised, lived; what he condemned, perished.

As Donatello grew old, his anxiety grew more powerful to know what the inspired eyes of the wonderful artist had detected in his great statue.

At length the immortal Florentine turned his eyes to his native republic.

Ah, death! can no worth ward thee? Must the inspired artist's eyes be dark, his hand motionless, his heart still, and his inventive brain as dull as the clay he models? Yes! Donatello lies stretched on his last couch, and the light of life is passing from his eyes; yet even in that awful hour his thoughts ran on the wishes of his past years, and he sent for the Florentine artist.

"I am going, Michael—my chisel is idle, my vision is dim; but I feel thy hand, my noble boy, and I hear thy kind breast sob. I glory in thy renown; I predicted it, and I bless my Creator that I have lived to see it. But before I sink into the tomb, I charge thee, on thy friendship, on thy religion, answer my question truly."

"As I am a man, I will."

"Then tell me, without equivocation, what it is that my St. George wants?"

"The gift of speech!" was the reply.

A gleam of sunshine fell across the old man's face.

The smile lingered on his lips long after he lay cold as the marble upon which he had so often stamped the conceptions of his genius. *Scottish Annual.*

THE BOAT RACE.

[ADAPTED.]

There are few pleasanter spots for a summer residence than by the shores of Cedar Lake. At the southern extremity stands Stoughton University; at the northern end is the Corouna Academy for young ladies; midway, and fringing the shore, lies the village of Arrow-head.

The attractions of this village are really remarkable—boating in summer, skating in winter, varied and lovely walks through the valley and up the hill-sides; houses sheltered from the north and east winds, and cooled in the hot summer days by the refreshing breeze which comes over the water. All this makes the frame for a pleasant picture of rest and happiness.

Then there is the annual boat race, rowed by a crew of eight young ladies from the Academy, and a crew of eight young students from the College.

The starting-point is opposite the village; the course, one mile to the south and back—two miles in all; distance allowed to the young ladies' boat, eight lengths.

The first of June last year was a delicious summer day, still and bright, the water as smooth as glass. All were on the tip-toe of expectation.

At last the students' boat shot out from the creek where she lay. It was a beautiful sight to see these eight young fellows in their suits of white flannel and blue caps, their brown, muscular arms bare, bending their backs to the oars as if they were parts of a single machine.

"The gals can't stand agin them fellers," said the old blacksmith.

"You jest wait till the gals git agoin'," said the old carpenter. "Ye ought tew see 'em climb ropes an' swing dumb-bells at the institootion. I reckon, Jake, them gals can row a mile in double-quick time."

"Wal, I dunno jest what tew say," said Jake, an old fisherman. "I've seed 'em both, often, when they was a prac*ti*sin', an' I tell you, thar wan't no slouch 'bout neither o' 'em ; but, ye see, the young fellers is nat'rally longer-winded than the gals."

And now the Corouna boat swept into view, with her eight rowers in dark-blue costumes and white straw hats.

If the sight of the College boat was beautiful, how lovely was this! Eight young girls (young ladies, for those who prefer that more dignified and less attractive expression), all in the flush of youth and vigorous health—every muscle taught its duty—each rower alert not to be a tenth of a second out of time, or let her oar dally with the water so as to lose an ounce of its propelling virtue—no rocking—no splashing—no apparent effort.

And now, "Take your places!" cries the umpire: the two boats feel their way slowly to their respective positions, the girls' eight lengths in front of the students'.

And now, there they are—bodies bent forward, arms outstretched, oars in the water—waiting for the word "Go!"

Away springs the *Corouna*, and, eight lengths behind her, leaps the College boat. And now, half the distance has been rowed: the girls' boat is rounding the buoy, the students' four lengths behind; but every minute she is gaining. Now there is but one length between them, when the captain of the students' boat turns his head and sees the coxswain of the *Corouna* bending forward at every stroke, as if *her* weight were of such mighty consequence that a few ounces might turn the scale of victory!

But he saw more—he caught a glimpse of the stroke-oar of the *Corouna*. What a flash of loveliness it was! Her face and neck like the reddest of June roses, with the strain and heat of expected triumph.

The captain of the students' boat was a stanch and steady rower; but he was human—the blade of his oar lingered a moment in the water: the boat, which seemed to possess all the life and nervousness of a Derby favourite, felt the check, and all her men bent with more vigour to their oars. The girls saw this movement, and made a spurt to keep their lead. It was of no use—slowly but surely the other boat was gaining on them.

The little coxswain of the *Corouna* now held aloft a lovely bouquet. "Look!" she cried, and flung it in front of the students' boat. The captain again looked round, and there, once more, was that lovely vision which had a minute ago bewitched him.

She must have thrown the bouquet. Yes! it was a challenge; he must accept it. He was sure of the race—he would sweep past the winning line in triumph with that bouquet at the bow of his boat—he stoops, and picks it up.

Now the students' bow creeps past the stern of the *Corouna*—now her bow is on a level with the fourth fair rower— now they are bow to bow—the winning line is only a few yards in front—every rower is straining desperately, madly, when, crack goes one of the students' oars, and up flash its splintered fragments, as the bow of the *Corouna* springs past the line eighteen inches ahead of the students' boat!

OLIVER WENDELL HOLMES.

THE DEATH OF PAUL DOMBEY.

(By permission of Messrs. CHAPMAN AND HALL.)

Paul had never risen from his little bed. He lay there, listening to the noises in the street, quite tranquilly; not caring much how the time went, but watching it, and watching everything about him, with observing eyes. When the sunbeams struck into his room through the rustling blinds, and quivered on the opposite wall like golden water, he knew that evening was coming on, and that the sky was red and beautiful. As the reflection died away, and a gloom went creeping up the wall, he watched it deepen, deepen, deepen into night. Then he thought how the long streets were dotted with lamps, and how the peaceful stars were shining overhead. His fancy had a strange tendency to wander to the river, which he knew was flowing through the great city; and now he thought how black it was, and how deep it would look, reflecting the hosts of stars—and more than all, how steadily it rolled away to meet the sea.

His only trouble was the swift and rapid river. He felt forced, sometimes, to try to stop it—to stem it with his childish hands, or choke its way with sand; and when he saw it coming on resistless, he cried out! But a word from his sister Florence, who was always at his side, restored him to himself; and leaning his poor head upon her breast, he told Floy of his dream, and smiled.

The people round him changed unaccountably—except Florence; Florence never changed—and what had been the doctor was now his father, sitting with his head upon his hand. And Paul was quite content to shut his eyes again, and see what happened next, without emotion. But this figure, with its head upon its hand, returned so often, and remained so long, and sat so still and solemn, never speaking, never being spoken to, and rarely lifting up its face, that Paul began to wonder, languidly, if it were real; and, in the night-time, saw it sitting there, with fear.

"Floy," he said, "what is that?"

"Where, dearest?"

"There! at the bottom of the bed."

"There's nothing there, except papa!"

The figure raised its head, and rose, and coming to the bedside, said, "My own boy, don't you know me?"

Paul looked it in the face, and thought, was this his father? But the face, so altered to his thinking, thrilled while he gazed, as if it were in pain; and, before he could reach out both his hands to take it between them, and draw it towards him, the figure turned away quickly from the little bed, and went out at the door.

How many times the golden water danced upon the wall; how many nights the dark, dark river rolled towards the sea in spite of him; Paul never sought to know. If their kindness, or his sense of it, could have increased, they were more kind and he more grateful every day; but whether they were many days, or few, appeared of little moment now to the gentle boy. One night he had been thinking of his mother, and her picture in the drawing-room downstairs. The train of thought suggested to him to inquire if he had ever seen his mother; for he could not remember whether they had told him yes or no—the river running very fast, and confusing his mind.

"Floy, did I ever see mamma?"

"No, darling; why?"

"Did I never see any kind face, like a mamma's, looking at me when I was a baby, Floy?" he asked incredulously, as if he had some vision of a face before him.

"Oh yes, dear!"

"Whose, Floy?"

"Your old nurse's, often."

"And where is my old nurse?" said Paul. "Is she dead too? Floy, are we *all* dead, except you?"

There was a hurry in the room, for an instant—longer, perhaps; but it seemed no more—then all was still again; and Florence, with her face quite colourless, but smiling, held his head upon her arm. Her arm trembled very much.

"Show me that old nurse, Floy, if you please!"

"She is not here, darling. She shall come to-morrow."

"Thank you, Floy!"

Little Dombey closed his eyes, and fell asleep. But he soon awoke—woke mind and body, and sat upright in his bed. He saw them now about him. There was no gray mist before them, as there had been sometimes in the night. He knew them every one, and called them by their names.

"And who is this? Is this my old nurse?" said the child, regarding with a radiant smile a figure coming in. Yes, yes! No other stranger would have shed those tears at sight of him, and called him her dear boy, her pretty boy, her own poor blighted child. No other woman would have stooped down by his bed, and taken up his wasted hand, and put it to her lips and breast, as one who had some right to fondle it. No other woman would have so forgotten everybody there but him and Floy, and been so full of tenderness and pity. "Floy, this is a kind good face. I am glad to see it again. Don't go away, old nurse! Stay here! Now lay me down; and, Floy, come close to me and let me see you!" Sister and brother wound their arms around each other, and the golden light came streaming in, and fell upon them, locked together. "How fast the river runs between its green banks and the rushes, Floy! But it's very near the sea. I hear the waves! They always said so." Presently he told her that the motion of the boat upon the stream was lulling him to rest. How green the banks were now, how bright the flowers growing on them, and how tall the rushes! Now the boat was out at sea, but gliding smoothly on; and now there was a shore before them. Who stood on the bank? He put his hands together, as he had been used to do at his prayers. He did not remove his arms to do it; but they saw him fold them so behind her neck. "Mamma is like you, Floy; I know her by the face! But tell them that the print upon the stairs is not divine enough. The light about the head is shining on me as I go!"

The golden ripple on the wall came back again, and nothing else stirred in the room...... The old, old fashion! The fashion that came in with our first parents, and will last unchanged until our race has run its course, and the wide firmament is rolled up like a scroll. The old, old fashion—Death! Oh, thank God, all who see it, for that older fashion yet, of Immortality! And look upon us, angels of young children, with regards not quite estranged, when the swift river bears us to the ocean!   DICKENS.

CALEB PLUMMER AND HIS BLIND DAUGHTER.
ADAPTED FROM "THE CRICKET ON THE HEARTH."

(*By permission of* Messrs. CHAPMAN AND HALL.)

John Peerybingle, the carrier, had just got home on a wild, tempestuous night of wind and rain.

"O John, what a state you are in!" said his little wife.

"I believe you, Dot; it ain't exactly summer weather, is it, Dot?"

"I wish you wouldn't call me Dot, John!"

"Why, little woman! what else are you and baby there but a dot and carry one?"

It was pleasant to see big, burly, honest John bending over the baby's cot, with the kind of puzzled look which an amiable mastiff might be supposed to show, if he, one day, found himself the father of a young canary.

"Isn't he beautiful, John? ain't he lovely in his sleep?"

"I believe you, Dot! He always *is* asleep, ain't he, Dot?"

"Good gracious, John, no!"

"Oh! I thought he was—see him winking! And I say, Dot, look at his mouth! Why, he's gasping like a gold and silver fish."

"Like a gold and silver fish indeed! You don't deserve to be a father, John, that you don't!"

"Hulloh, Dot, that's Caleb's knock.—Come in, Caleb, come in." And in came a little, meagre, thoughtful, dingy-faced man;

his outer garment was made of an old sack, on the back of which were these words, "Glass, with care."

"Good-evening, John! Good-evening, mum! Baby's pretty well, I hope, mum?"

"We're all very well, thank you, Caleb."

"And how's business, Caleb?"

"Pretty well, thank you, John; there's rather a run on Noah's arks at present. Anything in the parcel line for me, John?"

"Yes, Caleb, I have a small parcel for you—there you are."

"'For Caleb Plummer, with cash.' With cash, John! I don't think that's for me."

"With cash, Caleb! Where d'ye make out cash?—With care, Caleb, with care!"

"Oh, to be sure! with care. Yes, John, yes, that's for me. It's a box of dolls' eyes for my daughter's work. I wish it was her sight, in a box, John."

"I wish it was, Caleb, or could be."

"Thank'ee, John; you speak very kindly. What's the damage, John?"

"I'll damage *you*, Caleb, if you ask again."

"Thank'ee, John; it's your kind way. Well, I think I'd better be going.—By-the-by, mum, you couldn't have the goodness to pinch Boxer's tail for half a moment. Could you, mum?"

"Why, Caleb, what a question!"

"Oh, never mind, mum; perhaps Boxer wouldn't like it. We've a small order for barking dogs, and I'd like to come as near natur' as possible for sixpence."

At that moment, Mr. Tackleton, the toy merchant, Caleb's master, entered.

"Beastly night.—Oh, *you're* here, are you?—Peerybingle, have you a box for me?"

"There's a wedding-cake for you."

"Caleb, carry that box to my house—let it fall, and I'll murder you."

"Good-evening, mum."

"I'll see you out, Caleb."

"Thank'ee, mum. Good-evening, John."

"Good-night, Caleb, good-night."

"Peerybingle, a word with you. In three days I get married; you'll come to the wedding. We're in the same boat, you know."

"How in the same boat, Mr. Tackleton?"

"A leetle disparity—*you* understand. Here I am, Tackleton. I have the humour to marry a young wife, and a pretty wife; but as for love—bah! there's *your* wife—she honours and obeys, no doubt, but do you think now, Peerybingle, do you think there's anything more in't?"

"I think I'd kill the man who said there wasn't."

"Exactly so—to be sure—of course—I'm certain of it—good-night!"

Caleb Plummer and his blind daughter lived in a small nutshell of a wooden house. I ought to have said that Caleb lived there, and his blind daughter somewhere else. Caleb was no conjurer, but in the only magic art which still remains to us—the magic of devoted, deathless love—Nature had been his teacher, and from her teaching all the wonder came.

The blind girl never knew that round her rose bare, discoloured walls; the blind girl never knew that wood was rotting, iron rusting; the blind girl never knew that Caleb's scanty hairs were turning grayer and more gray before her sightless face; the blind girl never knew that Mr. Tackleton was a hard, selfish, cruel man.

"And so you were out last night, dear father, in your beautiful new great-coat!"

The old sack was hanging up to dry.

"Yes, Bertha, yes; but it's too good for me."

"Too good for you, dear father! What can be too good for you?"

"I'm half ashamed to wear it, though. When I hear the boys behind me say, 'Hulloh! here's a swell!' I don't know which way to look."

"I see you, father! I see you as plainly as if I had the eyes I never want when you are with me—a blue coat!"

"Bright blue, Bertha."

"Yes, yes, bright blue. The colour I can just remember in the blessed sky—a bright-blue coat!"

"Made loose to the figure, Bertha."

"Yes, yes, loose to the figure; and in it, you, dear father, looking so young and handsome!"

"Hulloh! hulloh! I shall be vain presently."

"I know you, father. I have found you out!"

"Yes, Bertha, yes, you have found me out."

"Father, you speak very softly! You're not tired?"

"Tired, Bertha, tired! I never was tired! I'll sing you a verse of your favourite song, Bertha:—

> 'There grew a little flower 'neath a great oak tree.
> When the tempest 'gan to lower little heeded she;
> No need had she to cower, for she dreaded not its power—
> She was happy in the bower of her great oak tree.
>
> > Sing, Heigh! lack-a-day!
> > Sing, Heigh! lack-a-day!
> > Let the tears fall free,
> For the pretty little flower and the great oak tree.
>
> > Sing, Heigh! lack-a-day!
> > Sing, Heigh! lack-a-day!
> > Sing, Heigh! lack-a-day!
> > Let the tears fall free,
> For the pretty little flower and the great oak tree.'"

"You're singing, are you?" said Mr. Tackleton, entering suddenly; "go it! *I* can't sing—I can't afford to sing. I hope you can afford to work too!"

"If you could only see Mr. Tackleton, Bertha—how he's winking at me! He's such a man to joke!"

"Well, Bertha, and how are you?"

"Quite well, thank you. As happy as even you can wish me to be."

("Poor idiot! No gleam of reason; not a gleam.) Shall I tell you a secret, Bertha?"

"If you will."

"In two days I marry May Fielding."

"Marry!"

("She's such a confounded idiot!) Ay, marry! Church, clerk, parson, bells, coach, favours, and all the rest of the tomfoolery. A wedding, you know, Bertha, a wedding."

"I know, I understand."

("Do you? It's more than I expected.) Well, you'll join the party; I'll expect you."

"Yes."

("Poor fool!) I'm off!"

And he slammed the door behind him.

"Father, I'm lonely in the dark. Tell me about May Fielding, and our friend, our benefactor, Mr. Tackleton. He's older than May."

"Yes, Bertha, yes; he's a little older.—Great Power! have I deceived her only to break her heart at last?—Bertha, my dear, I have a confession to make to you."

"A confession, father?"

"Yes, my darling: I have wandered from the truth, meaning to be kind to you; but I have been cruel, cruel!"

"You cruel to me, dear father!"

"Not meaning it, my child; but I have been, and I never knew it till to-day."

"Father, what do you mean?"

"Your road in life was rough, my poor one, and I meant to smooth it for you. I have altered objects, changed the characters of people, to make you happier. I have deceived you— God forgive me!—and surrounded you with fancies."

"But living people are not fancies? You can't change them!"

"I have done so, Bertha. Mr. Tackleton is a stern, selfish, grinding man; a hard master to you and me, my dear, these many years; ugly in his looks, cold and callous in his nature; unlike what I have made him to you in everything—in everything."

"Why, why did you do this? Why did you fill my heart so full, and then come in like death and tear away the objects of my love? O Heaven! how blind I am! how helpless and alone!"

"Not alone, dear Bertha," said the carrier's wife, who had just entered; "not alone."

"Sister—I may call you sister?"

"Yes, Bertha, yes."

"Tell me what my home is, what it really is."

"It is a poor place, Bertha; as roughly sheltered from the weather as your father in his sackcloth coat."

"My father in a sackcloth coat! You'll not deceive me?"

"No, Bertha, no."

"Look, then, where my father is, and tell me what you see."

"I see an old, gray-haired man, worn with care and work; I see him now, bowed down and sorrowful; but, Bertha, I have seen him, many times before, striving hard for one sacred object—your happiness—and I honour his gray head, and bless him!"

The blind girl broke away, and falling on her knees before him, took the gray head to her breast.

"It is my sight restored! There's not a gallant figure on this earth that I would love so dearly as this! There's not a furrow on this brow, not a gray hair on this dear head, that shall be forgotten in my prayers and thanks to Heaven!"

"The fresh, smart father in the blue coat, Bertha, he's gone!"

"Nothing is gone, dear father! The soul of all that was most dear to me is here—here with you; and I am not blind any longer—my eyes are opened!" CHARLES DICKENS.

ON THE DEATH OF PRESIDENT GARFIELD.

On the morning of Saturday, July 2nd, the President was a contented and happy man—not in an ordinary degree, but joyfully, almost boyishly happy. On his way to the railroad station, to which he drove slowly, in conscious enjoyment of the beautiful morning, with an unwonted sense of leisure, and a keen anticipation of pleasure, he felt that after four months of trial his administration was strong in its grasp of affairs, strong in popular favour, and destined to grow stronger; that grave difficulties confronting him at his inauguration had been safely passed; that trouble lay behind him, and not before him; that he was going to his Alma Mater to renew the most cherished associations of his young manhood, and to exchange greetings with those whose deepening interest had followed every step of his upward progress, from the day he entered upon his college course until he had attained the loftiest elevation in the gift of his countrymen.

Surely, if happiness can ever come from the honours or triumphs of this world, on that quiet July morning, James Garfield may well have been a happy man. No foreboding of evil haunted him; no slightest premonition of danger clouded his sky. His terrible fate was upon him in an instant. One moment he stood erect, strong, confident in the years stretching peacefully out before him; the next he lay wounded, bleeding, helpless, doomed to weary weeks of torture, to silence and the grave.

Great in life, he was surpassingly great in death. For no cause, in the very frenzy of wantonness and wickedness, by the red hand of murder, he was thrust from the full tide of this world's interest, from its hopes, its aspirations, its victories, into the visible presence of death—and he did not quail. Not alone for the one short moment in which, stunned and dazed, he could give up life, hardly aware of its relinquishment, but through days of deadly languor, through weeks of agony that was not less agony because silently borne, with clear sight and calm courage he looked into his open grave. What blight and ruin met his anguished eyes, whose lips may tell!—what brilliant broken plans, what baffled high ambitions, what sundering of strong, warm manhood's friendships, what bitter rending of sweet household ties! Behind him a proud, expectant nation, a great host of sustaining friends; a cherished and happy mother, wearing the full, rich honours of her early toil and tears; the wife of his youth, whose whole life lay in his; the little boys, not yet emerged from childhood's day of frolic; the fair young daughter, claiming every day and every day rewarding a father's love and care; and in his heart the eager, rejoicing power to meet all demands. Before him—desolation and great darkness! And his soul was not shaken. His countrymen were thrilled with instant, profound, universal sympathy. Masterful in his mortal weakness, he became the centre of a nation's love, enshrined in the prayers of a world. But all the love and all the sympathy could not share with him his suffering; he trod the wine-press alone. With unfaltering front he faced death. With unfailing tenderness he took leave of life. Above the demoniac hiss of the assassin's bullet he heard the voice of God. With simple resignation he bowed to the divine decree.

As the end drew near, his early craving for the sea returned. The stately mansion of power had been to him the wearisome hospital of pain; and he begged to be taken from its prison walls, from its oppressive stifling air, from its homelessness and its hopelessness. Gently, silently, the love of a great people bore the pale sufferer to the longed-for healing of the sea, to live or to die, as God should will, within sight of its heaving billows, within sound of its manifold voices. With wan, fevered face tenderly lifted to the cooling breeze, he looked out wistfully upon the ocean's changing wonders,—on its distant sails, whitening in the morning light; on its restless waves, rolling shoreward to break and die beneath the noonday sun; on the red clouds of evening, arching low to the horizon; on the serene and shining pathway of the stars. Let us think that his dying eyes read a mystic meaning which only the rapt and parting soul may know. Let us believe that in the silence of the receding world he heard the great waves breaking on a further shore, and felt already upon his wasted brow the breath of the eternal morning. JAMES G. BLAINE.

THE STORY OF LE FEVRE.

[ADAPTED.]

My Uncle Toby was sitting at supper one evening, when the landlord of the village inn entered the room with an empty phial in his hand, and begged for a glass or two of sack.

"'Tis for a poor gentleman, I think of the army, who has taken ill at my house. If I could neither beg, borrow, nor buy such a thing, I would almost steal it for the poor gentleman, he is so ill."

"Thou art a good-natured soul; I will answer for thee," said my Uncle Toby, "and thou shalt drink the gentleman's health in a glass of sack thyself; and take a couple of bottles, with my service, and tell him he is heartily welcome to them, and to a dozen more if they will do him any good."

The landlord had just left, when my Uncle Toby said to his old and faithful servant the corporal, "Step after him, Trim, and ask if he knows the gentleman's name."

"I have quite forgot his name, captain," said the landlord, coming back; "but I can ask his son again."

"Has he a son with him, then?"

"A boy about twelve years of age. Poor lad! he does nothing but mourn and lament for his father night and day."

When the landlord had gone, my Uncle Toby laid down his knife and fork, and the corporal, without being ordered, took his plate away, and brought him his pipe and tobacco.

THE STORY OF LE FEVRE.

"Corporal," said my Uncle Toby, after he had smoked about a dozen whiffs. The corporal came in front of his master, and made his bow. My Uncle Toby smoked on.

"Corporal," said my Uncle Toby. The corporal made his bow again. My Uncle Toby said no more, but finished his pipe.

"Trim, I have a project in my head of wrapping myself up warm in my roquelaure, and paying a visit to this poor gentleman."

"Your honour's roquelaure has not been on since the night your honour received your wound, when we mounted guard before the gate of St. Nicolas; besides, it is so cold and rainy a night that, what with the roquelaure, and what with the weather, 'twill be enough to give your honour your death."

"I fear so, Trim; but I am not at rest in my mind. I wish I had not heard so much of this affair, or that I had heard more of it; how shall we manage it, corporal?"

"Leave it, an' please your honour, to me. I'll go to the inn and reconnoitre, and bring your honour a full account in an hour."

"Thou shalt go, Trim."

It was not till my Uncle Toby had finished his three pipes that the corporal came back and gave the following account:—

"I despaired at first of being able to bring back your honour any kind of intelligence regarding the poor sick lieutenant."

"Is he in the army then, Trim?"

"He is."

"And in what regiment, Trim?"

"I'll tell your honour everything as it happened. I first asked where the lieutenant's servant was, and I was answered that he had no servant with him, and that he had come to the inn with hired horses. 'When I get better, my dear,' he said to his son, 'we can hire horses from hence.' 'But, alas!' said the landlady to me, 'the poor gentleman will never get from hence; and when he dies, his son will certainly die with him, for he is broken-hearted already.' I was hearing this account, when the boy came into the kitchen to get a slice of thin toast for his father. 'I will do it for my father myself,' said the lad.—'Pray let me save you the trouble,' said I.—'I believe, sir,' said he very modestly, 'I can please him best myself.'—'I am sure,' said I, 'his honour will not like the toast the worse for being toasted by an old soldier.' He took hold of my hand, and burst into tears."

"Poor lad!" said my Uncle Toby, "he has been brought up from a child in the army, and the name of a soldier, Trim, sounded in his ears like the name of a friend."

"I never, in the longest march, had so great a mind for my dinner as I had to cry with him for company. What could be the matter with him, an' please your honour?"

"Nothing in the world, Trim, but that thou art a good-natured fellow. Go on, Trim, go on."

"When I gave him the toast, I thought it was proper to tell him I was Captain Shandy's servant, and that your honour, though a stranger, was extremely concerned for his father, and if there was anything in your house he was heartily welcome to it. He made a very low bow (which was meant for your honour), but no answer, for his heart was full. 'I warrant you, my dear,' said I, as I opened the door for him, 'your father will be well soon.' The curate was smoking by the kitchen fire, but said not a word, good or bad, to comfort the poor lad. I thought it wrong."

"I think so, too," said my Uncle Toby.

"When the lieutenant had taken his glass of sack and toast, he sent down word that he should be glad to see me in a few minutes if I would step upstairs. 'I believe,' said the landlord, 'he is going to say his prayers.'—'I thought,' said the curate, 'you gentlemen of the army, Mr. Trim, never said prayers at all.'—'I heard the poor gentleman say his prayers last night, and very devoutly too,' said the landlady.—'Are you sure of it?' said the curate.—'A soldier, an' please your reverence,' said I, 'prays as often of his own accord as a parson; and when he is fighting for his king, ay, and for his honour too, he has the most reason to pray to God of any one in the whole world.'"

"'Twas well said of thee, Trim," said my Uncle Toby.

"'But when a soldier,' said I, 'an' please your reverence, has been standing for twelve hours up to his knees in cold water, or engaged,' said I, 'for months together in long and dangerous marches, detached here, countermanded there, benumbed in his joints, without straw, maybe, in his tent to kneel on, he must say his prayers how and when he can. I believe,' said I, for I was piqued for the reputation of the army, 'I believe, an' please your reverence, that when a soldier gets time to pray, he prays as heartily as a parson, though not with all his fuss and hypocrisy.'"

"Thou shouldst not have said that, Trim," said my Uncle Toby, "for God only knows who is a hypocrite and who is not. At the great and general review of us all, corporal, at the day of judgment, and not till then, it will be seen who have done their duties in this world and who have not. In the meantime, we may depend upon it that God Almighty is so good and just a governor of the world, that if we have but done our duties in it, it will never be inquired into whether we have done them in a red coat or a black one; but go on, Trim, with the story."

"The lad now came in and said that his father would be glad to see me. I went upstairs with him, and entered the lieutenant's room. He did not offer to speak to me till I had walked up to his bedside. 'If you are Captain Shandy's servant,' said he, 'you must present my compliments to your master for his courtesy to me. If he was in Flanders'—I told him your honour was—'then,' said he, 'I served three campaigns with him, but I had not the honour of his acquaintance. Please tell him my name is Le Fevre, a lieutenant in Angus's; but he knows me not—possibly he may know my story. Pray, tell the captain I was the ensign at Breda, whose

THE STORY OF LE FEVRE.

wife was most unfortunately killed by a musket-shot as she lay in my arms in my tent.'—'I remember the story, an' please your honour,' said I.—'Do you so?' said he; 'then well may I.' And taking a ring out of his bosom, which was tied to a black ribbon about his neck, he kissed it twice. 'Here, Billy,' said he to his boy, who flew across the room, and falling on his knees, took the ring and kissed it too."

"I wish, Trim," said my Uncle Toby, "I wish I was asleep. I remember the story of the ensign and his wife, and that he was universally pitied by the whole regiment; but finish the story."

"'Tis finished already, for I could stay no longer, so wished his honour a good night."

"Thou hast left this matter short, Trim, and I will tell thee in what. In the first place, when thou madest an offer of my services to Le Fevre, that thou didst not make an offer to him of my purse."

"Your honour knows I had no orders."

"True; thou didst very right as a soldier, Trim, but certainly very wrong as a man. In the second place—for which, indeed, thou hast the same excuse—when thou offeredst him whatever was *in* my house, thou shouldst have offered him my *house* too. A sick brother-officer should have the *best* quarters, Trim; and if we had him with us, we could tend and look to him. Thou art an excellent nurse thyself, Trim; and what with thy care of him, and his boy's, and mine together, we might set him on his legs again—in a fortnight or three weeks he might march."

"He will never march, an' please your honour, in this world," said the corporal.

"He shall march to his regiment!" said my Uncle Toby.

"He cannot stand it," said the corporal.

"He shall be supported!" said my Uncle Toby.

"He'll drop at last," said the corporal.

"He shall not drop!" said my Uncle Toby.

"Ah, well-a-day! do what we can for him, the poor soul will die."

"He shall not die, by heaven!"

The accusing spirit which flew up to heaven's chancery with the oath, blushed as he gave it in; and the recording angel, as he wrote it down, dropped a tear upon the word, and blotted it out for ever.

Rev. Lawrence Sterne.

ESCAPE OF SIR ARTHUR AND MISS WARDOUR.

[ADAPTED FROM "THE ANTIQUARY."]

Sir Arthur Wardour and his daughter had gone to dine with Mr. Jonathan Oldbuck, the antiquary. Being a lovely evening, they resolved to walk home by the shore. Following the windings of the beach, they found themselves under a huge extent of rocky headlands, which rose to the height of two or three hundred feet; when the sun became almost obscured, and a lurid shade of darkness blotted the serene light of a summer evening. The wind came out in wild and fitful gusts, and the mass of waters, so lately calm, now formed waves which burst upon the shore with a sound resembling distant thunder.

The rapid advance of the tide and this sudden change of weather appalled them. As they pressed forward they observed some one on the beach coming towards them. The advancing figure made many signs, but the haze of the atmosphere rendered them indistinct and incomprehensible. Some time before they met Sir Arthur recognized the old blue-gowned beggar, Edie Ochiltree.

"Turn back! turn back! Why didna ye turn when I waved tae ye?"

"We are going round by Halket Head, my good man."

"Halket Heid! Halket Heid! It was a' I could dae tae win roon' it twenty minutes since. The tide's comin' in three feet abreist. Back! back! it's oor only chance. I heard ye was here; an' when I lookit at the lift an' the rin o' the tide, I couldna bide tae think o' the dainty young leddy's danger, wha has aye been sae kind tae ilka forlorn heart that cam' near her. But I doubt, I doubt, I've been beguiled. Mak' haste, mak' haste, my winsome leddy. Tak' haud o' my airm, auld an' frail though it be, an' we may dae weel yet, for a' that's come an' gane."

They pressed back bravely, but when the breakers rose in foam against the dark brow of the precipice, old Edie exclaimed,—

"God hae mercy on us! We're lost!"

"My child! my child! to die such a death!"

"Dear father! And you, too, old man, have lost your life in trying to save ours!"

"That's no worth the coontin', my winsome leddy; here, or yonder, at the back o' a dyke, in a wreath o' snaw, or in the bosom o' a wave, what signifies whaur the auld gaberlunzie dees?"

"My good man, can you think of nothing—of no help? I'll give you a farm. I'll make you rich."

"Oor riches, Sir Arthur, will sune be equal. They are indeed sae already, for I hae nae land, an' ye would gie your haill barony for a square yard o' rock that would be dry for twal hours. I was a bauld craigsman ance in my days, but it's lang, lang since syne. No, no! Nae mortal could spiel thae rocks withoot a rape; an' if I had a rape, my e'esicht, an' my fute-step, an' my hand-grip hae a' failed me. There was a path here ance— His name be praised! There's some ane comin' doon the craig e'en noo! You're richt, sir! you're richt! That gate, that gate! Fasten the rape weel roon' auld Crummie's horn! That's yon muckle big stane there. That's it—that'll dae. Canny, canny! Guidsake! tak' time an' tak' tent. Vera weel! Noo, wi' your help an' the rape's thegither, I'll win at ye; an' we'll get up the young leddy an' Sir Arthur."

Young Lovel, for he it was, lowered the ends of two strong ropes he had with him, one of which old Edie secured around Miss Wardour, wrapping her first in his old blue gown. With the aid of the other rope, the brave old man now ascended the face of the precipice, and after one or two marvellous escapes stood safe beside young Lovel. They were now able to raise Miss Wardour. Lovel then descended to help Sir Arthur, and, mounting again, they raised him also beyond the reach of the billows, which even now overflowed the beach on which they had so lately stood. The spray flew as high as their place of refuge.

"The lassie," said old Edie, "the puir sweet lassie! Mony's the nicht like this *I* hae wather'd, but hoo can *she* ever win through't?"

"I'll climb up," said Lovel, "and get more assistance."

"Are ye mad?" said old Edie, "are ye mad? It's God's grace, an' a great miracle besides, that ye're no in the middle o' that roarin' sea; but tae venture up again, it's a mere an' a clear temptin' o' Providence."

"I have no fear, my friend; I'll go."

"Deil be in my feet then! if ye gang, I'll gang tae."

"No, no, we can't both go."

"Stay yoursell then an' I'll gang. Let death spare the green corn an' tak' the ripe."

"Stay both of you," said Miss Wardour, "I implore you. 1 can pass the night very well here."

"Hark!" said Lovel; "hark! what sound is that?"

"The skriegh o' a Tammie Norie; I ken the skirl weel."

"No! it was a human voice; and see! the gleam of torches."

On the verge of the cliff an anxious company had now assembled. The antiquary was the foremost, leaning over the very brink. "Hilli-ho! hilli-ho! I see them, Mucklebackit."

"I see them mysell weel eneugh," said Mucklebackit, an old smuggler. "D'ye think ye'll help them ony wi' skirlin' that gate? Steenie, lad, bring the mast here, an' we'll sune bouse them up."

The mast of a boat was soon fixed in the ground, with a yard across, a rope, and a block at each end; and, lastly, an arm-chair well secured was lowered to the sufferers. Miss Wardour was first tied to the chair with Lovel's neckcloth and old Edie's leathern belt.

"Now then, lads," cried the old smuggler, "bouse awa' wi' her! Canny, canny! Swerve the yard a bit. Hurrah! There she sits safe on dry land!"

The antiquary, in his exuberance of joy, took off his greatcoat to wrap round the young lady, and would have pulled off his under-coat and vest also had not Caxon, the old barber, withheld him.

"Haud a care, haud a care, Monkbarns! Your honour will be killed wi' the hoast, an' then there will be but ae wig left in the parish, an' that's but the minister's."

"You are right, you are right, my prince of barbers. Miss Wardour, let me convey you to the carriage."

"Not till I have seen my father safe."

"Right, right; that's right too. I should like to see him safe myself; and here he comes, here he comes. Welcome! welcome! my good old friend; though I can't say to warm land, or to dry land, yet to safe land. A cord for ever against fifty fathom of water! Sir Arthur, you have dangled at a rope's end for once in your life. What have we here? What patched and weather-beaten matter is this? What! is it thou, old Edie? Who, then, is the other?"

"Ane that's worth twa o' us, Monkbarns. He's behaved this blessed nicht as if he had three lives, and was willin' to lose them a' to save ither folk's."

Lovel was now safely landed. Sir Arthur and Miss Wardour at once drove home, Edie Ochiltree was hustled off to the old smuggler's house, the antiquary laid hold of Lovel.

"Why, man, you have been a hero—a perfect Sir William Wallace, by all accounts. You shall go home with me to Monkbarns."

"No, thanks; I must go back to Fairport."

"Not a step, not a pace, not an inch!"

"My dear sir, I am wet to the skin."

"Shalt have my dressing-gown and slippers, man, and catch the antiquarian fever, as men do the plague, by wearing infected garments. Shalt have the remains of a glorious chicken-pie, and a bottle of my oldest port."

"Nay, but really, my dear sir—"

"Nay, nay, nay! I'll take no denial. So come along, my young Sir William Wallace; come along, and welcome to Monkbarns." SIR WALTER SCOTT.

A WILD NIGHT AT SEA.

(*By permission of* Messrs. CHAPMAN AND HALL.)

A dark and dreary night: people nestling in their beds or circling late about the fire; Want, colder than Charity, shivering at the street corners; church-towers humming with the faint vibration of their own tongues, but newly resting from the ghostly preachment—"One!" The earth covered with a sable pall, as for the burial of Yesterday; the clumps of dark trees—its giant plumes of funeral feathers—waving sadly to and fro: all hushed, all noiseless, and in deep repose, save the swift clouds that skim across the moon; and the cautious wind, as, creeping after them upon the ground, it stops to listen, and goes rustling on, and stops again, and follows, like a savage on the trail.

Whither go the clouds and wind so eagerly? If, like guilty spirits, they repair to some dread conference with powers like themselves, in what wild region do the elements hold council, or where unbend in terrible disport?

Here! Free from that cramped prison called the earth, and out upon the waste of waters. Here, roaring, raging, shrieking, howling, all night long. Hither come the sounding voices from the caverns on the coast of that small island, sleeping a thousand miles away, so quietly, in the midst of **angry waves**; and hither, to meet them, rush the blasts from unknown desert places of the world. Here, in the fury of their unchecked liberty, they storm and buffet with each other, until the sea, lashed into passion like their own, leaps up in ravings mightier than theirs, and the whole scene is whirling madness.

On, on, on, over the countless miles of angry space, roll the long heaving billows. Mountains and caves are here, and yet are not; for what is now the one, is now the other; then all is but a boiling heap of rushing water. Pursuit, and flight, and mad return of wave on wave, and savage struggling, ending in a spouting up of foam that whitens the black night; incessant change of place, and form, and hue; constancy in nothing but eternal strife; on, on, on they roll, and darker grows the night, and louder howl the winds, and more clamorous and fierce become the million voices in the sea—when the wild cry goes forth upon the storm, "A ship!"

Onward she comes, in gallant combat with the elements, her tall masts trembling, and her timbers starting on the strain; onward she comes, now high upon the curling billows, now low down in the hollows of the sea, as hiding for the moment from its fury; and every storm-voice in the air and water cries more loudly yet, "A ship!"

Still she comes striving on: and at her boldness and the spreading cry, the angry waves rise up above each other's hoary heads to look; and round about the vessel, far as the mariners on her decks can pierce into the gloom, they press upon her, forcing each other down, and starting up, and rushing forward from afar, in dreadful curiosity. High over her they break, and round her surge and roar; and, giving place to others, moaningly depart, and dash themselves to fragments in their baffled anger. Still she comes onward bravely. And though the eager multitude crowd thick and fast upon her all the night, and dawn of day discovers the untiring train yet bearing down upon the ship in an eternity of troubled water, onward she comes, with dim lights burning in her hull, and people there asleep, as if no deadly element were peering in at every seam and chink, and no drowned seaman's grave, with but a plank to cover it, were yawning in the unfathomable depths below.

CHARLES DICKENS.

OLD SCROOGE.

[ADAPTED FROM "A CHRISTMAS CAROL."]

(*By permission of* Messrs. CHAPMAN AND HALL.)

Marley was dead to begin with—he was as dead as a door-nail. Scrooge knew he was dead—of course he did. Scrooge and he were partners for I don't know how many years! Scrooge was his sole executor—his sole residuary legatee—his sole friend—and sole mourner. Oh, but he was a tight-fisted hand at the grindstone was Scrooge—a grasping, wrenching, clutching, scraping, covetous old sinner.

Nobody ever stopped him in the street to say, "My dear Scrooge, how are you? When will you come to see me?" No beggars implored him for a trifle. No children asked him, "What it was o'clock?"

Even the blind-men's dogs appeared to know him, and when they saw him coming on, would tug their owners into doorways and up courts; and then would wag their tails, as though they said, "No eye at all is better than an evil eye, dark master." But what did Scrooge care? Bah! all this was the very thing he liked!

One day, of all the days of the year, on Christmas eve, old Scrooge sat busy in his counting-house. It was cold, bleak, biting weather—foggy withal; he could hear the people outside go wheezing up and down, beating their hands upon their breasts and stamping their feet upon the pavement stones to warm them.

The door of Scrooge's counting-house was open, that he might keep his eye upon his clerk, who, in a dismal little cell beyond

—a sort of tank—was copying letters. Scrooge had a very small fire; the clerk's fire was so very much smaller it looked like one coal, but he couldn't replenish it, because Scrooge kept the coal-box in his own room; wherefore, the clerk put on his white comforter, and tried to warm himself at the candle, in which effort, not being a man of a strong imagination, he failed.

"A merry Christmas, uncle!" said a cheerful voice: it was the voice of Scrooge's nephew, who had just entered.

"Bah!" said Scrooge. "Humbug!"

"Christmas a humbug! You don't mean that, uncle!"

"I do! Merry Christmas! Out upon merry Christmas! What's Christmas-time to you, but a time for finding yourself a year older but not an hour richer; a time for paying bills—without money. Merry Christmas! Keep Christmas in your own way, and let me keep it in mine."

"Keep it! Yes; but you don't keep it."

"Let me leave it alone then; much good may it do you! Much good it has ever done you."

"There are many things, uncle, from which I might have derived good, by which I have not benefited, I daresay—Christmas among the rest; but I am sure I have always thought of Christmas when it has come round—apart from the veneration due to its sacred name and origin, if anything belonging to it can be apart from that—as a good time, a kind, forgiving, loving, charitable time. And although, uncle, it has never put a scrap of gold or silver in my pocket, I believe it has done me good, and will do me good, and I say, God bless it!"

The clerk in the tank involuntarily applauded.

"Let me hear another sound from you," said Scrooge, "and you'll keep your Christmas—by losing your situation."

"Don't be angry, uncle! Come and dine with us to-morrow!"

"No—I won't!"

"But—why?—why?"

"Why did you get married?"

"Because I—well—because I fell in love."

"Because you fell in love! Good-afternoon!"

"We've never had a quarrel, uncle, to which I have been a party; why can't we be friends?"

"Good-afternoon!"

"Well, I'll keep my Christmas humour to the last—so a merry Christmas, uncle!"

"Good-afternoon!"

"And a happy new year!"

"Good-afternoon!"

Foggier yet, and colder—piercing, searching, biting cold. The owner of one scant young nose, gnawed and mumbled by the cold, as bones are gnawed by dogs, stooped down at Scrooge's keyhole to regale him with a Christmas carol; but at the first sounds of

Felix   "God bless you, merry gentleman,
             May nothing you dismay,"

Scrooge seized the ruler with such alacrity that the singer fled in terror, leaving the keyhole to the fog and even more congenial frost.

At length the hour of shutting up the counting-house arrived. With an ill-will Scrooge dismounted from his stool, and tacitly admitted the fact to the expectant clerk in the tank, who instantly snuffed his candle out, and put on his hat.

"You'll want all day to-morrow, I suppose!" said Scrooge.

"If quite convenient, sir."

"But it's *not* convenient—and it's not fair. If I was to stop half-a-crown for it, you'd think yourself ill-used, I'll be bound!—(The clerk smiled faintly.)—And yet you don't think *me* ill-used when I pay a day's wages for no work."

The clerk observed that it was only once a year.

"A poor excuse for picking a man's pocket every twenty-fifth of December," said Scrooge, buttoning his greatcoat to the chin. "But I suppose you *must* have the whole day. Be here all the earlier next morning."

The clerk promised that he would, and Scrooge walked out with a growl. CHARLES DICKENS.

MARLEY'S GHOST.

[ADAPTED FROM "A CHRISTMAS CAROL."]

(By permission of Messrs. CHAPMAN AND HALL.)

Scrooge took his usual melancholy dinner, in his usual melancholy tavern, and having read all the newspapers, and beguiled the rest of the evening with his banker's book, went home to bed.

Now it is a fact that there was nothing at all particular about the knocker on the door, except that it was very large. Let any one explain then, if he can, how it happened that Scrooge, having his key in the lock of the door, saw in the knocker, not a knocker, but Marley's face! Marley's face!

As Scrooge looked fixedly at this phenomenon, it was a knocker again.

To say that he was not startled would be untrue, but he put his hand on the key he had relinquished—turned it sturdily—walked in—and lit his candle.

He then went through his rooms to see that all was right—sitting-room, bed-room, lumber-room—all as they should be. Nobody under the table; nobody under the sofa. A small fire in the grate. Spoon and basin ready—the little saucepan of gruel (Scrooge had a cold in his head) upon the hob. Nobody under the bed; nobody in the closet.

Quite satisfied, he locked himself in; double-locked himself in, which was not his custom.

Thus secured against surprise, he took off his cravat, put on his dressing-gown, slippers, and his night-cap, and sat down before the fire to take his gruel.

As Scrooge leaned back in his chair, he heard a clanking noise deep down below, as if some one were dragging a heavy chain over the casks in the wine merchant's cellar.

The cellar door flew open with a booming sound!

Then he heard the noise much louder!

Then coming up the stair! Then coming straight towards his door!

"It's humbug!" said Scrooge; "I won't believe it!"

His colour changed though when, without a pause, it came on through the heavy door, and passed into the room before his eyes!

The same face! the very same!

Marley in his pig-tail, usual waistcoat, tights, and boots.

His body was transparent, so that Scrooge, observing him, and looking through his waistcoat, could see the two buttons on the coat behind.

"How, now!" said Scrooge; "what do you want with me?"

"Much!"

"Who are you?"

"Ask me who I *was?*"

"Who *were* you then? you're particular—for a shade."

He was going to say "*to* a shade," but altered the word as more appropriate.

"In life I was your partner, Jacob Marley."

"Can you sit down?"

"I can."

"Do it then."

Scrooge asked the question because he didn't know that a ghost so transparent might find himself in a condition to take a chair. But the ghost sat down as if he were quite used to it.

"You don't believe in me?"

"I don't."

"Why do you doubt your senses?"

"Because a little thing affects them; a slight disorder of the stomach makes 'em cheats. You may be a blot of mustard—a crumb of cheese—a fragment of an under-done potato. There's more of *gravy* than of *grave* about you, whatever you are. Humbug, I tell you! Humbug!"

At this the spectre raised such a frightful cry that Scrooge held on tight to his chair, to save himself from falling in a swoon.

"Mercy!" he cried, "dreadful apparition! Why do you trouble me?"

"Man of the worldly mind, do you believe in me or not?"

"I do! I must! But why do spirits walk the earth? and why do they come to me?"

"It is required of every man that the spirit within him should walk abroad among his fellow-men, and if that spirit go not forth in life, it is condemned to do so after death. It is doomed to wander through the world, and witness what it cannot share, but might have shared on earth, and turned to happiness."

"Jacob! old Jacob Marley," said Scrooge, "tell me more —speak comfort to me, Jacob!"

"I have none to give—it comes from other regions, Ebenezer Scrooge, and is conveyed by *other* ministers to *other* kinds of men. I cannot rest—I cannot linger anywhere; in life, my spirit never roved beyond the limits of our money-changing hole, and weary journeys lie before me."

"You must have been very slow about it, Jacob! Seven years dead! and travelling all the time?"

"The whole time. No rest! no peace! incessant torture of remorse."

"You travel fast?"

"On the wings of the wind."

"You might have got over a great quantity of ground in seven years, Jacob!"

"O captive-bound! and double-ironed! not to know that any Christian spirit, working kindly in its little sphere, what- ever it may be, will find its mortal life too short for its vast means of usefulness—not to know that no space of regret can make amends for one life's day misused."

"But you were always a good man of business, Jacob!"

"Business! Mankind was my business. The common welfare was my business. Charity, mercy, forbearance, benevolence, were all my business. The dealings of my trade were but a drop of water in the comprehensive ocean of my business. Why did I walk through crowds of fellow-beings, with my eyes turned down, and never raise them to that blessed Star which led the wise men to a poor abode? Were there no poor homes to which its light would have conducted *me?* Hear me! my time is nearly gone."

"I will—I will—but don't be hard upon me! don't be flowery, Jacob!"

"I am here to-night to warn you that you have yet a chance and hope of escaping my fate, Ebenezer."

"You were always a good friend to me, Jacob; thank'ee."

"Look to see me no more, and look that, for your own sake, you remember what has passed between us."

CHARLES DICKENS.

AN IRISHMAN'S LOVE FOR HIS CHILDREN.

[ADAPTED.]

Some years ago, on our passage to New York, we had on board a number of emigrants, among whom was an Irishman with his wife and three children, the eldest, a girl, about seven years of age.

They were very poor, but the beauty and intelligence of the children quite won the heart of a lady passenger, and, now and again, she would have them brought into the cabin and their hunger appeased.

Gleesome, bright-eyed little creatures, they were all life and happiness, and in blissful ignorance of the poverty by which they were surrounded.

AN IRISHMAN'S LOVE FOR HIS CHILDREN.

One day they were in the cabin, when this lady said to me, "I wonder if those poor people would part with one of these darlings. I should much like to adopt one."

"I don't know," I said; "suppose we make the inquiry."

The father was sent for. "My good friend," said the lady, "you are very poor, are you not?" His answer was peculiarly Irish.

"Is it poor, mi lady? If there's a poorer man than misilf troublin' the world, Hiven pity both of uz, fur we'd be about aqual!"

"Then," said I, "you must find it no easy matter to support your children."

"Is it to support thim, sir? I niver supported thim; they git supported, somehow or other; they've niver been hungry yit. Whin they are, it'll be toime enough to complain."

"Well, then," I continued, "would it not be a relief to you to part with one of them?"

He started, turned pale, and with a wild glare in his eye passionately said, "A relaif! what d'ye mean, sir? Wud it be a relaif, d'ye think, to have mi hand chopped from mi body, or mi heart torn out of mi breast?"

"Oh, you don't understand us," said my lady friend. "Suppose you were enabled to place one of your children in ease and comfort, would you interfere with its well-doing?"

The tact of women! She had touched the chord of paternal affection. The poor fellow was silent and all bewildered. At last he said, "God bliss ye, mi lady! Hiven knows I'd be right glad to better the child—it isn't in regard to misilf; but hadn't I better go an' spake to Mary—she's the mother of thim—an' 'twould be onraisonable to be givin' away her children behind her back."

"Very well," I said; "off you go to Mary, and hear what she says."

In about an hour he came back, his eyes red and swollen. "Well," said I, "what success?"

"'Twas no aisy matter, sir, but it's for the child's good, and Hiven give us stringth to bear it!"

"Well, and which are we to have?"

"Well, sir, I've been spakin' to Mary, an' she thinks as Nora there is the ouldest—she's siven past—she wouldn't miss the mother so much; an' if ye'll jist let her take a partin' kiss, she'd give her to ye wid a blissin'."

So he took away his three children, to look at one of them for the last time.

When he returned he was leading the *second* eldest, a little girl about five.

"How is this? have you changed your mind?"

"Well, no; I haven't exackly changed mi moind, sir, but I've changed the child. Ye see, sir, I've been spakin' to Mary, an' whin it came to the ind, sir, she couldn't part wid Nora at all, at all! But here's little Biddy—an' if she'll do as well?"

"Yes, yes; we'll take Biddy."

"Hiven be her guardian! God be kind to thim that's kind to you!" Then he went away, and all that night little Biddy remained with us. But early next morning he reappeared, and this time he had his *youngest* child—a mere baby—in his arms.

"What's the matter now?" I said.

"Well, sir, ye see, I've been spakin' to Mary, an' whin I begude to think of Biddy's eyes—look at thim, sir; they're the image of her mother's—I couldn't let her go. But here's little Paudeen; he won't be much bother to any one, for if he takes after his mother, he'll have the brightest eyes an' the softest heart in creation; an' if he takes after his father, he'll have a purty hard fist an' a broad pair of shoulders to push his way in the world. Take *him*, sir, an' gi' me back Biddy."

He left the baby, and took away his pet Biddy.

I wasn't at all surprised when, a few minutes afterwards, he rushed into the cabin and caught up little Paudeen in his arms.

"Look at him, sir! look at him! It's the youngest—only two years ould. You wouldn't have the heart to keep him from uz. The long an' the short of it is, sir, I've been spakin' to Mary—*she* couldn't part wid Nora, an' *I* couldn't part wid Biddy, but naither of uz could live half a day widout little Paudeen! No, sir, no! we can bear the bitterness of poverty, but we can't part wid our children—unless it be the will of Hiven to take them from uz!"

A CITY BY NIGHT.

That stifled hum of Midnight, when Traffic has lain down to rest; and the chariot-wheels of Vanity, still rolling here and there through distant streets, are bearing her to Halls roofed-in, and lighted to the due pitch for her; and only Vice and Misery, to prowl or to moan like nightbirds, are abroad: that hum, I say, like the stertorous, unquiet slumber of sick Life, is heard in Heaven! The joyful and the sorrowful are there; men are dying there, men are being born; men are praying,—on the other side of a brick partition men are cursing: and around them all is the vast, void Night. The proud Grandee still lingers in his perfumed saloons, or reposes within damask curtains; Wretchedness cowers into truckle-beds, or shivers hunger-stricken into its lair of straw: in obscure cellars *Rouge-et-Noir* languidly emits its voice-of-destiny to haggard, hungry Villains; while Councillors of State sit plotting, and playing their high chess-game, whereof the pawns are Men. The Lover whispers his mistress that the coach is ready; and she, full of hope and fear, glides down, to fly with him over the borders: the Thief, still more silently, sets-to his picklocks and crowbars, or lurks in wait till the watchmen first snore in their boxes. Gay mansions, with supper-rooms and dancing-rooms, are full of light, and music, and high-swelling hearts; but in the Condemned Cell the pulse of life beats tremulous and faint, and bloodshot eyes look out through the darkness, which is around and within, for the light of a stern last morning. Upwards of five-hundred-thousand two-legged animals without feathers lie round us, in horizontal positions; their heads full of the foolishest dreams. Riot cries aloud, and staggers and swaggers in his rank dens of shame; and the Mother, with streaming hair, kneels over her pallid dying infant, whose cracked lips only her tears now moisten.—All these heaped and huddled together, with nothing but a little carpentry and masonry between them; —crammed in like salted fish in their barrel;—or weltering, shall I say, like an Egyptian pitcher of tamed vipers, each struggling to get its *head above* the others : *such* work goes on under that smoke counterpane!—But I sit above it all; I am alone with the Stars. CARLYLE.

OLD PARSON RAYNE.

(By permission of the Author.)

There is a quaint, old-fashioned parsonage standing on the great high road that leads from Audrey End to London—from the sleepiest village in all Hertfordshire to the mighty Babylon. In the summer, when the roses twine about the porch, and the sweet, old-fashioned flowers in the little front garden scent the air, passing strangers, dusty with travel, stop and lean over the low stone wall, and gaze admiringly at the picture before them; but in the winter, when the roses are gone, when the fierce wind shrieks among the leafless trees, and the snow lies thick around, the traveller passes on, and thrusts his hands deeper than ever into his greatcoat pockets, for the sight of the lonely house chills him to the marrow.

There is a story about the parsonage, and any man, woman, or child in Audrey End will tell it you. Eight years ago, one Christmas eve, old Parson Rayne stood with his white face pressed against the great bow-window, and saw his only son, his brave Eric, stride along the broad road, his face turned Londonwards. They had parted in anger—parted with never a farewell, with never a God-speed—and from that day to this no Eric had returned out of the gray haze that hangs, autumn and winter, like a veil over the brow of Audrey Hill.

It was the old story of youthful folly—of hot blood in young veins, and scrape after scrape, until at last a forgiving father would forgive no more. Fierce words were spoken, and a proud lad, his handsome face distorted with passion, cast aside home and kindred in his mad infatuation, and left the old home, vowing that it should know him no more.

Old Parson Rayne, in his passion, had uttered words which stung the lad to the quick. He bade his son begone and disgrace him no more. And the son took him at his hasty word, and went.

From that hour the parson had been an altered man. He was alone—alone in the great house with old Scotch Janet, who had been his faithful servant thirty years, who had taken baby Eric from the poor dead mother's arms, and loved him as her "ain bairn."

There is a picture which hangs over the fireplace in the sitting-room. It is the portrait of a blue-eyed, golden-haired boy of six, and old Janet looks at that picture often till her eyes are red, for that is her bairn—her bonny lad, that she loved as her own. That is the pretty boy who grew to be a handsome lad, and broke his father's heart, went away to London, and was heard of no more.

Old Janet had her hands full now, or perhaps she would have broken her heart too, for year by year the old master grew more and more strange and absent in his mind. The neighbours nodded their heads when the parson's sermons seemed confused, and when he made slips in the service.

"He's thinking about his son," they said; "his mind's going."

The neighbours were right. Slowly but surely the old parson's mind was going.

At home he would sit for hours lost in thought, heeding not

Janet, who tried to coax him out of his reverie, or to tempt him to the table with the old Scotch dishes she could cook so well, which once the master had relished so much.

It was sad and weary work for the good soul as the years went by, and the dear old master grew daily more feeble, more absent-minded, and more lost in the past. His white face, watching from the window for the son that never came, grew a familiar sight to the folks of Audrey End; and the children coming home from school would look askance as they passed the house, for it was whispered that the parson was "queer" and "odd," and "not right," and the little ones, catching the whispered remarks, grew to look upon the minister as something uncanny, and to be avoided.

At last the talk of the strangeness of Parson Rayne spread in wider circles, and all the county heard it, and the gossips at the village ale-house carried the story from place to place, with ever-growing additions, until the old minister of Audrey End was known far and near as the Mad Parson.

Janet heard it in the village on the afternoon of Christmas eve, and she shuddered. She had hidden the worst from herself. She had tried to think that she was mistaken, that the master was only fretting and absent-minded; but now everybody saw it, she could be blind no longer. What would they do with the poor dear if he went quite out of his mind? They would take him away to some horrible place, where strangers would be cruel to him, and he would end his days in misery—a prisoner, tended by harsh keepers!

Old Janet hurried out of the shop where the thoughtless words had been spoken, and her eyes were red and swollen when she reached the Parsonage. She had known for months what must be the end, and yet she had never realized it as she did now.

For months the Rev. Eric Rayne had not officiated. The curate had done all the work latterly; and hard work it was, for the church at Audrey End was the church for half-a-dozen outlying hamlets, and visiting the parishioners meant a considerable amount of physical exertion.

The curate was a good-hearted, manly young fellow, and he never shirked the extra work that fell upon him. He came to the Parsonage every day to see how the old gentleman was, and always had a kindly, cheery word for him. But of late he, too, had begun to look grave and to shake his head. When Janet came back from the village the curate was with her master.

The old gentleman raised his head as Janet entered, and he looked at her eagerly, with a strange light in his generally dull eyes.

"Ha!" he exclaimed; "it's not Eric. I thought it was. He'll come to-night."

Janet looked at the curate for advice.

"Humour him," he whispered. "I don't like his appearance at all."

"What are you whispering for?" exclaimed the old gentleman fiercely, half rising in his easy-chair. "I tell you Eric is coming to-night—over the seas—thousands of miles—my Eric is coming to-night. Janet, take me to the window. I'll watch for him."

The arm-chair was wheeled to the window, and the passing villagers saw the white face of the old parson still watching—watching with eager eyes for the boy that was to come back at last.

The curate, bidding Janet not leave her master alone, for this new fancy boded no good, gave a last glance at the motionless figure in the great bow-window, and stole softly out, for he had a cross-country journey to make to an outlying farmhouse ere his day's work was done.

The gray shadows deepened over the snow-clad country, and the labourers coming from the farms passed onward to the village in the gloaming—home to their wives and children.

And never a one but as he passed looked up at the bow-window and muttered a kindly word of sympathy as he saw, in the twilight, the white face of the old parson pressed to the window-pane, and watching for his boy to come out of the darkness that had fallen on Audrey Hill.

Old Janet busied herself with preparations for the morrow, but the tears trickled down her furrowed cheeks as she hung the holly in the hall. Where would her poor old master spend his next Christmas?

That was the thought that harassed old Janet, and made her so wretched that she set-to and scolded the little village girl who had come in to help with the housework, and nearly frightened the child out of her wits.

Janet was sorry directly afterwards, and loaded the child with good things and caresses.

"Janet!"

It was the master's voice. Janet heard it, for she had left the sitting-room door ajar while she was in the kitchen.

She found the old parson still by the window, but the darkness had fallen upon the world without, and he could watch the London road no longer.

"Janet," he said feebly, "put me by the fire; I'm going to sleep. Wake me when Master Eric comes. He'll come to-night; he'll come to-night!"

Old Janet's lips trembled as she wheeled her master's chair in front of the fire, drew the red curtains across the window, and lit the lamp.

"Yes, dearie," she said soothingly. "Maybe he will—maybe he will."

"See, Janet!" exclaimed Parson Rayne, lifting his arm and pointing with his trembling finger to the picture of the golden-haired boy that hung above the mantel-shelf. "That's my Eric. Do you remember him, Janet? It's a hundred years since he went away."

Janet said never a word, but went out of the room lest her full heart should overflow, and her master should see her grief.

Parson Rayne sat back in his easy-chair, with his hands folded across his breast, and his eyes fixed upon little Eric— his Eric, his blue-eyed, golden-haired boy that was coming home to-night.

Gradually his eyes closed, and a deep sleep came upon him.

The clock ticked on, and still he slept. In his sleep he muttered "Eric" now and then for the child had passed from the painter's inanimate canvas to the living canvas of his brain, and in his dream he sat with the laughing boy upon his knee.

Old Janet stole softly in and out, and finding her master asleep, would not disturb him.

It was about seven o'clock when a gentle knock came at the door.

Janet opened it quietly, lest she should disturb the parson.

There were three persons standing in the darkness—a gentleman, a lady, and a little boy.

The gentleman was the young curate.

"Let us speak with you alone, Mistress Janet," he said. "Where is the vicar?"

"In the sittin'-room, asleep," answered Janet, wondering what visitors the curate had brought so late at night.

The curate held the door open, and motioned to the lady to follow him. And Janet, astonished, led the way to the kitchen.

Janet started when the little group stood in the light, and she saw the face of the little boy, who clung timidly to the lady's dress.

She rubbed her eyes, and then, with a white face and staring eyes, fell upon her knees. "Is it a wraith," she cried, "that you've brought wi' ye the nicht, or have my old eyes seen one face in memory so long that every child's face seems like it?"

"Hush, Janet," said the young clergyman; "it is a strange story which this lady has to tell. I met her in the village, asking her way here. This little one is the lost Eric's son; this lady is his wife."

"And he—my bonny bairn—where is he?" cried Janet

seizing the lady's hand. "Say he's waitin' out yonder for his faither to forgie him—say he's there! Ye dinna speak—tell me where he is! Oh my bairn—my bonny bairn—say he's there!"

The lady lifted her veil, and Janet saw that her face was wet with tears.

"Alas," she said with a little sob, "my husband is dead!"

Old Janet sat back in her chair, and buried her face in her hands.

"Listen, Janet," said the lady, rising and taking the old servant's hand gently in hers—"listen, my good Janet. Eric has told me of you—how you were more than a mother to him. For you I have his dying message, and almost his dying kiss; the last one that he gave me is for his father."

"Dead!" sobbed Janet, rocking herself to and fro. "Dead! and the maister has hoped on a' thae weary years, and I hae hoped too. And we'll never see him again this side o' the grave. Oh my bairn—my bonny bairn!"

"I come to-night with a message from him, with the last words his lips ever uttered," whispered the lady. "I have come over leagues of water, from a far-off land, to tell Eric's father how, dying, he blessed him and prayed for him. It was when his last illness was upon him that he told me for the first time the story of his parting with his father."

"Why did he never write? why did he never write?" cried Janet, still with her apron to her eyes.

"He would not. He swore that his father should never see or hear of him again. It was cruel and wicked. Had I known it, it should never have been. On his death-bed his pride broke down, the old memories of home conquered, and with his dying breath he bade me bring my child to England and place him on his grandfather's knee."

Mrs. Rayne lifted her child upon her own knee as she spoke, loosed the wrapper from his throat, and took his little hat off, and, as she did so, a shower of golden curls fell over the boy's shoulders.

The clergyman started, and Janet's red eyes were fixed upon the child as though he were a vision.

"It's my bairn," she murmured; "it's my bairn! Ye hae seen the picture in the sittin'-room, sir; is it no my bonny bairn himsell?"

"The likeness is marvellous," answered the clergyman, looking intently at the child—"most marvellous. He might have stepped from the canvas."

Then Janet told Eric's widow how the parson was asleep, how his mind was wandering, and how he had said that his Eric would come that night.

The young clergyman sat for a moment in deep thought. He was wondering how best to break the news of the son's death to the old parson—how best to tell him that beneath his roof were the wanderer's widow and child.

"Gie the bairn to me," said Janet, taking little Eric in her arms and kissing him passionately, "and bide ye here. I'll tak' him tae the maister."

Mrs. Rayne consented to Janet's proposition, and bade the child not be frightened, but go with the kind lady and see his grandpa.

Little Eric had heard of the poor grandpa he was coming to see, and many a time, as the great ship ploughed its way across the Atlantic, the child had asked when it would be England, where grandpa lived.

So, kissing his little hand to his mother, he let Janet carry him tenderly in her loving arms into the sitting-room where grandpa was sleeping.

Softly the old servant crept in with her precious burden in her arms; and as her eyes sought eagerly the picture of little Eric above the mantel-piece, she stooped and pressed a fervent kiss upon the little one's rosy lips, for the father lived again in the son.

Parson Rayne still slept. Gently Janet placed the little boy beside his knee, and bade him not speak till grandpapa awoke.

Then she sat herself down by the fire, as she used to do in the days when her Eric was a little one, and her old voice piped out, in a sweet mellow tone, an old Scotch song that had been a favourite with the child.

Presently the minister muttered as if in his sleep. The words of the old familiar song were flooding across his brain, working themselves into his troubled dream, as external sounds will at times.

"Sing to him, Janet," he murmured; "sing to him. Sing to Eric."

The boy looked up at hearing his name, and gently touched his grandfather's hand. Slowly the heavy lids were lifted, and the eyes looked down.

For one moment the old parson seemed dazed; then he raised his trembling hands and rubbed his eyes, and looked in wonder at the child who stood beside his knee.

"My Eric!" he cried, lifting the child up, and clasping him to his breast. "My Eric—at last! at last!"

Then the tears flowed fast from his eyes, and burying his face in the boy's golden curls, he sobbed like a child.

Eric, frightened, gave a little cry.

"My darling, my boy!" said the old parson, lifting his head; "you are my Eric, are you not? I have been dreaming—a bad, dreadful dream. I dreamt you were grown to be a man, and had left your poor old father to die. But you are Eric, aren't you? Speak—speak! Let me hear it is not some vision come to mock me!"

"My name is Eric Rayne. Are you my gan'pa?"

"Grandpa!"

The old man sat with his trembling hand upon the child's head, and glanced upward at the picture above the mantelpiece.

Janet, who had stood a silent spectator of the scene, came quietly forward.

"Maister," she said, laying her hand upon his shoulder,

"this is our bairn's bairn. His faither has sent him across the sea to you. You said your Eric would come the nicht. God sends you this ane, and is he no Eric? Is he no the blue-eyed, golden-haired bairn his faither was?"

The old parson's white face was flushed with emotion, his dull eyes were bright. The sudden joy, the strange meeting, had aroused the long-torpid brain. Gradually the truth dawned upon him.

"I know now," he said softly. "My Eric is dead; this is his son."

Gently old Janet crept from the room and left the child and the old man together.

That night all was told. That night the old parson, the impending veil lifted from his reason, heard from the lips of his daughter-in-law the strange story of Eric Rayne's flight from home, and subsequent life.

Edith Rayne told how she had met Eric in America. Soon after their marriage they went to California, and there her husband made money in a mining adventure which had since become world-famous.

There little Eric was born; and there her husband was seized with the illness which proved fatal to him.

"On his death-bed Eric told me all, and how, in his pride, he had never repented the vow he made that you should hear of him no more. But, lying there, knowing that the end was near, his heart melted, and he yearned to see you again and crave your forgiveness. 'Take little Eric, Edith,' he whispered, 'when I am gone, and go to England to the village where my father's house is, and tell him that I died blessing him and asking his forgiveness.' Then he had the little one lifted up to him, and kissed him, bidding him carry that kiss across the sea to his grandpapa, and say that Eric sent it."

Edith Rayne, as she spoke, lifted her boy on to his grandfather's knee, and the lips of the child and the old man met.

* * * * * *

It is summer, and the roses bloom about the porch of the old Parsonage that stands upon the London Road.

The air is full of the scent of flowers, and the dusty road is flooded with golden sunlight.

Pressed against the bow-window of the Parsonage is a face familiar to all the country-side. It is the face of old Parson Rayne, but it is not the white, drawn face of old; the cheeks are full and pink, and the lips are parted in a smile.

Parson Rayne is watching for Eric, and he does not watch in vain. Bareheaded, his golden curls dancing in the sunlight, the little one comes running towards the house, his hands full of flowers which the cottagers have given him.

And behind him, walking more sedately, comes Edith Rayne, his mother.

Then grandpa hurries to the gate and lifts the child up and kisses him, and presently the old house rings with childish laughter and the clatter of little feet.

It is a happy home now, and old Janet is quite contented to hand over the keys to the sweet lady who has brought sunshine to it from across the seas, and is a daughter to the old master, who for eight long years was childless.

Eric is dead; but Eric's wife and Eric's son came one Christmas eve out of the haze that hung over Audrey Hill, and with them came reason and happiness once more to old Parson Rayne.

GEORGE R. SIMS.

CHRISTMAS EVE IN A BELFRY.

[ADAPTED.]

We were a merry party at Uncle George's house one Christmas eve, a good many years ago now.

Uncle George was a widower, with three daughters. Polly, the youngest, was a merry-eyed, laughter-loving girl of eighteen.

"Polly," said I, at the end of a dance, "how very quiet

some people are to-night. I'll wager a dozen pairs of gloves I know what you're thinking about."

"Some people are very smart to-night; pray, what am I thinking about?"

"How tremendously warm it is!" broke in Uncle George. "Christmas eve! Why, it's hot enough for July. Tom, open the lawn-door and let in some fresh air."

I opened the door, and returned to Polly. "What do you say to a turn round the garden?"

"Oh, I should so enjoy it!"

"Well, throw your shawl over your shoulders, and on the first move we'll slip out unobserved."

In a few minutes we strolled quietly out by the lawn-door.

"What a delightful evening! Look at that lovely moon! isn't it beautiful?"

"Glorious! It reminds me of a poem I read some time ago. Let me see; it begins—

'When the pale orb of Diana shines over the sea,
When nature's reposing—reposing—'

I forget what comes next; I know the line ends with he—or she—or be. Oh, I say, Polly, shall we have a turn round the old church?"

We now arrived at the church tower. The door was open; I peeped in. "Shall we mount to the belfry and view the village by moonlight? You won't be frightened?"

"Frightened! No. What a charming adventure for Christmas eve. Come along, Tom."

Half way up the stair we came to an iron door: how fortunate! it was open also.

We now gained the summit, and were standing just under the chime of bells.

"How beautiful! Look at the lights in the village—and see, yonder's our house; I wonder if they've—"

There was a sudden gust of wind, and then a loud bang. I

ran down the stair. The middle door was blown to; we were securely fastened in! There we were, shut up in the belfry of an old Norman church tower, just before midnight on Christmas eve!

"What are we to do, Tom? whatever will become of us?"

"Be calm, Polly; compose yourself. I've a box of vesuvians. I'll light them one by one, and throw out signals of distress."

"But who is to see them? It's not twelve o'clock yet! Must we stay here all night?"

"Polly!"

"Oh, bother! do something! I would, if I were a man. I shall die before morning!"

"Never mind, Polly; I'll not desert you. At least, we shall die together!"

"Thank you; you're too kind. I'm catching an awful—cold."

"Oh, that's nothing! No, no, I don't mean that, but—hush! don't you hear voices?"

"Yes, yes; it's old Giles and his man David! They ring the chimes on Christmas eve."

The bells now began to swing slowly to and fro. *Ding-dong! ding-dong! ding-dong!*

I ran down to the iron door. "Hullo there! Giles, I say! Giles, we're shut in!"

"Mussy on uz! wot be that, David? didn't ye 'ear zummat?"

"No, I 'eard nowt!"

"Giles, I say! Giles, open the door! We're shut in!" and I rattled at the door.

"Eh! Giles, Giles! it be a ghost! Coom away, man! Coom away!"

"Don't run away wi'out me, David! Don't leave me 'ere alone, ye coward! Don't!"

And away ran the two old men towards the village, shouting, 'A ghost! a ghost!"

"Here's a nice kettle of fish, Polly; these two old idiots have taken me for a ghost, and they'll raise the village. Well, never mind; here goes."

And seizing a rope, I began to ring one of the bells.

"What on earth are you doing, Tom?"

"Sounding the tocsin, Polly. (*Ding-dong!*) Ringing the alarm-bell, Polly!" (*Ding-dong!*)

And now "there was a sound of revelry" below. Looking down we could see a small army of villagers, armed with shovels, rakes, and pitchforks. Then we heard Uncle George say, "A ghost! humbug! A sovereign to the first man who mounts the belfry!"

"Ah'll go, squire!"

"That's right, my man; I'll join you," said Uncle George. "It's all fancy; there's no one up there."

We heard them mount the stairs, and rattle at the iron door. "Who is up there?" To which I replied by a long, loud, unearthly yell.

Uncle George sprang downstairs, three steps at a time, followed by his *stanch* supporters.

"Five sovereigns to the man who breaks open that door!"

"Give uz 'old o' your shovel, Jacob; ghost or no ghost, ah'll av' 'um out!"

The door was now attacked with heavy blows by the besiegers.

A little afraid for Polly, I said, "Go upstairs while I capitulate." Then I shouted, "Hullo, you ruffians! What's all this noise about?"

"Bless me! that's Tom's voice."

"Of course it is, uncle; and Polly's here as well.—Come downstairs, Polly."

The door was at last forced open, and Polly rushed into her father's arms.

"Don't be angry, papa; we couldn't help it."

"Angry, my dear, no, no! But what's this your wrapped up in? Ha, ha, ha! You are a beauty now, and no mistake!"

Polly did cut rather a queer figure, enveloped as she was in an old sack I had found in the belfry, while her hands and face were covered with black dust.

"It's a shame to laugh at you, my dear, but really—ha, ha, ha!—I can't help it. Bless me, how cold you are! Put on my ulster, and we'll run the whole way home."

And thus ended our adventure on Christmas eve in a belfry.

MOSLEY.

HOUP-LA.

(By permission of Messrs. FREDERICK WARNE AND Co.)

"Now, come, young shaver, look alive! Be quick, or—" and Mr. Frisco cracked his long white whip—"it'll be worse for you. D'ye hear?"

"Yes, yes, Mr. Frisco."

There was a moment of intense silence in the deserted circus-ring, lighted only by one flaring gas jet, and such daylight as could flicker feebly through the ventilation apertures at the top of the tent.

The boy, an ill-fed, meagre-faced, undersized lad of twelve years old or so, with thin, trembling lips, tightened by a life of misery and fear, and big, bright eyes, unnaturally keen and quick, stood ready to mount the ladder leading to the trapeze swings high up above their heads.

Poor little chap! He had been many days now trying hard to achieve a difficult and dangerous trapeze leap, which was, in fact, utterly beyond his strength to perform.

That leap was never absent from his thoughts for a single instant during his waking hours, and night after night he dreamt with horror of his morning's rush through the air.

"Come, up you go!" shouted the ring-master savagely.

So up he went, took the leap, and, missing the bar, fell into the net below. There was a quiver and a crack of the long white whip, followed by a piercing shriek from the poor boy.

"Come, up you go again! Fail this time, and you'll do it without the net."

"I'll be killed, Mr. Frisco!"

"It's all your worth! Up you go!"

Up he toiled once more, took the leap, and fell again.

The white thong flew out with a hiss, and curled once more round the limbs of the helpless boy.

"You shall do it now without the net," the ring-master shouted, and he flung down the whip and kicked the boy aside; but the next instant he had measured his length upon the ground, and lay biting the sawdust of the ring.

"Do it without the net! No, he will not, you miserable coward," shouted a voice in his ears. "As I live, you shall have a taste of your own treatment! Get up!"

As the bully regained his feet, the thong of his own whip whizzed through the air and caught him neatly in a double circle round the limbs, and fell again and again in sharp, cutting strokes, until his brawny body had, pretty nearly every inch of it, paid the dearest penalty of his cowardice. At last he fell writhing to the ground again. Then the new-comer stayed his arm and drew the long white thong through his left hand, as if it had done good service and he was grateful to it.

A lithe, handsome fellow he was—soldier all over him—cool as ice, too, as he surveyed the writhing, howling Mr. Frisco with infinite amusement in his steady blue eyes.

"Now, stop that noise! Do you hear? Or do you want another taste of this? Get up!"

Very slowly and unwillingly the ring-master rose.

"Are you this boy's father?"

"No."

"Where is his father?"

"He's dead."

"And his mother?"

"She's dead too."

"Who looks after him?"

"I do."

"Oh, you do! Nice way you've got of doing it! Well, if you want him back again, you can apply to the magistrates; meantime, I shall give the police orders to look after you. —Come along, my lad."

"He's my apprentice—he's bound to me—he has cost me pounds and pounds, and—"

"Yes; you can tell all that to the magistrates, you know. Here is my card, though you know me well enough without it."

He made a gesture to the boy to go before him, and left the circus, still carrying the whip in his hand. He hailed a cab and drove to the barracks.

"Are you cold, my boy?"

"Ay, sir."

"Well, never mind, you'll be warm by-and-by. What's your name?"

"They call me Houp-La."

"Houp-La! A very likely name for you. But what is your real name?"

"Tom Snow."

"How old are you?"

"Twelve, goin' on thirteen, sir."

"Can you read or write?"

"No; but I can do the snake-trick an' the wrigglin'-dodge."

"Yes, I know. I've seen you do both."

Lieutenant Lacy found the favourite of the regiment—which Bootles was to a man, from commanding officer down to the last-joined subaltern and most lately enlisted recruit—sitting in a big chair before the fire, watching the boy, who was sitting on a skin rug, luxuriating in the heat and warm light of the bright flames which blazed half-way up the chimney.

"Where did you pick him up?"

"At the circus, Lacy; that brute Frisco was teaching him a new trapeze trick with the aid of that whip, and I stopped him and brought young Houp-La away. That's all."

"And how did Mr. Fwrisco come off?"

"'E wolloped 'im."

" Ah! wolloped him, did he? And what did Mr. Fwrisco say to that?"

"'E 'owled! Wen 'e come in and see wot 'e were up to, 'e sends 'im flyin' among the sawdust; and then 'e says, 'Get up!' and 'e 'ad to get up, and then the capting 'e give 'im proper. I never see such a wollopin'—wi' 'is own whip, too, that was the best o' it. But the capting ain't never goin' to let me go back to 'im—never no more. I'll never do nothin' wot'll vex you—I never will—no, not if I was to swing for it."

It was surprising how soon young Houp-La settled down into his new life. He was popular, too, with everybody, high and low.

More than two years had passed away when the Scarlet Lancers received orders for active service. On that last day, when home lay at one end of the journey, and Egypt at the other—when war stood out grim and ghastly—there was scarcely a really light heart to be found in the entire strength of the gay and gallant regiment.

Young Houp-La came in to say good-bye to his mistress.

"You are very young for this service, my boy."

"Yes, mum."

"But I know you will do your very best to make the captain comfortable."

"I will, mum, I will; you may depend on me."

And she drew the poor little circus waif to her heart, and asked God to bless him.

One evening, when the Scarlet Lancers had left Alexandria behind them, Captain Ferrars was summoned to the colonel's tent. Tom, who was outside, heard the order and followed his master. With his sharp young ear held close to the tent, he heard the details of a dangerous mission which Captain Ferrars had been chosen to perform. The order was given in the simplest words—he was to carry a despatch to a body of troops lying about five miles from the Scarlet Lancers' camp. To reach the other British camp, the envoy must pass through the rebel lines. And young Tom heard it all—every word.

"Why couldn't they send some duffer as wouldn't be missed?—there's plenty on 'em about. If only I was a man. I never wanted to be a man before—I was proud o' my littleness; but now—now—I'd give the world, if I 'ad it, to be as big as my master. The world—ay, my life, for that matter."

He now saw the despatch given to his master; saw him put it in his pocket-book.

"Why shouldn't I give my life? The capt'n 'ud make a big hole in the regiment, but who'd ever miss me? If I get back, well and good; if I don't, it won't make a deal o' matter. Ay, I'll do it."

He now saw his master walk quickly to his own tent, and followed him.

"Is that you, Tom?"

"Yes, sir."

"Take my flask on the chest there to the mess-tent and get it filled with brandy, and be quick."

"Yes, sir."

Tom had seen the moment he entered the tent that Captain Ferrars had laid down his pocket-book on the chest. Quick as thought Tom snatched it up with the flask, and ran out. Once outside, he threw the flask to the winds, and made for the outposts.

By means of the snake-trick, on which he had so prided himself of old, he wriggled past the various sentries with the stealth and noiselessness of an Indian scout, took out the despatch, threw the pocket-book away, and with a last look at the camp, turned his face towards the five miles of difficulty and danger which lay before him.

The lad's brave spirit never failed him for an instant. He never thought of the harm he might be doing, still less of the risk he was running.

"What a long time that boy is! My pocket-book! the despatch!—I put it there—I'm certain of it—I could swear to it."

He turned all his pockets out, tossed everything over and over; pocket-book and despatch were not to be found.

The colonel must be told at once; so, with a mighty effort, he pulled himself together and went out, with a sinking heart, to tell the tale of his own shame and dishonour.

After he had given up his sword and his parole of honour, and then had passed the night in his tent alone, it all came out. His flask had been found as soon as morning light broke over the camp not twenty yards from his tent; his pocket-book had been found just outside the most advanced outposts; and Tom was missing.

That Tom had taken the despatch seemed beyond all doubt, but Captain Ferrars declared his firm belief in Tom's faithfulness.

That evening electric lights flashed these words, in cypher, from the other camp,—

"*All right! Got your message! Will act as you direct!*"

"Ask who took the message?"

The reply came back,—

"*A boy! Left camp—on return journey—with reply—before daybreak!*"

The news spread through the camp in next to no time. Captain Ferrars went straight to the colonel and asked that a searching-party might be sent out at once.

"Certainly, certainly! And go yourself, if you care to do it, Ferrars. I have much pleasure in returning your sword. I sincerely hope the lad has come to no harm; he is the hero of the campaign."

A mile from the rebel outposts they found him. Captain Ferrars heard a low moan, and, in a moment, was down upon his knees beside the half-unconscious boy.

"Tell the capt'n I got there safe—the answer's in my wes'coat pocket. I couldn't get back as well. One o' them Arabs shot me. I crawled as far's I could, but I couldn't get no furder. Is that you, sir?"

"Where are you hurt, my boy?"

"It's all over wi' me now, sir."

And now strong but gentle hands bore him tenderly back to the captain's tent. He bade them send for the colonel, that he might give the despatch into his own hands.

"I knew the capt'n couldn't go safe—where I could; an' I thought as 'ow it wouldn't matter so much—if aught 'appened to me. You're not angry wi' me, are you, sir?"

"No, my boy; certainly not. You're the bravest lad in the army. I am proud of you—very proud."

"You'll tell the missis, capt'n—as 'ow I kep' my word—an' took care of you, sir?"

"I wish she were here now, my boy. She would thank you as I cannot do, and comfort you as I don't know how."

The minutes passed slowly away, and intense silence reigned throughout the tent. Suddenly Tom spoke again.

"I ain't in no pain now, sir—but I'm orful tired."

"Try and sleep a little, Tom."

"Yes, I think I'll try—I'm orful tired."

Then there was silence again—a silence longer, deeper, more profound than that which had been before—broken only by the sound of the boy's sharp-drawn breath.

Captain Ferrars held the slight form close in his arms; held it till the last faint sigh had fluttered through the whitened lips; held it, even though he knew that the brave hero-soul had slipped away.

"You'd better come away now, old fellow," said Lacy. "You can't do the poor little chap any good now."

Captain Ferrars slowly unloosed his hold, and looked down upon the brave, white face of the little circus waif who had been faithful even to the very end.

"I knew he hadn't sold me—God bless him! He loved me better than himself." Then he turned away, and strode out into the darkness alone.   JOHN STRANGE WINTER.

ONE NICHE THE HIGHEST.

The scene opens with a view of the great Natural Bridge in Virginia. There are three or four lads standing in the channel below, looking up with awe to that vast arch of unhewn rocks which the Almighty bridged over these everlasting butments, "when the morning stars sang together." The little piece of sky spanning those measureless piers is full of stars, although it is mid-day. It is almost five hundred feet from where they stand, up those perpendicular bulwarks of limestone to the key of that vast arch, which appears to them only of the size of a man's hand. The silence of death is rendered more impressive by the little stream that falls from rock to rock down the channel. The sun is darkened; and the boys have uncovered their heads, as if standing in the presence-chamber of the Majesty of the whole earth. At last this feeling begins to wear away; they look around them, and find that others have been there before them. They see the names of hundreds cut in the limestone butments. A new feeling comes over their young hearts, and their knives are in their hands in an instant. "What man has done, man can do," is their watchword, while they draw themselves up, and carve their name a foot above those of a hundred full-grown men who have been there before them.

They are all satisfied with this feat of physical exertion except one, whose example illustrates perfectly the forgotten truth that there is "no royal road to learning." This ambitious youth sees a name just above his reach—a name which will be green in the memory of the world when those of Alexander, Cæsar, and Bonaparte will rot in oblivion. It was the name of Washington. Before he marched with Braddock to that fatal field, he had been there, and left his name a foot above any of his predecessors. It was a glorious thought to write his name side by side with that great father of his country. He grasps his knife with a firmer hand, and clinging to a little jutting crag, he cuts again into the limestone, about a foot above where he stands; he then reaches up and cuts another for his hands. 'Tis a dangerous adventure; but as he puts his feet and hands into those gains, and draws himself up carefully to his full length, he finds himself a foot above every name chronicled in that mighty wall. While his companions are regarding him with concern and admiration, he cuts his name in wide capitals large and deep into that flinty album. His knife is still in his hand, and strength in his sinews, and a new created aspiration in his heart. Again he cuts another niche, and again he carves his name in larger capitals. This is not enough. Heedless of the entreaties of his companions, he cuts and climbs again. The gradations of his ascending scale grow wider apart: he measures his length at every gain he cuts. The voices of his friends wax weaker and weaker, till their words are finally lost on his ear. He now for the first time casts a look beneath him. Had that glance lasted a moment, that moment would have been his last. He clings with a convulsive shudder to his little niche in the rock. An awful abyss awaits his almost certain fall. He is faint with severe exertion, and trembling from the sudden view of the dreadful destruction to which he is exposed. His knife is worn half-way to the haft. He can hear the voices, but not the words, of his terror-stricken companions below. What a moment! what a meagre chance to escape destruction! There is no retracing his steps. It is impossible to put his hands into the same niche with his feet, and retain his slender hold a moment. His companions instantly perceive this new and fearful dilemma, and await his fall with emotions that "freeze their young blood." He is too high to ask for his father and mother, his brothers and sisters, to come and witness or avert his destruction. But one of his companions anticipates his desire. Swift as the wind, he bounds down the channel, and the situation of the fated boy is told upon his father's hearth-stone. Minutes of almost eternal length roll on, and there are hundreds standing in that rocky channel, and hundreds on the bridge above, all holding their breath, and awaiting the fearful catastrophe. The poor boy hears the hum of new and numerous voices both above and below. He can just distinguish the tones of his father, who is shouting with all the energy of despair, "William, William! don't look down! Your mother and Henry and Harriet are all here praying for you! Don't look down! Keep your eye towards the top!" The boy didn't look down. His eye is fixed like a flint towards heaven, and his young heart on Him who reigns there. He grasps again his knife. He cuts another niche, and another foot is added to the hundreds that remove him from the reach of human help from below. How carefully he uses his wasting blade! How anxiously he selects the softest places in that vast pier! How he avoids every flinty grain! How he economizes his physical powers, resting a moment at each gain he cuts. How every motion is watched from below! There stand his father, mother, brother, and sister, on the very spot where, if he falls, he will not fall alone.

The sun is half-way down in the west. The lad has made fifty additional niches in that mighty wall, and now finds himself directly under the middle of that vast arch of rock, earth, and trees. He must cut his way in a new direction to get from this overhanging mountain. The inspiration of hope is in his bosom; its vital heat is fed by the increasing shouts of hundreds perched upon cliffs and trees, and of others who stand with ropes in their hands upon the bridge above, or with ladders below. Fifty more gains must be cut before the longest rope can reach him. His wasting blade strikes again into the limestone. The boy is emerging painfully foot by foot from under that lofty arch. Spliced ropes are in the hands of those who are leaning over the outer edge of the bridge. Two minutes more and all will be over. That blade is worn to the last half inch. The boy's head reels; his eyes are starting from their sockets. His last hope is dying in his heart, his life must hang upon the next gain he cuts. That niche is his last. At the last flint-gash he makes, his knife—his faithful knife—falls from his nerveless hand, and ringing along the precipice, falls at his mother's feet. An involuntary groan of despair runs like a death-knell through the channel below, and all is still as the grave. At the height of nearly three hundred feet, the devoted boy lifts his hopeless heart and closing eyes to commend his soul to God. 'Tis but a moment—there! one foot swings off!—he is reeling—trembling—toppling over into eternity. Hark! a shout falls on his ears from above! The man who is lying with half of his length over the bridge has caught a glimpse of the boy's head and shoulders. Quick as thought the noosed rope is within reach of the sinking youth. No one breathes. With a faint, convulsive effort, the swooning boy drops his arm into the noose. Darkness comes over him, and with the words "God!" and "mother!" whispered on his lips just loud enough to be heard in heaven, the tightening rope lifts him out of his last shallow niche. Not a lip moves while he is dangling over that fearful abyss; but when a sturdy Virginian reaches down and draws up the lad, and holds him up in his arms before the tearful, breathless multitude—such shouting and such leaping and weeping for joy never greeted a human being so recovered from the yawning gulf of eternity.

ELIHU BURRITT.

THE MOTHER AND HER DEAD CHILD.

There sat a mother with a little child. She was so downcast, so afraid that it should die! It was so pale; the small eyes had closed themselves; it drew its breath so softly, and now and then with a deep respiration, as if it sighed, and the mother looked still more sorrowfully on the little creature.

Then a knocking was heard at the door, and in came a poor old man wrapped up as in a large horse-cloth, for it warms one, and he needed it, as it was the cold winter season. Everything

THE MOTHER AND HER DEAD CHILD.

out of doors was covered with ice and snow, and the wind blew so that it cut the face.

As the old man trembled with cold, and the little child slept a moment, the mother went and poured some ale into a pint-pot and set it on the stove that it might be warm for him. The old man sat and rocked the cradle; and the mother sat down on a chair close by him, looked at her little sick child that drew its breath so deep, and raised its little hand.

"Do you think that I shall save him?" said she. "Our Lord will not take him from me?"

And the old man—it was Death himself—he nodded so strangely, it could just as well signify Yes as No. And the mother looked down in her lap, and the tears ran down over her cheeks. Her head became so heavy—she had not closed her eyes for three days and nights; and now she slept, but only for a minute, when she started up and trembled with cold. "What is that?" said she, and looked on all sides; but the old man was gone, and her little child had gone—he had taken it with him; and the old clock in the corner burred, and burred, the great leaden weight ran down to the floor, bump! and then the clock also stood still.

But the poor mother ran out of the house and cried aloud for her child.

Out there, in the midst of the snow, there sat a woman in long, black clothes; and she said, "Death has been in thy chamber, and I saw him hasten away with thy little child. He goes faster than the wind, and he never brings back what he takes."

"Oh, only tell me which way he went!" said the mother. "Tell me the way, and I shall find him!"

"I know it!" said the woman in black clothes; "but before I tell it, thou must sing for me all the songs thou hast sung to thy child. I am fond of them; I have heard them before. I am Night; I saw thy tears whilst thou sangst them."

"I will sing them all—all!" said the mother; "but do not stop me now—I may overtake him—I may find my child."

THE MOTHER AND HER DEAD CHILD.

But Night stood still and mute. Then the mother wrung her hands, sang, and wept. And there were many songs, but yet many more tears; and then Night said, "Go to the right, into the dark pine forest: thither I saw Death take his way with thy little child."

The roads crossed each other in the depths of the forest, and she knew no longer whither she should go. Then there stood a thorn-bush; there was neither leaf nor flower on it. It was also in the cold winter season, and ice-flakes hung on the branches.

"Hast thou seen Death go past with my little child?" said the mother.

"Yes," said the thorn-bush; "but I will not tell thee which way he took, unless thou wilt first warm me up at thy heart. I am freezing to death; I shall become a lump of ice."

And she pressed the thorn-bush to her breast so firmly, that it might be thoroughly warmed; and the thorns went right into her flesh, and her blood flowed in large drops. But the thorn-bush shot forth fresh green leaves, and there came flowers on it in the cold winter night, the heart of the afflicted mother was so warm; and the thorn-bush told her the way she should go.

She then came to a large lake, where there was neither ship nor boat. The lake was not frozen sufficiently to bear her; neither was it open or low enough that she could wade through it; and across it she must go if she would find her child. Then she lay down to drink up the lake; and that was an impossibility for a human being, but the afflicted mother thought that a miracle might happen nevertheless.

"Oh, what would I not give to come to my child!" said the weeping mother; and she wept still more, and her eyes sank down into the depths of the waters and became two precious pearls. But the water bore her up, as if she sat on a swing, and she flew on the rocking waves to the shore on the opposite side, where there stood a mile-broad, strange house—one knew not if it were a mountain with forests and caverns, or if it were built up; but the poor mother could not see it, she had wept her eyes out.

"Where shall I find Death, who took away my little child?" said she.

"He has not come here yet," said the old grave-woman, who was appointed to look after Death's great greenhouse. "How have you been able to find your way hither? and who has helped you?"

"Our Lord has helped me," said she. "He is merciful, and you will also be so. Where shall I find my little child?"

"Nay, I know not," said the woman, "and you cannot see! Many flowers and trees have withered this night. Death will soon come and plant them over again. You certainly know that every person has his or her life's tree or flower, just as every one happens to be settled. They look like other plants, but have pulsations of the heart. Children's hearts can also beat. Go after yours, perhaps you may know your child's; but what will you give me, if I tell you what you shall do more?"

"I have nothing to give," said the afflicted mother, "but I will go to the world's end for you."

"Nay, I have nothing to do there," said the woman; "but you can give me your long black hair. You know yourself that it is fine, and that I like it. You shall have my white hair instead; that's always something."

"Do you demand nothing else?" said she;—"that I will gladly give you." And she gave her fine black hair, and got the old woman's snow-white hair instead.

So they went into Death's great greenhouse, where flowers and trees grew strangely into one another. There stood fine hyacinths under glass bells, and there stood strong-stemmed peonies. There grew water-plants, some so fresh, others half-sick; the water-snakes lay down on them, and black crabs pinched their stalks. There stood beautiful palm trees, oaks, and plantains; there stood parsley and flowering thyme. Every tree and every flower had its name. Each of them was a human life, and the human frame still lived—one in China and another in Greenland—round about in the world. There were large trees in small pots, so that they stood so stunted in growth, and ready to burst the pots; in other places there was a little dull flower in rich mould, with moss round about it, and it was so petted and nursed. But the distressed mother bent down over all the smallest plants, and heard within them how the human heart beat; and amongst millions she knew her child's.

"There it is!" cried she, and stretched her hands out over a little blue crocus, that hung quite sickly on one side.

"Don't touch the flower!" said the old woman; "but place yourself here, and when Death comes—I expect him every moment—do not let him pluck the flower up, but threaten him that you will do the same with the others. Then he will be afraid. He is responsible for them to our Lord, and no one dares to pluck them up before He gives leave."

All at once an icy cold rushed through the great hall, and the blind mother could feel that it was Death that came.

"How hast thou been able to find thy way hither?" he asked. "How couldst thou come quicker than I?"

"I am a mother," said she.

And Death stretched out his long hand towards the fine little flower; but she held her hands fast round his, so tight, and yet afraid that she should touch one of the leaves. Then Death blew on her hands, and she felt that it was colder than the wind, and her hands fell down powerless.

"Thou canst not do anything against me!" said Death.

"But our Lord can!" said she.

"I only do his bidding!" said Death. "I am his gardener: I take all his flowers and trees, and plant them out in the great garden of Paradise, in the unknown land; but how they grow there, and how it is there, I dare not tell thee."

"Give me back my child!" said the mother, and she wept and prayed. At once she seized hold of two beautiful flowers close by, with each hand, and cried out to Death, "I will tear all thy flowers off, for I am in despair."

"Touch them not!" said Death. "Thou say'st that thou art so unhappy, and now thou wilt make another mother equally unhappy."

"Another mother!" said the poor woman, and directly let go her hold of both the flowers.

"There, thou hast thine eyes," said Death. "I fished them up from the lake. They shone so bright; but I knew not they were thine. Take them again; they are now brighter than before. Now look down into the deep well close by: I shall tell thee the names of the two flowers thou wouldst have torn up, and thou wilt see their whole future life—their whole human existence. See what thou wast about to disturb and destroy!"

And she looked down into the well, and it was a happiness to see how the one became a blessing to the world, to see how much happiness and joy were felt everywhere. And she saw the other's life, and it was sorrow and distress, horror and wretchedness.

"Both of them are God's will!" said Death.

"Which of them is Misfortune's flower? and which is that of Happiness?" asked she.

"That I will not tell thee," said Death; "but this thou shalt know from me, that the one flower was thy own child; it was thy child's fate thou saw'st—thy own child's future life!"

Then the mother screamed with terror: "Which of them was my child? Tell it me! save the innocent! save my child from all that misery! rather take it away! take it into God's kingdom! Forget my tears, forget my prayers, and all that I have done!"

"I do not understand thee," said Death. "Wilt thou have thy child again? or shall I go with it there, where thou dost not know?"

Then the mother wrung her hands, fell on her knees, and

prayed to our Lord, "Oh, hear me not when I pray against Thy will, which is the best! hear me not! hear me not!"

And she bowed her head down in her lap, and Death took her child and went with it into the unknown land.

HANS CHRISTIAN ANDERSEN.

A NOBLE REVENGE.

A young officer had so far forgotten himself, in a moment of irritation, as to strike a private soldier. The inexorable laws of military discipline forbade to the injured soldier any practical redress. He could look for no retaliation by acts. Words only were at his command, and in a tumult of indignation, as he turned away, the soldier said to his officer that he would "make him repent it." This, wearing the shape of a menace, naturally rekindled the officer's anger, and intercepted any disposition which might be rising within him towards a sentiment of remorse; and thus the irritation between the two young men grew hotter than before.

Suppose yourself a spectator, looking down into a valley occupied by two armies. They are facing each other, you see, in martial array,-but it is no more than a skirmish which is going on, in the course of which, however, an occasion suddenly arises for a desperate service. A redoubt, which has fallen into the enemy's hands, must be recaptured at any price, and under circumstances of all but hopeless difficulty. A strong party has volunteered for the service; there is a cry for somebody to head them; you see a soldier step out from the ranks to assume this dangerous leadership; the party moves rapidly forward; in a few minutes it is swallowed up in clouds of smoke; for half-an-hour from behind these clouds you receive hieroglyphic reports of bloody strife—fierce repeating signals, flashes from the guns, rolling musketry, and exulting hurrahs, advancing or receding, slackening or redoubling.

A NOBLE REVENGE.

At length all is over: the redoubt has been recovered; that which was lost is found again; the jewel which had been made captive is ransomed with blood. Crimsoned with glorious gore, the wreck of the conquering party is relieved, and at liberty to return. From the river you see it ascending. The plume-crested officer in command rushes forward, with his left hand raising his hat in homage to the blackened fragments of what once was a flag, whilst with his right hand he seizes that of the leader, though no more than a private from the ranks. *That* perplexes you not; mystery you see none in *that*, for distinctions of order perish, ranks are confounded, "high and low" are words without a meaning, and to wreck goes every notion of feeling that divides the noble from the noble, or the brave man from the brave. But wherefore is it that now, when suddenly they wheel into mutual recognition, suddenly they pause? This soldier, this officer—who are they? Once before they had stood face to face; once again they are meeting, and the gaze of armies is upon them. If, for a moment, a doubt divides them, in a moment the doubt has perished. One glance exchanged between them publishes the forgiveness that is sealed for ever. As one who recovers a brother whom he had accounted dead, the officer sprang forward, threw his arms around the neck of the soldier, and kissed him, as if he were some martyr, glorified by that shadow of death from which he was returning; whilst on *his* part, the soldier, stepping back and saluting his officer, makes this immortal answer—that answer which shut up for ever the memory of the indignity offered to him, even whilst, for the last time, alluding to it, "Sir," he said, "I told you before that I would make you repent it."

THOMAS DE QUINCEY.

SELECTIONS IN POETRY.

THE GAIN OF GIVING.

"He that findeth his life shall lose it," was the minister's text that day, and Eleanor seemed to listen, though her thoughts were far away : in a week it would be holiday-time, and she longed for the time to come that would take her away from the city to her beautiful seaside home.

"He that loseth his life shall find it." Though the words bore a meaning plain, they had none for the child who heard them with restless eyes and brain ; but the sermon at last was ended, and the preacher slowly said, "Our contribution this morning will be for the Children's Aid."

Eleanor's heart beat faster, her face wore a troubled look, as her hand closed softly over her little pocket-book, where she carried a birthday present, a bright new piece of gold, and the look of trouble deepened while her hand took a firmer hold.

"I can't give this," she was thinking, "though it's all I have to give, and I wish that the children all could go to a pleasant place to live." But she saw with a little trembling sob that the bag was on its way, and when it passed her the gold piece in the midst of the silver lay.

'Twas an August day at the sea-shore, and Eleanor raced along where the heavy waves were rolling, and the tide was running strong. She stooped for a sea-shell lying on the hard and shining sand, when a mighty breaker caught her, and swept her away from land.

But before she could cry or struggle, she was seized by a little lad, who dragged her out of the water with all the strength he had; and he said, to her look of wonder, as soon as he'd breath to speak, "I'm one of the Fresh Air children, staying here for a week."

Eleanor thought of the gold piece she had sadly given away: "Why, perhaps, if I'd kept that money he wouldn't be here to-day!—Weren't you afraid of drowning?" He slowly shook his head: "I didn't think of myself at all, but of saving you," he said.

And she suddenly thought of the sermon; its meaning grew clear and plain, about the finding and losing, the giving that's greatest gain—that the life which is lived for others is the only life to lead, and, instead of our vain self-seeking, we should care for another's need. *From "The Young Pilgrim."*

THE KING'S TEMPLE.

A mighty king on his couch reclined, with a haughty thought in his lonely mind: "Has not God prospered me more than all? A nation would rise at my single call, and its fairest maid would be proud to wear a crown by the side of my crowned gray hair. I'll rear Him a house for my greatness' sake, and nobody's aid will I claim or take; from the gilded spire to the great crypt stone it shall be my offering, and mine alone."

Then the site was chosen, the builders wrought to find a shape for the monarch's thought. Soon the abbey rose 'gainst the calm blue sky, and they built it broad, and they built it high; but if any offered, with spade or hod, to give his labour for naught to God, then the poor man's mite by the king was spurned, and he paid him for every stone he turned.

Till at last, on a gorgeous autumn day, all the solemn priests in their white array, with prayers, and anthems, and censers came, and opened the abbey in God's great name.

THE KING'S TEMPLE.

Now there lay in the chancel a great white stone, with the king's name on it, and his alone; and the king stood near it with haughty brow, and pondered, "The future will know me now by the glorious temple I have made, unsullied by any plebeian aid."

And far away, where the melody came but softly, there lingered an aged dame; her garment was worn, and her hair was thin, and she looked like the last of all her kin—who had none to love, who had none to blame, who would start at the sound of her Christian name. Yet she said, as the music o'er her passed, "Thank God that his house is complete at last!"

*   *   *   *

The monarch, that night, on his couch reclined, with a proud content in his lonely mind; but when he slept he strangely dreamed—in the abbey chancel alone he seemed, and he sought his own royal name to read, but lo! another was there instead. 'Twas a woman's name he never had heard, and his heart with wonder and wrath was stirred.

And when he awoke, throughout his land by mouth of heralds he sent command, if a woman bearing a certain name, within a month to his presence came, she should have a cup with a jewelled rim, besides the honour of seeing him.

On the second day, as he sat alone, the courtiers who stood about his throne informed him the woman was at the gate; and they thought, of course, she would have to wait (for even so did the royal kin) for the kingly pleasure to let her in; but he stamped his foot with a stern "Begone! and straightway bring her, and leave us alone." So a great lord brought her, and that lord swore that the king awaited her at the door!

Then, slowly and trembling, in there came, in her poor best weeds, a poor old dame, and the king himself (there were none to stare) kindly led her up to a velvet chair; and when she grew used to the splendid place, and found she could gaze on the royal face, he begged, if she could, she would make it known why he dreamed her name on the chancel stone.

"For what work have *you* done?" the monarch said; "*I've* built all the abbey, and asked no aid."

And the old dame lifted her streaming eyes, and held up her hands in her great surprise. "My liege," she answered, "how much could I do at a great, good work that was meet for you? 'If the king had asked us,' I often thought, 'I could not have given, for I have naught.' But in works for God, how it seems his plan, there's something to do that any one can; so when the builders were ready to sink, I carried some water and gave them to drink."

The king said nothing. Ere morning shone, *his* name was gone from the chancel stone; and with looks of wonder the courtiers read the name of the *woman* writ there instead.

ANON.

THE GIFT OF TRITEMIUS.

Tritemius of Herbipolis one day, while kneeling at the altar's foot to pray alone with God, as was his pious choice, heard from beneath a miserable voice—a sound that seemed of all sad things to tell, as of a lost soul crying out of hell.

Thereat the abbot rose, the chain whereby his thoughts went upward broken by that cry, and, looking from the casement, saw below a wretched woman with gray hair aflow, and withered hands stretched up to him, who cried for alms as one who might not be denied.

She cried, "For the dear love of Him who gave His life for ours, my child from bondage save—my beautiful, brave firstborn, chained with slaves in the Moor's galley, where the sunsmit waves lap the white walls of Tunis!"

"What I can I give," Tritemius said—"my prayers?"

"O man of God!" she cried, for grief had made her bold, "mock me not so. I ask not prayers, but gold; words cannot serve me, alms alone suffice. Even while I plead, perchance my first-born dies!"

"Woman!" Tritemius answered, "from our door none go unfed; hence are we always poor. A single soldo is our only store. Thou hast our prayers; what can we give thee more?"

"Give me," she said, "the silver candlesticks on either side of the great crucifix; God well may spare them on his errands sped, or he can give you golden ones instead."

Then said Tritemius, "Even as thy word, woman, so be it; and our gracious Lord, who loveth mercy more than sacrifice, pardon me if a human soul I prize above the gifts upon his altar piled! Take what thou askest, and redeem thy child."

But his hand trembled as the holy alms he laid within the beggar's eager palms; and as she vanished down the linden shade, he bowed his head and for forgiveness prayed.

So the day passed, and when the twilight came he rose to find the chapel all a-flame, and, dumb with grateful wonder, to behold upon the altar—candlesticks of gold!

J. G. WHITTIER.

A LITTLE HELP WORTH A GREAT DEAL OF PITY.

I have seen a blind man walking along the busy street; I have heard the people talking as they watched his shambling feet; I have marked their words of pity as they saw him pass along through the overcrowded city, 'mid the ever-busy throng. And I've seen a bright-eyed schoolboy leave his brothers at their play to help the sightless stranger across the busy way. Ah! the *pity* was not worthless, though it lent no kindly hand; but that little *help* outvalued all the pity in the land.

I have seen a little orphan left without a mother's care; I have heard the words of sorrow that the neighbours had to spare. I have known them say, "The workhouse is just meant for such as she;" and though very sorry for her, "Well, she has no claim on me." And I've seen a toiling widow, with children half a score, take the little lonely orphan to her hospitable door. There were fifty folks who pitied, there was only one to aid; but the one excelled the fifty as the shine excels the shade.

I have heard a schoolboy sighing o'er his lessons home from school; I have seen him vainly trying to master some new rule; I have marked the words of pity that a brother's lip supplied; and I've seen the dewy tear-drop that yet remained undried. Then I've seen a mother gently take the blunder-covered slate, and with loving effort help him make the crooked answers straight. That pity, though a brother's, was forgotten in a day; but that loving help of mother's will never pass away.

I have seen a little two-year-old stand crying by a brook; and I've marked a country maiden deep buried in a book. I have known her rise up quickly, lay the treasured work aside, lift the little fellow gently o'er the water clear and wide; and I've seen the merry sunshine light up his face at last, which if she had *only* pitied would have still been overcast.

Oh! let pity lead to *action*, for the world is full of need; there are many eyes that water, there are many hearts that bleed. The blind man on the causeway, the orphan with its fears, the schoolboy in his troubles, the baby in its tears, are like a thousand others, whom to help if we but try, we shall "scatter seeds of kindness for the reaping by-and-by." Let us ever act as brothers, ne'er with pity be content, always doing good to others both in *action* and *intent*. Though the pity may be useful, 'tis but little if 'tis all, and the smallest piece of kindly help is better than it all.   A. H. MILES.

KING JOHN AND THE ABBOT OF CANTERBURY.

An ancient story I'll tell you anon of a notable prince that was called King John; and he ruled England with main and with might, for he did great wrong, and maintained little right.

And I'll tell you a story, a story so merry, concerning the

Abbot of Canterbury; how for his house-keeping, and high renown, they rode post for him to fair London town.

An hundred men, the king did hear say, the abbot kept in his house every day; and fifty gold chains, without any doubt, in velvet coats waited the abbot about.

"How now, Father Abbot, I hear it of thee thou keepest a far better house than me; and for thy house-keeping and high renown, I fear thou work'st treason against my crown."

"My liege," quoth the abbot, "I would it were known, I never spend nothing but what is my own; and I trust your Grace will do me no deere, for spending of my own true-gotten gear."

"Ay, ay, Father Abbot, thy fault it is high, and now for the same thou needest must die; for except thou canst answer me questions three, thy head shall be smitten from thy bodie.

"And first," quoth the king, "when I'm in this stead, with my crown of gold so fair on my head, among all my liege-men so noble of birth, thou must tell me, to one penny, what I am worth.

"Secondly, tell me, without any doubt, how soon I may ride the whole world about. And at the third question thou must not shrink, but tell me here truly what I do think."

"Oh, these are hard questions for my shallow wit, nor I cannot answer your Grace as yet; but if you will give me but three weeks' space, I'll do my endeavour to answer your Grace."

"Now three weeks' space to thee will I give, and that is the longest time thou hast to live; for if thou dost not answer my questions three, thy lands and thy livings are forfeit to me."

Away rode the abbot, all sad at that word, and he rode to Cambridge and Oxenford; but never a doctor there was so wise, that could with his learning an answer devise.

Then home rode the abbot of comfort so cold, and he met his shepherd a-going to fold: "How now, my Lord Abbot, you are welcome home; what news do you bring us from good King John?"

"Sad news, sad news, shepherd, I must give : that I have but three days more to live ; for if I do not answer him questions three, my head will be smitten from my bodie.

"The first is to tell him there in that stead, with his crown of gold so fair on his head, among all his liege-men so noble of birth, to within one penny of what he is worth.

"The second, to tell him, without any doubt, how soon he may ride the whole world about. And at the third question I must not shrink, but tell him there truly what he does think."

"Now cheer up, Sir Abbot, did you never hear yet that a fool may learn a wise man wit? Lend me horse, and serving-men, and your apparel, and I'll ride to London to answer your quarrel.

"Nay, frown not, if it hath been told unto me, I am like your lordship as ever may be ; and if you will but lend me your gown, there is none shall know us at fair London town."

"Now horses and serving-men thou shalt have, with sumptuous array most gallant and brave ; with crozier, and mitre, and rochet, and cope, fit to appear 'fore our father the Pope."

* * * * *

"Now welcome, Sir Abbot," the king he did say, "'tis well thou'rt come back to keep thy day ; for, and if thou canst answer my questions three, thy life and thy living both savèd shall be.

"And first, when thou seest me here in this stead, with my crown of gold so fair on my head, among all my liege-men so noble of birth, tell me to one penny what I am worth."

"For thirty pence our Saviour was sold among the false Jews, as I have been told ; and twenty-nine is the worth of thee, for I think thou art one penny worser than he."

The king he laughed, and swore by St. Bittel, "I did not think I had been worth so little!—Now secondly tell me, without any doubt, how soon I may ride the whole world about."

"You must rise with the sun, and ride with the same, until the next morning he riseth again ; and then your Grace need not make any doubt but in twenty-four hours you'll ride it about."

The king he laughed, and swore by St. John, "I did not think it could be done so soon!—Now from the third question thou must not shrink, but tell me here truly what do I think."

"Yea, that shall I do, and make your Grace merry: you think I'm the Abbot of Canterbury; but I'm his poor shepherd, as plain you may see, that am come to beg pardon for him and for me."

The king he laughed, and swore by the mass, "I'll make thee Lord Abbot this day in his place!"

"Now nay, my liege, be not in such speed, for alack! I can neither write nor read."

"Four nobles a week, then, I will give thee for this merry jest thou hast shown unto me; and tell the old abbot, when thou comest home, thou hast brought him a pardon from good King John."

Old Ballad.

ROBERT OF LINCOLN.

Merrily swinging on brier and weed, near to the nest of his little dame, over the mountain-side or mead, Robert of Lincoln is telling his name: "Bob-o'-link, Bob-o'-link, spink, spank, spink; snug and safe is that nest of ours, hidden among the summer flowers. Chee, chee, chee."

Robert of Lincoln is gaily dressed, wearing a bright black wedding coat; white are his shoulders and white his crest: hear him call in his merry note, "Bob-o'-link, Bob-o'-link, spink, spank, spink; look what a nice new coat is mine, sure there was never a bird so fine. Chee, chee, chee."

Robert of Lincoln's Quaker wife, pretty and quiet, with plain brown wings, passing at home a patient life, broods in the grass while her husband sings, "Bob-o'-link, Bob-o'-link, spink, spank, spink; brood, kind creature; you need not fear thieves, and robbers while I am here. Chee, chee, chee."

Modest and shy as a nun is she, one weak 'chirp is her only note; braggart and prince of braggarts is he, pouring boasts from his little throat: " Bob-o'-link, Bob-o'-link, spink, spank, spink; never was I afraid of man; catch me, cowardly knaves, if you can. Chee, chee, chee."

Six white eggs on a bed of hay, flecked with purple, a pretty sight! There, as the mother sits all day, Robert is singing with all his might, " Bob-o'-link, Bob-o'-link, spink, spank, spink; nice good wife that never goes out, keeping house while I frolic about. Chee, chee, chee."

Soon as the little ones chip the shell, six wide mouths are open for food; Robert of Lincoln bestirs him well, gathering seed for the hungry brood: " Bob-o'-link, Bob-o'-link, spink, spank, spink; this new life is likely to be hard for a gay young fellow like me. Chee, chee, chee."

Robert of Lincoln at length is made sober with work and silent with care; off is his holiday garment laid, half-forgotten that merry air, " Bob-o'-link, Bob-o'-link, spink, spank, spink; nobody knows but my mate and I where our nest and our nestlings lie. Chee, chee, chee."

Summer wanes; the children are grown; fun and frolic no more he knows; Robert of Lincoln's a humdrum crone. Off he flies, and we sing as he goes, " Bob-o'-link, Bob-o'-link, spink, spank, spink; when you can pipe that merry old strain, Robert of Lincoln, come back again. Chee, chee, chee."

W. C. BRYANT.

THE CHARCOAL MAN.

Though rudely blows the wintry blast, and sifting snows fall white and fast, Mark Haley drives along the street, perched high upon his waggon seat; his sombre face the storm defies, and thus from morn till eve he cries,—" Charco'! charco'!" while echo faint and far replies,—" Hark, O! hark, O!" " Charco'!"—" Hark, O!"—Such cheery sounds attend him on his daily rounds.

The dust begrimes his ancient hat; his coat is darker far

than that; 'tis odd to see his sooty form all speckled with the feathery storm: yet in his honest bosom lies nor spot nor speck,—though still he cries,—" Charco'! charco'!" and many a roguish lad replies,—" Ark, ho! ark, ho!" "Charco'!"— " Ark, ho!"—Such various sounds announce Mark Haley's morning rounds.

Thus all the cold and wintry day he labours much for little pay; yet feels no less of happiness than many a richer man, I guess, when through the shades of eve he spies the light of his own home and cries,—" Charco' charco'!" and Martha from the door replies,—" Mark, ho! Mark, ho!" "Charco'!"— " Mark, ho!"—Such joy abounds when he has closed his daily rounds.

The hearth is warm, the fire is bright, and while his hand, washed clean and white, holds Martha's tender hand once more, his glowing face bends fondly o'er the crib wherein his darling lies, and in a coaxing tone he cries,—" Charco'! charco'!" and baby with a laugh replies,—" Ah, go! ah, go!" "Charco'!" —" Ah, go!"—while at the sounds the mother's heart with gladness bounds.

Then honoured be the charcoal man! though dusky as an African; 'tis not for you that chance to be a little better clad than he, his honest manhood to despise, although from morn till eve he cries,—" Charco'! charco'!" While mocking echo still replies,—" Hark, O! hark, O!" "Charco'!"—" Hark, O!"—Long may the sounds proclaim Mark Haley's daily rounds!

J. T. TROWBRIDGE.

THE NIGHT BEFORE CHRISTMAS.

'Twas the night before Christmas, when all through the house
Not a creature was stirring, not even a mouse;
The stockings were hung by the chimney with care,
In hopes that St. Nicholas soon would be there:
The children were nestled all snug in their beds,

THE NIGHT BEFORE CHRISTMAS.

While visions of sugar-plums danced in their heads;
And mamma in her kerchief, and I in my cap,
Had just settled our brains for a long winter's nap,—
When out on the lawn there arose such a clatter,
I sprang from my bed to see what was the matter.
Away to the window I flew like a flash,
Tore open the shutters and threw up the sash.
The moon on the breast of the new-fallen snow
Gave a lustre of mid-day to objects below;
When, what to my wondering eyes should appear,
But a miniature sleigh and eight tiny reindeer,
With a little old driver, so lively and quick
I knew in a moment it must be St. Nick.
More rapid than eagles his coursers they came,
And he whistled and shouted and called them by name:
" Now, Dasher! now, Dancer! now, Prancer and Vixen!
On, Comet! on, Cupid! on, Donner and Blitzen!
To the top of the porch, to the top of the wall!
Now, dash away, dash away, dash away all!"
As dry leaves that before the wild hurricane fly,
When they meet with an obstacle, mount to the sky,
So up to the house-top the coursers they flew,
With the sleigh full of toys,—and St. Nicholas too.
And then in a twinkling I heard on the roof
The prancing and pawing of each little hoof.
As I drew in my head and was turning around,
Down the chimney St. Nicholas came with a bound.
He was dressed all in fur from his head to his foot,
And his clothes were all tarnished with ashes and soot;
A bundle of toys he had flung on his back,
And he looked like a peddler just opening his pack.
His eyes how they twinkled! his dimples how merry!
His cheeks were like roses, his nose like a cherry;
His droll little mouth was drawn up like a bow,
And the beard on his chin was as white as the snow.

The stump of a pipe he held tight in his teeth,
And the smoke it encircled his head like a wreath.
He was chubby and plump—a right jolly old elf;
And I laughed, when I saw him, in spite of myself.
A wink of his eye and a twist of his head
Soon gave me to know I had nothing to dread.
He spoke not a word, but went straight to his work,
And filled all the stockings; then turned with a jerk,
And laying his finger aside of his nose,
And giving a nod, up the chimney he rose.
He sprang to his sleigh, to his team gave a whistle,
And away they all flew like the down of a thistle;
But I heard him exclaim, ere he drove out of sight,
"Happy Christmas to all, and to all a good-night!"

C. S. MOORE.

MARJORIE'S ALMANAC.

Robins in the tree-tops,
    Blossoms in the grass,
Green things are growing
    Everywhere you pass;
Sudden little breezes,
    Showers of silver dew;
Black bough and bent twig
    Budding out anew;
Pine tree and willow tree,
    Fringed elm and larch—
Don't you think that Maytime's
    Pleasanter than March?

Apples in the orchard,
    Mellowing one by one;
Strawberries upturning
    Soft cheeks to the sun;

MARJORIE'S ALMANAC.

Roses faint with sweetness,
  Lilies fair of face ;
Drowsy sense and murmurs
  Haunting every place ;
Lengths of golden sunshine,
  Moonlight bright as day—
Don't you think that Summer's
  Pleasanter than May ?

Roger in the corn-patch
  Whistling negro songs ;
Pussy by the hearth-side
  Romping with the tongs ;
Chestnuts in the ashes
  Burning through the rind ;
Red leaf and gold leaf
  Rustling down the wind ;
Mother " doing " peaches
  All the afternoon—
Don't you think that Autumn's
  Pleasanter than June ?

Little fairy snowflakes
  Dancing in the flue ;
Old Mr. Santa Claus,
  What is keeping you ?
Twilight and firelight,
  Shadows come and go ;
Merry chime of sleigh bells
  Tinkling through the snow ;
Mother's knitting stockings,
  Pussy's got the ball—
Don't you think that Winter's
  Pleasanter than all ?

                J. B. ALDRICH.

A CATASTROPHE.

No human being who saw that sight but felt a shudder of pale affright. He sat in a window three stories high, a little baby with no one nigh. A stranger saw him, and stopped to stare; a crowd soon gathered to watch him there.

A gleam—a flutter! in airy flight came past the window a butterfly bright. From fields of clover and perfumed air, wayfaring insect, what brought you there? The baby saw it, and eagerly reached out to catch it, crowing with glee.

With fat pink fingers, reached out—and fell! The awful horror, no tongue can tell! Poor little baby, so sweet and bright! Pale faces quivered, lips grew white, weak women fainted, strong men grew weak; up rose one woman's heart-piercing shriek.

Hurrah for the awning! upon the fly it caught the youngster, and tossed him high. The bounce prodigious made baby scowl; he caught his breath, and set up a howl. All blessed the awning that had no flaw;—but a madder baby you never saw.

P. Arkwright.

A MODEST WIT.

A supercilious nabob of the East—haughty, being great—purse proud, being rich—a governor, or general, at the least, I have forgotten which—had in his family a humble youth, who went from England in his patron's suite; an unassuming boy, and, in truth, a lad of decent parts, and good repute. This youth had sense and spirit; but yet, with all his sense, excessive diffidence obscured his merit.

One day, at table, flushed with pride and wine, his honour, proudly free, severely merry, conceived it would be vastly fine to crack a joke upon his secretary.

"Young man," he said, "by what art, craft, or trade, did your good father gain a livelihood?"

"He was a saddler, sir," Modestus said; "and in his time was reckoned good."

"A saddler, eh! and taught you Greek, instead of teaching you to sew! Pray, why did not your father make a saddler, sir, of you?"

Each parasite, then, as in duty bound, the joke applauded, and the laugh went round. At length Modestus, bowing low, said, "I crave pardon if too free I make, sir; by your leave, I fain would know your father's trade!"

"My father's trade! Bless me, that's too bad! My father's trade! Why, blockhead, are you mad? My father, sir, did never stoop so low—he was a gentleman, I'd have you know."

"Excuse the liberty I take," Modestus said, with archness on his brow; "pray, why did not your father make a gentleman of you?" ANON.

THE GLOVE AND THE LIONS.

King Francis was a hearty king, and loved a royal sport;
And one day, as his lions fought, sat looking on the court:
The nobles filled the benches round, the ladies by their side,
And 'mongst them sat the Count de Lorge, with one for whom
    he sighed;
And truly 'twas a gallant thing to see that crowning show—
Valour and love, and a king above, and the royal beasts below.

Ramped and roared the lions, with horrid laughing jaws;
They bit, they glared, gave blows like beams—a wind went
    with their paws;
With wallowing might and stifled roar, they rolled on one
    another,
Till all the pit, with sand and mane, was in a thunderous smother;
The gory foam, above the bars, came whizzing through the air;
Said Francis then, "Faith! gentlemen, we're better here than
    there!"

De Lorge's love o'erheard the king,—a beauteous lively dame,
With smiling lips and sharp bright eyes, which always seemed
 the same.
She thought, "The count my lover is brave as brave can be—
He surely would do wondrous things to show his love of me :
King, ladies, lovers, all look on ; the occasion is divine !
I'll drop my glove, to prove his love : great glory will be mine !"

She dropped her glove—to prove his love ; then looked at him
 —and smiled :
He bowed, and in a moment leaped among the lions wild.
The leap was quick—return was quick—he has regained his
 place,—
Then threw the glove—but not with love—right in the lady's
 face !
" In truth," cried Francis, " rightly done !" and he rose from
 where he sat ;
" Not love," quoth he, " but vanity, sets love a task like that !"
LEIGH HUNT.

LOCHINVAR.

Oh, young Lochinvar is come out of the west !
Through all the wide Border his steed was the best ;
And, save his good broadsword, he weapon had none,
He rode all unarmed, and he rode all alone.
So faithful in love, and so dauntless in war,
 There never was knight like the young Lochinvar !

He stayed not for brake, and he stopped not for stone,
He swam the Esk river where ford there was none ;
But, ere he alighted at Netherby gate,
The bride had consented !—the gallant came late !
For a laggard in love, and a dastard in war,
 Was to wed the fair Ellen of brave Lochinvar !

So boldly he entered the Netherby Hall,
Among bride's-men, and kinsmen, and brothers, and all:
Then spoke the bride's father, his hand on his sword—
For the poor craven bridegroom said never a word—
"Oh, come ye in peace here, or come ye in war,
Or to dance at our bridal, young Lord Lochinvar?"

"I long wooed your daughter, my suit you denied:
Love swells like the Solway, but ebbs like its tide!
And now am I come, with this lost love of mine
To lead but one measure, drink one cup of wine!—
There are maidens in Scotland, more lovely by far,
That would gladly be bride to the young Lochinvar!"

The bride kissed the goblet; the knight took it up,
He quaffed off the wine, and he threw down the cup!
She looked down to blush, and she looked up to sigh,
With a smile on her lips and a tear in her eye;
He took her soft hand, ere her mother could bar,—
"Now tread we a measure!" said young Lochinvar.

So stately his form, and so lovely her face,
That never a hall such a galliard did grace!
While her mother did fret, and her father did fume,
And the bridegroom stood dangling his bonnet and plume;
And the bride-maidens whispered, "'Twere better by far
To have matched our fair cousin with young Lochinvar!"

One touch to her hand, and one word in her ear,
When they reached the hall-door, and the charger stood near.
So light to the croupe the fair lady he swung,
So light to the saddle before her he sprung!
"She is won! we are gone, over bank, bush, and scaur!
They'll have fleet steeds that follow!" quoth young Lochinvar.

There was mounting 'mong Græmes of the Netherby clan;
Fosters, Fenwicks, and Musgraves, they rode and they ran;
There was racing and chasing on Cannobie Lea—
But the lost bride of Netherby ne'er did they see!
So daring in love, and so dauntless in war,
Have ye e'er heard of gallant like young Lochinvar?

Sir Walter Scott.

THE RIDE OF JENNIE MACNEAL.

Paul Revere was a rider bold—well has his valorous deed been told; Sheridan's ride was a glorious one—oft it has been dwelt upon. But why should *men* do all the deeds on which the love of a patriot feeds? Hearken to me, while I reveal the dashing ride of Jennie Macneal.

On a spot as pretty as might be found in the dangerous length of the Neutral Ground, in a cottage, cosy, and all their own, she and her mother lived alone. Safe were the two, with their frugal store, from all of the many who passed their door; for Jennie's mother was strange to fears, and Jennie was tall for fifteen years; with fun her eyes were glistening, her hair was the hue of the blackbird's wing. And while the friends who knew her well, the sweetness of her heart could tell; a gun that hung on the kitchen wall, looked solemnly quick to heed her call; and they who were evil-minded knew her nerve was strong and her aim was true.

One night, when the sun had crept to bed, and rain-clouds lingered overhead, soon after a knock at the outer door, there entered a dozen dragoons or more. The captain his hostess bent to greet, saying, "Madam, please give us a bit to eat; we will pay you well. Then we must dash ten miles ahead, to catch a rebel colonel abed. He is visiting home, it doth appear; we will make his pleasure cost him dear."

Now, the gray-haired colonel they hovered near, had been Jennie's true friend, kind and dear; and oft, in her younger days, had he right proudly perched her upon his knee. She had hunted by his fatherly side; he had taught her how to fence and ride; and once had said, "The time may be your skill and courage may stand by me."

With never a thought or a moment more, bareheaded she slipped from the cottage door; ran out where the horses were left to feed, unhitched and mounted the captain's steed; and down the hilly and rock-strown way she urged the fiery horse of gray. Around her slender and cloakless form pattered and moaned the ceaseless storm; secure and tight, a gloveless hand grasped the reins with stern command; and on she rushed for the colonel's weal, brave, fearless-hearted Jennie Macneal.

Hark! from the hills, a moment mute, came a clatter of hoofs in hot pursuit; and a cry from the foremost trooper said, "Halt! or your blood be on your head!" She heeded it not, and not in vain she lashed the horse with the bridle-rein. Into the night the gray horse strode; his shoes struck fire from the rocky road; and the high-born courage, that never dies, flashed from his rider's coal-black eyes. The pebbles flew from the fearful race; the raindrops splashed on her glowing face. "On—on, brave horse!" with loud appeal, cried eager, resolute Jennie Macneal.

"Halt!" once more came that voice of dread; "halt! or your blood be on your head!" But no one answering to the calls, sped after her a volley of balls. They passed her in her rapid flight; they screamed to her left, they screamed to her right. But, rushing still o'er the slippery track, she sent no token of answer back.

The gray horse did his duty well, till all at once he stumbled and fell—himself escaping the nets of harm, but flinging the girl with a broken arm. Still undismayed by the numbing pain, she clung to the horse's bridle-rein, and gently bidding him to stand, patted him with her able hand; then sprang again to the saddle-bow, "Good horse! one more trial now!"

As if ashamed of the heedless fall, he gathered his strength once more for all; and galloping down a hillside steep, gained on the troopers at every leap. They were a furlong behind or more, when the girl burst through the colonel's door—her poor arm, helpless, hanging with pain, and she all drabbled and drenched with rain; but her cheeks as red as firebrands are, and her eyes as bright as a blazing star—and shouted, "Quick! be quick, I say! They come! they come! Away! away!" Then fainting on the floor she sank.

The startled colonel pressed his wife and children to his breast, and turned away from his fireside bright, and glided into the stormy night; then soon and safely made his way to where the patriot army lay. But first he bent, in the warm firelight, and kissed the forehead cold and white.

The girl roused up at the martial din, just as the troopers came rushing in; and laughed, even in the midst of a moan, saying, "Good sirs, your bird has flown. 'Twas I who scared him from his nest; so deal with me now as you think best."

But the gallant young captain bowed, and said, "Of womankind I must crown you queen; so brave a girl I have never seen. Wear this gold ring as your valour's due; and when peace comes, I'll come for you."

But Jennie's face an arch smile wore: "There's a lad in Putnam's corps told me the same a long time ago; you two would never agree, I know. I promised my love to be true as steel," said brave, true-hearted Jennie Macneal.

WILL CARLETON.

THE BATTLE OF BLENHEIM.

It was a summer evening, old Kaspar's work was done, and he before his cottage door was sitting in the sun; and by him sported on the green his little grandchild, Wilhelmine. She saw her brother Peterkin roll something large and round, which he beside the rivulet in playing there had found: he came to ask what he had found, that was so large, and smooth, and round.

Old Kaspar took it from the boy, who stood expectant by; and then the old man shook his head, and with a natural sigh, "'Tis some poor fellow's skull," said he, "who fell in the great victory. I find them in the garden, for there's many here about; and often, when I go to plough, the ploughshare turns them out: for many thousand men," said he, "were slain in that great victory."

"Now tell us what 'twas all about," young Peterkin he cries; and little Wilhelmine looks up with wonder-waiting eyes: "Now tell us all about the war, and what they fought each other for."

"It was the English," Kaspar cried, "who put the French to rout; but what they fought each other for, I could not well make out: but everybody said," quoth he, "that 'twas a famous victory. My father lived at Blenheim then, yon little stream hard by: they burned his dwelling to the ground, and he was forced to fly; so with his wife and child he fled, nor had he where to rest his head. With fire and sword the country round was wasted far and wide, and many a widowed mother then, and new-born baby, died! But things like that, you know, must be at every famous victory. Great praise the Duke of Marlbro' won, and our good Prince Eugene."

"Why, 'twas a very wicked thing!" said little Wilhelmine.

"Nay—nay, my little girl," quoth he, "it was a famous victory. And everybody praised the Duke, who this great fight did win."

"But what good came of it at last?" quoth little Peterkin.

"Why, that I cannot tell," said he; "but 'twas a famous victory!" SOUTHEY.

PAPA'S LETTER.

I was sitting in my study writing letters, when I heard—
" Please, dear mamma, Mary told me mamma mustn't be disturbed;

But I'se tired of the kitty, want some ozzer sing to do.
Witing letters is 'ou, mamma? Tan't I wite a letter too?"

"Not now, darling! mamma's busy; run and play with kitty now."
"No, no, mamma! me wite letter, mamma, you will show me how."
I would paint my darling's portrait, as his sweet eyes searched my face—
Hair of gold and eyes of azure, form of childish witching grace.

But the eager face was clouded, as I slowly shook my head,
Till I said, "I'll make a letter of *you*, darling boy, instead."
So I parted back the tresses from his forehead high and white,
And a stamp, in sport, I pasted 'mid its waves of golden light.

Then I said, "Now, little letter, go away and bear good news;"
And I smiled as down the staircase clattered loud the little shoes.
Leaving me, the darling hurried down to Mary, in his glee:
"Mamma's witing lots of letters; *I'se* a letter, Mary, see."

No one heard the little prattler, as once more he climbed the stair,
Reached his little cap and tippet, standing on the table there;
No one heard the front door open, no one saw the golden hair,
As it floated o'er his shoulders on the crisp October air.

Down the street the baby hastened, till he reached the office door,
"I'se a letter, Mr. Postman, is there room for any more?
'Cause this letter's going to papa; papa lives with God, 'ou know;
Mamma sent me for a letter: does 'ou sink 'at I can go?"

But the clerk, in wonder, answered, "Not to-day, my little
   man."
" Den I'll find anozzer office, 'cause I must go if I can."
Fain the clerk would have detained him, but the pleading
   face was gone,
And the little feet were hastening, by the busy crowd swept
   on.

Suddenly the crowd was parted, people fled to left and right,
As a pair of maddened horses at that moment dashed in
   sight.
No one saw the baby figure, no one saw the golden hair,
Till a voice of frightened sweetness rang out on the autumn
   air.

'Twas too late! A moment only stood the beauteous vision
   there ;
Then the little face lay lifeless, covered o'er with golden
   hair.
Reverently they raised my darling, brushed away the curls
   of gold,
Saw the stamp upon the forehead, growing now so icy cold.

Not a mark the face disfigured, showing where a hoof had
   trod ;
But the little life was ended—" papa's letter " was with God !
ANON.

THE CAPTAIN'S CHILD.

There was a child whose early home was on the rolling deep ;
the waters sung his lullaby, and rocked him to his sleep. He
was the captain's only child ; and when his mother died, he
would not to her kindred send the prattler from his side. And
so the little boy grew up, a dweller on the sea : for feats of

horsemanship, he learned to climb the tall mast tree. The song of birds at early morn it was not his to hear; but the ocean breeze, that swept the seas, was music in his ear. Yet was the ship a rugged school for one so fair and young; and harshly in his hearing oft his father's accents rung. For dearly as he loved the boy, that love was never shown in fond endearment, but in care of discipline alone. Yet Harry was a merry boy, brimful of fearless fun, and blithely, with a shipboy's skill, could up the rigging run. Oh, but the sailors loved him well; the sunshine of his smile, with memories of their childish days did home-sick hearts beguile. All household loves on him were showered, as in their sight he grew; and so the captain's child became the darling of the crew.

Now of a monkey I must tell, a droll and knavish elf, the sailors' pet, and Harry's plague, a mimic of himself; a grinning, chattering ape it was, and mischievous full oft. One day he clutched the cap from Harry's head, and darted up aloft. Up in the rigging with his prize the thievish monkey flew; now here, now there, it dodged about, and Harry followed too. At first it was a merry chase, and blithely all looked on; but many a weather-beaten face paled ere the cap was won. The eager boy, without a thought of danger or of dread, had reached at length the topmost pole where scarce was room to tread. Where none could turn, and none could bend, he stood in dizzy trance, beyond the reach of others' help, nor dared to downward glance. Breathless with fear, the crew looked up; none spoke, no one stirred, not even when the captain's tread upon the deck was heard. "What is the matter now, my men? why stand ye moonstruck there?" None answered him—one look above revealed the speechless fear. Pale with his agony, the boy is trembling, ere he fall upon the deck with murderous crash;—the captain saw it all. But not a nerve or muscle yet with quivering anguish shook. "Bring me my fowling-piece," he said, and steadfast aim he took. Then stern, and loud. and trumpet-clear he cried, "Attend to me! This moment, sir, I fire, unless you jump into the sea." A life-long agony compressed throbs in the breasts of all. Not on the deck, not on the deck, resounds the dreadful fall! Off at his father's word he sprang, far in the yielding wave; and many a sailor overboard dashed after him to save. Safe! safe! now quickly on the deck the rescued boy they bear. Then failed at once the father's heart, he might not linger there. No, ere his trembling arms enfold the child to life restored, locked in his cabin, all alone, his heart-felt thanks are poured. Calm in the might of prayer, at length he bade them bring his boy, and clasped him to his yearning heart with all a father's joy. I tell not of the interview, which none beside might share: the love of father and of son, what language can declare? Yet from my story, you, dear friends, may of obedience learn, and how the truest love may wear an aspect strange and stern.

Mrs. Leeson.

THE DRUM.

Yonder is a little drum, hanging on the wall;
Dusty wreaths, and tattered flags, round about it fall.
A shepherd youth on Cheviot's hills watched the sheep whose skin
A cunning workman wrought, and gave the little drum its din.

Oh, pleasant are fair Cheviot's hills, with velvet verdure spread,
And pleasant 'tis, among its heath, to make your summer bed;
And sweet and clear are Cheviot's rills that trickle to its vales,
And balmily its tiny flowers breathe on the passing gales.
And thus hath felt the shepherd-boy whilst tending of his fold;
Nor thought there was, in all the world, a spot like Cheviot's wold.

And so it was for many a day!—but change with time will
    come!
And he—(alas for him the day!) he heard—the little drum!
"Follow," said the drummer-boy, "would you live in story!
For he who strikes a foeman down, wins a wreath of glory."
"Rub-a-dub!" and "rub-a-dub!" the drummer beats away—
The shepherd lets his bleating flock o'er Cheviot wildly stray.

On Egypt's arid wastes of sand the shepherd now is lying;
Around him many a parching tongue for "Water!" faintly
    crying:
Oh, that he were on Cheviot's hills, with velvet verdure spread,
Or lying 'mid the blooming heath where oft he made his bed;
Or could he drink of those sweet rills that trickle to its vales,
Or breathe once more the balminess of Cheviot's mountain gales!

At length, upon his wearied eyes the mists of slumber come,
And he is in his home again—till wakened by the drum!
"Take arms! take arms!" his leader cries, "the hated foeman's
    nigh!"
Guns loudly roar—steel clanks on steel, and thousands fall to
    die.
The shepherd's blood makes red the sand: "Oh! water—give
    me some!
My voice might reach a friendly ear, but for that little drum!"

'Mid moaning men, and dying men, the drummer kept his way,
And many a one by "glory" lured did curse the drum that day.
"Rub-a-dub!" and "rub-a-dub!" the drummer beat aloud—
The shepherd died! and, ere the morn, the hot sand was his
    shroud.
—And this is "glory"?—Yes; and still will man the tempter
    follow,
Nor learn that glory, like its drum, is but a sound—and hollow!

                        DOUGLAS JERROLD'S *Magazine*.

THE NEWS-BOY'S DEBT.

One day, last year, at Christmas time, while walking down a busy street, I saw a tiny ill-clad boy, one of the many that we meet. As ragged as a boy could be, with half a coat, and one whole shoe, mere patches to keep out the wind—I felt the wind blew keenly too. A news-boy, with a news-boy's lungs, a square Scotch face, an honest brow—a news-boy, hawking his last sheets, shouting his "extras" o'er and o'er: "Papers, sir, *The Evenin' News.*" He brushed away a tear and said, "Oh please, sir, don't refuse."

"How many have you? Never mind—don't stop to count —I'll take them all." He thanked me with a happy smile, a look half wondering, and half glad. I fumbled for the proper change, and said, "You seem a little lad to rough it in the street like this."

"I'm ten year old on Christmas day."

"Your name?"

"Jim Hanley."

"I haven't change—stay, here's a crown—you'll get change there across the way—five shillings. When you've got the change, come to my office—that's the place. Now, wait a bit— there's time enough, you needn't run a headlong race. Where do you live?"

"Most anywhere."

"And are you cold?"

"Ay, just a bit; I don't mind cold."

"Well, that is strange." He smiled again, and darted off to get the change.

Then, with a half-unconscious sigh, I sought my office-desk again; an hour or more, my busy brain found work enough with book and pen. But when the office-clock struck eight, I started, with a sudden thought, for there—beside my hat and gloves, lay those six papers I had bought. Why, where's the boy, and where's the change he should have brought an hour ago? Ah well! ah well! they're all alike; I was a fool to tempt him so. Dishonest! Well, I might have known, and yet—his face seemed honest too. But caution often comes too late. And so I took my homeward way, deeming distrust of humankind the only lesson of the day.

Just two days after, as I sat half-dozing in my office-chair, I heard a timid knock, and called out sharply, "Who is there?"

An urchin entered, barely seven—the same Scotch face, the same blue eyes. "Sir, if you please, my brother Jim, the one you gave the crown, you know, he couldn't bring the money, sir, because his back was hurted so; he got runned over, up the street—"

"Got run over, do you say?"

"Yes, sir, they picked him up for dead; an' all that day, an' yesterday, he wasn't rightly in his head. They took him to the 'ospital; I went, too, because you see we two is brothers, Jim an' me. He had your money in his hand, an' never saw it any more; indeed, he didn't mean to steal, Jim never stole a pin before. When he gets well—it won't be long—if you will call the money lent, he says he'll work his fingers off until he pays you ev'ry cent. He made me fetch his jacket here—it's torn, and dirtied pretty bad; it's only fit to sell for rags; but then, you know, it's all Jim had."

"No, no, my boy! take back the coat,—your brother's badly hurt, you say? Run out—hail a cab—and wait for me.— (Why! I'd give a thousand pounds for such a boy as he.")......

A half-hour after this we stood together in the crowded wards, and the nurse checked the hasty steps that fell too loudly on the boards. I thought him smiling in his sleep, and scarce believed her when she said, smoothing away the tangled hair from brow and cheek, "The boy is dead!" "Dead?"— dead! how fair he looked, one beam of sunshine on his hair. Poor lad!—well it's warm in heaven; no need of change and jackets there. Poor little Jim!—I turned away, and left a tear upon his sunburned cheek. *Harper's Magazine.*

A "LAPSUS LINGUÆ."

It chanced one day, so I've been told (the story is not very old), as Will and Tom, two servants able, were waiting at their master's table, Tom brought a fine fat turkey in, the sumptuous dinner to begin. Then Will appeared—superbly cooked, a tongue upon the platter smoked; when, oh! sad fate! he struck the door, and tumbled flat upon the floor. The servants stared, the guests looked down, when quick uprising with a frown, the master cried, "Sirra! I say, begone, nor wait a single day, you stupid cur! you've spoiled the feast; how can another tongue be dressed?" While thus the master stormed and roared, Will, who with wit was somewhat stored (for he by no means was a fool; some Latin, too, he'd learned at school), said (thinking he might change disgrace for laughter, and thus save his place), "Oh! call me not a stupid cur; 'twas but a *lapsus linguæ*, sir." "A *lapsus linguæ?*" one guest cries. "A pun!" another straight replies. The joke was caught—the laugh went round, nor could a serious face be found. The master, when the uproar ceased, finding his guests were all well pleased, forgave the servant's slippery feet, and quick revoked his former threat.

Now Tom had all this time stood still, and heard the applause bestowed on Will; delighted he had seen the fun of what his comrade late had done, and thought, should he but do the same, an equal share of praise he'd claim. As soon as told the meat to fetch in, bolted like lightning to the kitchen, and seizing there a leg of lamb (I am not certain, perhaps 'twas ham—no matter which), without delay off to the parlour marched away, and stumbling as he turned him round, twirled joint and dish upon the ground. For this my lord was ill-prepared; again the astonished servants stared. Tom grinned—but seeing no one stir, "Another *lapsus linguæ*, sir!" loud he exclaimed. No laugh was raised, no "clever fellow's" wit was praised. Confounded, yet not knowing why *his* wit could not one laugh supply, and fearing lest he had mistook the words, again thus loudly spoke (thinking again it might be tried) : "'Twas but a *lapsæ linguus*," cried. My lord, who long had quiet sat, now clearly saw what he was at. In wrath this warning now he gave—" When next thou triest, unlettered knave, to give, as thine, another's wit, mind well thou knowest what's meant by it; nor let a *lapsus linguæ* slip from out thy pert, assuming lip, till well thou knowest thy stolen song, nor think a leg of lamb a tongue." ANON.

EXCELSIOR.

The shades of night were falling fast, as through an Alpine village passed a youth, who bore, 'mid snow and ice, a banner with the strange device, " Excelsior!" His brow was sad; his eye beneath flashed like a falchion from its sheath; and like a silver clarion rung the accents of that unknown tongue, " Excelsior!" In happy homes he saw the light of household fires gleam warm and bright; above, the spectral glaciers shone: and from his lips escaped a groan, " Excelsior!"

"Try not the pass," the old man said; "dark lowers the tempest overhead; the roaring torrent is deep and wide!"

And loud that clarion voice replied, " Excelsior!"

"Oh, stay," the maiden said, " and rest thy weary head upon this breast!"

A tear stood in his bright blue eye; but still he answered, with a sigh, " Excelsior!"

"Beware the pine-tree's withered branch! beware the awful avalanche!" this was the peasant's last good night.

A voice replied, far up the height, " Excelsior!"

At break of day, as, heavenward, the pious monks of Saint Bernard uttered the oft-repeated prayer, a voice cried through the startled air, " Excelsior!" A traveller, by the faithful hound, half-buried in the snow was found, still grasping in his

hand of ice the banner with the strange device, "Excelsior!"
There, in the twilight, cold and gray, lifeless, but beautiful he
lay; and from the sky, serene and far, a voice fell, like a falling
star, "Excelsior!"   LONGFELLOW.

MEASURING THE BABY.

We measured the riotous baby against the cottage wall—
A lily grew at the threshold, and the boy was just as tall;
A royal tiger-lily, with spots of purple and gold,
And the heart of a jewelled chalice the fragrant dew to hold.

Without, the blue-birds whistled high up in the old roof-trees;
And to and fro at the window the red rose rocked her bees;
And the wee pink fists of the baby were never a moment still,
Snatching at shine and shadow that danced at the lattice-sill.

His eyes were as wide as blue-bells, his mouth like a flower unblown,
Two little bare feet, like funny white mice, peeped out from his snowy gown;
And we thought with a thrill of rapture, that yet had a touch of pain,
When June rolls round with her roses we'll measure the boy again.

Ah me! in a darkened chamber, with the sunshine shut away,
Through tears that fell like a bitter rain, we measured the boy to-day;
And the little bare feet that were dimpled and sweet as a budding rose
Lay side by side together, in the hush of a long repose.

Up from the dainty pillow, white as the risen dawn,
The fair little face lay smiling, with the light of heaven thereon;

And the dear little hands, like rose-leaves dropped from a rose,
    lay still,
Never to catch at the sunshine that crept to the shrouded sill.

We measured the sleeping baby with ribbons white as snow,
For the shining rosewood casket that waited him below ;
And out of the darkened chamber we went with a childless
    moan :—
. To the height of the sinless angels our little one had grown !

E. A. BROWN.

BARBARA FRIETCHIE.

Up from the meadows rich with corn, clear in the cool September morn, the clustered spires of Frederick stand, green-walled by the hills of Maryland. Round about them orchards sweep—apple and peach tree fruited deep ; fair as a garden of the Lord to the eyes of the famished rebel horde. On that pleasant morn of the early fall, when Lee marched over the mountain-wall—over the mountains winding down, horse and foot, into Frederick town.

Forty flags with their silver stars, forty flags with their crimson bars, flapped in the morning wind : the sun of noon looked down, and saw not one. Up rose old Barbara Frietchie then, bowed with her fourscore years and ten ; bravest of all in Frederick town, she took up the flag the men hauled down. In her attic window the staff she set, to show that one heart was loyal yet.

Up the street came the rebel tread, Stonewall Jackson riding ahead. Under his slouched hat left and right he glanced : the old flag met his sight. "Halt !"—the dust-brown ranks stood fast. "Fire !"—out blazed the rifle-blast. It shivered the window, pane and sash ; it rent the banner with seam and gash. Quick as it fell from the broken staff, Dame Barbara snatched the silken scarf ; she leaned far out on the windowsill, and shook it forth with a royal will. "Shoot, if you must, this old gray head, but spare your country's flag!" she said.

A shade of sadness, a blush of shame, over the face of the leader came; the nobler nature within him stirred to life at that woman's deed and word. "Who touches a hair of yon gray head, dies like a dog! March on!" he said.

All day long through Frederick street sounded the tread of marching feet; all day long that free flag tossed over the heads of the rebel host. Ever its torn folds rose and fell on the loyal winds that loved it well; and, through the hill-gaps, sunset light shone over it with a warm good-night.

Barbara Frietchie's work is o'er, and the rebel rides on his raids no more. Honour to her!—and let a tear fall, for her sake, on Stonewall's bier! Over Barbara Frietchie's grave, flag of Freedom and Union, wave! Peace, and order, and beauty, draw round thy symbol of light and law; and ever the stars above look down on thy stars below, in Frederick town!

J. G. Whittier.

A MOTHER'S ANSWER.

Over the lofty Ben Lomond the charm of the sunset fell;
And sweet in the purple twilight the chime of the old kirk bell.
And lo! in the grassy kirkyard was the white-haired dominie;
Men and women on either hand, and the children at his knee.

And there, in the still, warm evening, low sitting among the dead,
The good man took the Sacred Book, and the trial of Abraham read,
Until, in the solemn shadows, the sorrow grew wondrous near—
Fathers looked at their own bright sons, and the mothers dropped a tear.

Thoughtful all sat a little space, and then the dominie said,
"David, couldst thou have done this thing?" And the old
man bowed his head,
And standing up, with lifted face, answered, "I think I
could,
For I have found through eighty years that the Lord our
God is good!"

"Janet, Janet, could your faith have stood this test?"
She raised her grandchild in her arms, and held it to her
breast.
"God knows a mother's love," she said, while the tears dropped
from her eyes,
"And He never from a mother's heart would have asked such
sacrifice."

"Oh, mother wise!" the preacher said, "oh, mother wise and
good!
A sweeter depth than man can reach thy heart hath understood.
Take Janet's sermon with you, friends, and, as your years
go by,
Believe 'our Father' no poor soul beyond its strength will
try." L. E. BARR.

THE PIED PIPER OF HAMELIN.

(*By permission of the Author.*)

Hamelin town's in Brunswick, by famous Hanover city; the river Weser, deep and wide, washes its walls on the southern side: a pleasanter spot you never spied; but, when begins my ditty, almost five hundred years ago, to see the townsfolk suffer so from vermin, was a pity. Rats! They fought the dogs and killed the cats, and bit the babies in the cradles, split open the kegs of salted sprats, made nests inside men's Sunday hats; and even spoiled the w<u>o</u>men's chats, by drowning their speaking with shrieking and squeaking in fifty different sharps and flats.

At last the people in a body to the Town Hall came flocking. "'Tis clear," cried they, "our Mayor's a noddy; and as for our Corporation—shocking—rouse up, sirs! give your brains a racking, to find the <u>remedy</u> we're lacking, or, sure as fate, we'll send you packing!" At this the Mayor and Corporation quaked with a mighty consternation.

An hour they sat in council; at length the Mayor broke silence: "It's easy to bid one rack one's brain—I'm sure my poor head <u>aches</u> again, I've scratched it so, and all in vain. Oh for a trap, a trap, a trap!" Just as he said this, what should hap at the chamber door but a gentle tap! "Bless us!" cried the Mayor, "what's that? Only a scraping of shoes on the mat? Anything like the sound of a rat makes my heart go pit-a-pat! Come in!" cried the Mayor, looking bigger; and in did come the strangest figure. His queer, long coat from heel to head was half of yellow and half of red; and he himself was tall and thin, with sharp blue eyes, each like a pin, and light loose hair, yet swarthy skin, no tuft on cheek nor beard on chin, but lips where smiles went out and in: there was no guessing his kith and kin; and nobody could enough admire the tall man and his quaint attire. He advanced to the council-table, and, "Please your honours," said he, "I'm able, by means of a secret charm, to draw all creatures living beneath the sun, that creep, or swim, or fly, or run, after me so as you never saw! And I chiefly use my charm on creatures that do people harm—the mole, and toad, and newt, and viper; and people call me the Pied Piper." (And here they noticed round his neck a scarf of red and yellow stripe, and at the scarf's end hung a pipe; and his fingers, they noticed, were ever straying, as if impatient to be pl<u>aying</u> upon this p<u>ipe</u>, as low it dangled over his vesture so old-fangled.)

THE PIED PIPER OF HAMELIN.

"If I can rid your town of rats, will you give me a thousand guilders?"

"One?—fifty thousand!" was the exclamation of the astonished Mayor and Corporation.

Into the street the Piper stepped, smiling first a little smile, as if he knew what magic slept in his quiet pipe the while; and ere three shrill notes the pipe uttered, you heard as if an army muttered; and the muttering grew to a grumbling; and the grumbling grew to a mighty rumbling; and out of the houses the rats came tumbling. Great rats, small rats, lean rats, brawny rats; brown rats, black rats, gray rats, tawny rats; fathers, mothers, uncles, cousins; families by tens and dozens; brothers, sisters, husbands, wives—followed the Piper for their lives. From street to street he piped advancing, and step for step they followed dancing, until they came to the river Weser, wherein all plunged, and perished.

You should have heard the Hamelin people ringing the bells till they rocked the steeple.

"Go," cried the Mayor, "and get long poles; poke out the nests, and block up the holes; consult with carpenters and builders, and leave in our town not even a trace of the rats!"—when suddenly up the face of the Piper perked in the market-place, with a, "First, if you please, my thousand guilders!"

A thousand guilders! The Mayor looked blue; so did the Corporation too. To pay this sum to a wandering fellow with a gipsy coat of red and yellow! "Besides," quoth the Mayor, with a knowing wink, "our business was done at the river's brink; we saw with our eyes the vermin sink, and what's dead can't come to life, *I* think. So, friend, we're not the folks to shrink from the duty of giving you something to drink, and a matter of money to put in your poke; but as for the guilders, what we spoke of them, as you very well know, was in joke. A thousand guilders! come, take fifty!"

The Piper's face fell, and he cried, "No trifling! I'll not bate a stiver; and folks who put me in a passion may find me pipe to another fashion!"

"How?" cried the Mayor, "you lazy ribald, with idle pipe and vesture piebald, you threaten us, fellow? Do your worst, blow your pipe there till you burst!"

Once more he stepped into the street, and to his lips again laid his long pipe of smooth, straight cane; and ere he blew three notes (such sweet soft notes as yet musician's cunning never gave the enraptured air), there was a rustling that seemed like a bustling of merry crowds justling at pitching and hustling, small feet pattering, wooden shoes clattering, little hands clapping, little tongues chattering, and, like fowls in a farm-yard when barley is scattering, out came the children running—all the little boys and girls, with rosy cheeks and flaxen curls, and sparkling eyes and teeth like pearls, tripping and skipping, ran merrily after the wonderful music, with shouting and laughter.

The Mayor was dumb, and the Council stood as if they were changed into blocks of wood, unable to move a step, or cry to the children merrily skipping by—and could only follow with the eye that joyous crowd at the Piper's back. But how the Mayor was on the rack, and the wretched Council's bosoms beat, as the Piper turned from the High Street to where the Weser rolled its waters right in the way of their sons and daughters!

However, he turned from south to west, and to Koppelberg Hill his steps addressed, and after him the children pressed: great was the joy in every breast. "He never can cross that mighty top; he's forced to let the piping drop, and we shall see our children stop!" When, lo! as they reached the mountain's side, a wondrous portal opened wide, as if a cavern was suddenly hollowed; and the Piper advanced, and the children followed, and when all were in to the very last, the door in the mountain-side shut fast.

Alas! alas! for Hamelin! There came into many a burgher's

pate a text which says, that heaven's gate opes to the rich at as easy rate as the needle's eye takes a camel in!

The Mayor sent east, west, north, and south, to offer the Piper by word of mouth, wherever it was men's lot to find him, silver and gold to his heart's content, if he'd only return the way he went, and bring the children behind him. But soon they saw 'twas a lost endeavour, Piper and dancers were gone for ever!

ROBERT BROWNING.

DIMES AND DOLLARS.

"Dimes and dollars! dollars and dimes!" thus an old miser rang the chimes, as he sat by the side of an open box, with ironed angles and massive locks; and he heaped the glittering coin on high, and cried in delirious ecstasy—"Dimes and dollars! dollars and dimes! ye are the ladders by which man climbs over his fellows. Musical chimes! dimes and dollars! dollars and dimes!"

A sound on the gong, and the miser rose, and his laden coffer did quickly close and locked secure. "These are the times for a man to look after his dollars and dimes. A letter! Ha! from my prodigal son. The old tale—poverty—pshaw, begone!—Why did he marry when I forbade? 'She was so sweet, and her lot so sad!' As he has sown, so he must reap; but I my dollars secure will keep. 'A sickly wife and starving times!'—he should have wed with dollars and dimes."

Thickly the hour of midnight fell; doors and windows were bolted well. "Ha!" chuckled the miser, "not so bad! a thousand guineas to-day I've made. Money makes money; these are the times to double and treble the dollars and dimes. Now to sleep, and to-morrow to plan; rest is sweet to a wearied man." And he fell asleep with the midnight chimes, dreaming of glittering dollars and dimes.

The sun rose high, and its beaming ray into the miser's room found way. It moved from the foot till it lit the head of the miser's low uncurtained bed; and it seemed to say to him, "Sluggard, awake; thou hast a thousand dollars to make! Up, man, up!" How still was the place, as the bright ray fell on the miser's face! Ah! the old miser is dead; dreaming of gold, his spirit fled, and left behind but an earthly clod, akin to the dross that he made his god.

What now avail the chinking chimes of "dimes and dollars! dollars and dimes"? Men of the times, men of the times! content may not rest with dollars and dimes. Use them well, and their use sublimes the mineral dross of dollars and dimes. Use them ill, and a thousand crimes spring from a coffer of dollars and dimes. Men of the times, men of the times! let charity dwell with your dollars and dimes. HENRY MILLS.

ELKANO AND THE WIDOW.

(By permission of the Proprietors of " Harper's Magazine.")

  His window is over the factory flume,
  And Elkano, there, in his counting-room
   Sits hugging a littered table.
  He is setting forth in column and row
  Whatever a penny of gain can show—
  Mortgages, dividends, and rents;
  City bonds, and governments;
  A factory here, and a tannery there;
  Good bank stock and railway share:
  Thinks he, "It's a good round sum I make,
  Don't seem much like I was goin' to break."
  And he looked again, as he poised his pen;
  But just as he gave the pen a shake,
  He said, "Ho, ho!" at a strange mistake
   He found himself on the brink of.

ELKANO AND THE WIDOW.

"Wal, I declare! Thar's Widow Brown
In the cottage over at Tannery town;
The family had the house rent-free,
Long as her husband worked for me—
A good, smart, faithful chap was Jim—
Wish I'd forty as good as him;
But he died one day, an' left her thar,
An' I put the place in the parson's care—
    (Good old Parson Emery!)
To see that the house don't run away,
An' collect the rent she agreed to pay—
I'll send a letter this very day
    To jog the old man's memory."
The letter was straightway penned, and sent;
It preached hard times to a dreary extent,
And thus concluded the document:—
"You may, if you please, remit the rent
    Jim's widow owes for the cottage."
On Christmas morn the answer came.
"The parson's prompt; but what in the name?"
He said, as he opened and read the same:—
"Dear, noble, generous, honoured friend!"
Were terms he couldn't quite comprehend.
"What on earth's the old fool ravin' about?
He's crazy, beyond a shadow o' doubt;
A-writin' to me, as if I was a saint!—
Wal, maybe I be, an' maybe I ain't.
An' what's his argument?—Why, to be sure,
That 'I'm a merciful man to the poor.'
    Blamed old Dunderhead!
An' here he goes on in a gushin' mood—
'You've been so exceedin'ly good
To pity the widow's condition,
An' give me the blessed authority to
Remit the rent that is due.'

ELKANO AND THE WIDOW.

Remit! why don't he remit, then?—Wish I knew!
Place o' that, here's more o' his hullabaloo:—
'The widow begs to thank you for the remission.'
Remission! remit!—oh, the stupid old dunce!"—
    And he went for a dictionary;
It having occurred to him, all at once,
    That the meanings sometimes vary
Of even the simplest words we write,
And that a prosy old parson might use *one*,
And a man of business quite *another* vocabulary.
Finger and eye ran down the page,
" *RA—RE* "—he was flushed with rage—
" *Remember—Remind—Remit—
Send back* "—of course; but hulloh! what's this?
" *To release, to forgive, as a sin, or a debt.*"
'Twas so—'twas strange—'twas very absurd
That thus from a phrase, or a single word,
With equal reason, could be inferred
    Collection of debt—or quittance;
And so the simple old parson
Had given the widow remission,
    Instead of sending Elkano's remittance.
He glared a moment, then seized his pen;
Tore one letter, and wrote again,
Till, too impatient to brook delay,
Swung on his ulster, and swooped away
Toward Tannery town, and the Widow Brown,
    And the good, old, blundering minister.
As out by the forenoon train he went,
    He had ample time to consider.
" It's a leetle rough on a plain old gent
    Who never was known to give a cent
    (Say nothin' o' seventy dollars rent)
        To *any*body's widow.
They'll wonder what sort o' a man I be

When I tell 'em, right out, how it seems to me
Sich a stupid, ridikilous, fool's idee
That I should forgive a debtor.—
 It's very warm!
What makes 'em keep the cars so hot?—
Must be I'm fond o' parson's society;
For what else under the canopy
I'm makin' the trip for, I can't see.
It's an awkward mess, I do declare!
The widow, she'll cry; the parson, he'll stare;
Shouldn't wonder if somebody else'll swear!
Wish I was back in my office-chair.
For why should I go twelve miles or so,
 An' lose my time, an' my dinner,
To prove to their faces, beyond a doubt,
That I ain't no saint as they make out,
 But a hardened sort o' a sinner?"—
"Tannery town!" "Wal, here I be."
With gathering frown and firm-set teeth
He straight made his way to the parson's gate;
Though, after all, he approached the spot
Outwardly cold and inwardly hot—
As a brave man goes to be hanged or shot,
 Or whatever else is not the best thing for his
  constitution.
And when this answer he received,
"Parson ain't at home," will it be believed
He felt like the very same man reprieved
 At the moment of execution?
"No train back till half-past two;
 What on earth am I to do?"
He thought of his rent, and the Widow Brown,
And this is what he *did* do:—
He turned his feet up the snowy street,
And went to call on the widow.

When he arrived at the cottage door,
  He reached for the old bell-handle;
But paused a moment, amazed and grim,
For he heard such a racket, as seemed to him,
In the home of the late lamented Jim,
  Sufficient cause for scandal.
A short, sharp ring, then a hurried noise
Of whispering, scampering girls and boys.
The door was opened a little space,
Through which peered out, with a bashful grace,
A timidly-smiling, fair, young face;
And Elkano caught from the room beyond
A savoury sniff, a wonderful whiff
  Of most delicious cooking.
He sees a table with neat cloth spread,
Steaming dishes, and cream-white bread,
Cranberry sauce, and thick squash pies;
And the curly heads and wondering eyes
  Of the imps who had made the clatter.
A crabbed old man, to whom the sight
Of happy children gave small delight;
A hungry old man, an iron-fisted miser,
Confronting the widow, there he stood,
  Glowering under his vizor;
And it certainly seemed that his presence there
Would, to say the least, surprise her.
And he said to himself, "Her means are all spent,
She hasn't a penny to pay the rent;
While this is the way she gorges her brats!
I'll let her know that I understand
  Whose money pays for the orgies."
The widow, seeing him standing there,
Perceiving only his thin, white hair,
And his almost venerable air,
Asked him in, and placed a chair

With a charmingly natural action.
"Sir, I'm glad you've come
To see what happiness you've given us all.
Since you were so good—"
"Not I, Mrs. Brown; I never was good."—
"It seems a trifle to you, no doubt,
Such kindness as yours."—Here he burst out,—
"I tell you, woman, you're talking about
A thing that has no existence!"
"*You* may say that, but I could not, after all I know,
Permit *another* to wrong you so."
Then up spoke one of the younger crew,—
"You may bet your dollars on that, it's true!
For only yesterday, I tell you,
Wasn't she in high dudgeon,
At hearing you called by Deacon Shaw
The keenest old skinflint ever he saw,
And a stingy, hard carmudgeon!"
"Did he say that—say that 'bout me?
Why, he's harder hisself than the bark o' a tree!"
"Ah, sir, he has more heart than he lets folk see.
A little like you in that," says she.
"Ho, ho! ha, ha! That's a queer idee!
That's a curious calkilation!"
"But when the deacon heard what a friend you had been,
He expressed sincere repentance
For having misjudged you so till now."
"Mrs. Brown, I tell you—Mrs. Brown, I vow—"
But somehow he couldn't complete the sentence.
"Deacon Shaw was here at half-past one;
The goose was brought by the deacon's son;
And then it seemed as if every one
Must do as the deacon and you had done."
"Yes, sir," says Jamie; "and wasn't it fun?
It was ring, ring, ring! it was run, run, run!"

ELKANO AND THE WIDOW.

"It came to us in our sorest need,"
　The widow resumed; "and all are agreed
　'Twas the harvest of which you sowed the seed."
"I sowed the seed! Wal, I *am* beat!"
"And now, kind sir, will you sit by and not despise
　The bounty which Heaven, through you, supplies?"
"Mrs. Brown, you do take me by surprise."
　She smilingly reached for his coat and his hat;
　And the goose was fragrant, the goose was fat.
"I hope you will stay!"—"Wal, as to that—
　　I don't dine out very often—
　I called to explain; but never mind—
　Fact is, Mrs. Brown, I haven't dined,
　An' if you insist—since you *air* so kind—
　Don't care if I do;" and down he sat.
　The goose *was* fragrant, the goose *was* fat—
　　The old man did the carving;
　And the plates around that little board
　Were filled in a manner which didn't afford
　　The slightest hint of starving.
　With hope in her breast, and her children near,
　　The widow smiled contented;
　Even Elkano ceased to be
　Greatly scandalized, to see
　Cheerful faces and childish glee,
　　In the home of the late lamented.
　The widow talked, and told her plans:
"The parson has got my boys a chance
　To blow the organ the coming year;
　The girls will help me more and more;
　I'll sew—but what a change for them and me.
　If only my poor, dear husband—"
　Mrs. Brown here, for some reason,
　　Quite broke down.
"Wal, Mrs. Brown, it's a pretty tough case"

(He made a motion with his hand, but drew it back)
" I must say you've got a knack—
  You're gettin' along, an' I'm awful glad.
  No more; no 'thank'ee, ma'am "
(Down *again* went the uncertain hand).
" Your children are well, an' growin'.
  In a few years your boys'll be rich men—
    May be they will; no knowin'.
    So late? I'd no idee; train won't wait.
    Guess I'll have to be goin'."
" There was something," says Jamie, " you came to
    explain."
" Ah, yes; by the way, a leetle mistake;
    But that's all right.
  The parson didn't take in, not quite,
  My full intent regardin' the rent.
    Don't be the least bit worried
    'Bout that, for certain another year.—
  Bless me! that's the train I hear;
    Good-day!" and off he hurried.
" Wal, I declare, if that ain't old Emery comin' thar!
  Good thing me an' him didn't meet an hour ago;
    Good thing all round—shouldn't wonder."
The parson came panting up the hill,
  Hands out, all smiles, serenely unconscious still
    Of his most amazing blunder.
" How can I thank you, dear, noble, generous!—"
" No more o' that; please understand
    I've seen Jim's widow.
  Remit her rent the comin' year;
  An' I'd like to *remit* to her now this here.—
  By the way," drawls he, with a sidelong leer,
" Did ye ever notice, Em'ry, it's kind o' queer,
    That there's *two* ways o' remittin'?"

J. T. TROWBRIDGE.

MAUD MÜLLER.

Maud Müller, on a summer's day, raked the meadow, sweet with hay. Beneath her torn hat glowed the wealth of simple beauty and rustic health. Singing, she wrought, and her merry glee the mocking-bird echoed from his tree. But, when she glanced to the far-off town, white from its hill-slope looking down, the sweet song died; and a vague unrest and a nameless longing filled her breast—a wish, that she hardly dared to own, for something better than she had known!

The judge rode slowly down the lane, smoothing his horse's chestnut mane. He drew his bridle in the shade of the apple-trees to greet the maid, and ask a draught from the spring that flowed through the meadows, across the road. She stooped where the cool spring bubbled up, and filled for him her small tin cup; and blushed as she gave it, looking down on her feet so bare, and her tattered gown.

"Thanks!" said the judge; "a sweeter draught from a fairer hand was never quaffed."

He spoke of the grass, and flowers, and trees, of the singing birds and the humming bees; then talked of the haying, and wondered whether the cloud in the west would bring foul weather. And Maud forgot her brier-torn gown, and her graceful ankles bare and brown; and listened, while a pleased surprise looked from her long-lashed hazel eyes. At last, like one who for delay seeks a vain excuse, he rode away!

Maud Müller looked and sighed: "Ah me! that I the judge's bride might be! He would dress me up in silks so fine, and praise and toast me at his wine. My father should wear a broadcloth coat; my brother should sail a painted boat. I'd dress my mother so grand and gay! and the baby should have a new toy each day. And I'd feed the hungry and clothe the poor; and all should bless me who left our door."

The judge looked back as he climbed the hill, and saw Maud Müller standing still. "A form more fair, a face more sweet, ne'er hath it been my lot to meet. And her modest answer and graceful air, show her wise and good as she is fair. Would she were mine! and I to-day, like her, a harvester of hay: no doubtful balance of rights and wrongs, and weary lawyers with endless tongues; but low of cattle and song of birds, and health of quiet and loving words." Then he thought of his sister, proud and cold; and his mother, vain of her rank and gold. So, closing his heart, the judge rode on; and Maud was left in the field alone. But the lawyers smiled that afternoon, when he hummed in court an old love tune; and the young girl mused beside the well, till the rain on the unraked clover fell.

He wedded a wife of richest dower, who lived for fashion, as he for power. Yet oft in his marble hearth's bright glow, he watched a picture come and go; and sweet Maud Müller's hazel eyes looked out in their innocent surprise. Oft when the wine in his glass was red, he longed for the wayside-well instead; and closed his eyes on his garnished rooms, to dream of meadows and clover blooms. And the proud man sighed, with a secret pain: "Ah, that I were free again! free as when I rode that day, where the barefoot maiden raked her hay."

She wedded a man unlearned and poor, and many children played round her door. But care and sorrow, and household pain, left their traces on heart and brain. And oft when the summer sun shone hot on the new-mown hay in the meadow lot, in the shade of the apple-tree, again she saw a rider draw his rein; and, gazing down with timid grace, she felt his pleased eyes read her face. Sometimes her narrow kitchen walls stretched away into stately halls; the weary wheel to a spinnet turned, the tallow candle an astral burned; and for him who sat by the chimney lug, dozing and grumbling o'er pipe and mug, a manly form at her side she saw,—and joy was duty, and love was law!......Then she took up her burden of life again, saying only, "It might have been!"

Alas! for maiden, alas! for judge; for rich repiner and household drudge! God pity them both! and pity us all! who

vainly the dreams of youth recall. For of all sad words of tongue or pen, the saddest are these, "It might have been!" Ah, well for us all, some sweet hope lies deeply buried from human eyes; and in the hereafter, angels may roll the stone from its grave away.
J. G. WHITTIER.

CURFEW MUST NOT RING TO-NIGHT.

England's sun was slowly setting o'er the hills so far away,
Filling all the land with beauty, at the close of one sad day.
And his last rays kissed the forehead of a man, and maiden fair,
He with step so slow and weary, she with sunny floating hair;
He with bowed head, sad and thoughtful, she with lips so cold and white,
Struggling to keep back the murmur, "Curfew must not ring to-night."

"Sexton," Bessie's white lips faltered, pointing to the prison old,
With its walls so dark and gloomy, walls so dark, and damp, and cold,—
"I've a lover in that prison, doomed this very night to die
At the ringing of the curfew, and no earthly help is nigh—
Cromwell will not come till sunset," and her face grew strangely white,
As she spoke in husky whispers, "Curfew must not ring to-night."

" Bessie," calmly spoke the sexton,
"Long, long years I've rung the curfew from that gloomy shadowed tower;
Every evening, just at sunset, it has told the twilight hour.
I have done my duty ever, tried to do it just and right,
Now I'm old—I will not miss it; girl! the curfew rings to-night."

Wild her eyes, and pale her features, stern and white her thoughtful brow,
And within her heart's deep centre Bessie made a solemn vow ;
And her breath came fast and faster, and her eyes grew large and bright,
One low murmur, scarcely spoken, "Curfew must *not* ring to-night."

She with light steps bounded forward, sprang within the old church door,
Left the old man, coming slowly, paths he'd trod so oft before.
Not one moment paused the maiden ; but with cheek and brow aglow,
Staggered up the gloomy tower, where the bell swung to and fro ;
Then she climbed the slimy ladder, dark—without one ray of light,
Upward still, her pale lips saying, "Curfew *shall* not ring to-night."

She has reached the topmost ladder ; o'er her hangs the great, dark bell,
And the awful gloom beneath her—like the pathway down to hell—
See ! the ponderous tongue is swinging, 'tis the hour of curfew —*Now !*
And the sight has chilled her bosom, stopped her breath, and paled her brow ;
Shall she *let* it ring ? No, never ! her eyes flash with sudden light,
As she springs, and grasps it firmly, "Curfew shall *not* ring to-night."

Out she swung—far out—the city seemed a tiny speck below,
There, 'twixt heaven and earth suspended, as the bell swung to and fro ;

And the half-deaf sexton, ringing; years he had not heard the bell,
Thought the twilight curfew rang young Basil's funeral knell.

It was o'er, the bell ceased swaying, and the maiden stepped once more
Firmly on the damp old ladder, where, for hundred years before,
Human foot had not been planted.

O'er the distant hills came Cromwell; Bessie saw him, and her brow
Lately white with sickening horror, glows with sudden beauty now:
At his feet she told her story, he saw her hands all bruised and torn,
And her sweet young face so haggard, with a look so sad and worn;
Touched his heart with sudden pity, lit his eyes with misty light—
"Go—your lover lives," said Cromwell; "curfew *shall* not ring to-night."

Wide they flung the massive portal, led the prisoner forth to die,
All his bright young life before him—'neath the dark'ning English sky.
Bessie comes with flying footstep—eyes aglow with love-light sweet—
Kneeling on the turf beside him, lays his pardon at his feet.

In his strong, brave arms he clasped her, kissed the face upturned and white;
Whispered, "Darling, *you* have saved me, curfew *did* not ring to-night."

ROSE HARTWICK THORPE.

JANE CONQUEST.

'Twas about the time of Christmas, a many years ago,
When the sky was black with wrath and rack, and the earth was white with snow,
When loudly rang the tumult of winds and waves at strife,
In her home by the sea, with her babe on her knee, sat Harry Conquest's wife.
And he was on the waters—she knew not, knew not where,
For never a lip could tell of the ship to lighten her heart's despair.
And her babe was dying, dying—the pulse in the tiny wrist
Was all but still, and the brow was chill and pale as the white sea mist.
Jane Conquest's heart was hopeless; she could only weep, and pray
That the Shepherd mild would take the child painlessly away.
The night grew deep and deeper, and the storm had a stronger will,
And buried in deep and dreamless sleep lay the hamlet under the hill;
And the fire was dead on the hearth-stone within Jane Conquest's room,
And still sat she with her babe on her knee, at prayer amid the gloom,—
When, borne above the tempest, a sound fell on her ear,
Thrilling her through, for well she knew 'twas a voice of mortal fear;
And a light leapt in at the lattice, sudden and swift and red,
Crimsoning all the whited wall, and the floor and the roof o'erhead.
It shone with a radiant glory on the face of the dying child,
Like a fair first ray of the shadowless day of the land of the undefiled;
And it lit up the mother's features with a glow so strange and new,

JANE CONQUEST.

That the white despair that had gathered there seemed changed to hope's own hue.
For one brief moment, heedless of the babe upon her knee,
With the frenzied start of a frightened heart, up to her feet rose she;
And through the quaint old casement she looked upon the sea—
Thank God that the sight she saw that night so rare a sight should be!
Hemmed in by hungry billows, whose madness foamed at lip,
Half a mile from the shore, or hardly more, she saw a gallant ship
Aflame from deck to topmast, aflame from stem to stern,
For there seemed no speck on all the wreck where the fierce fire did not burn.
And the night was like a sunset, and the sea like a sea of blood,
And the rocks and the shore were bathed all o'er as by some gory flood.
She looked and looked, till the terror crept cold through every limb,
And her breath came quick, and her heart turned sick, and her sight grew dizzy and dim;
Till once more that cry of anguish thrilled through the tempest's strife,
And it stirred again in her heart and brain the active, thinking life;
And the light of an inspiration leapt to her brightened eye,
And on lip and brow was written now a purpose pure and high.
Swiftly she turned, and softly she crossed the chamber floor,
And, faltering not, in his tiny cot she laid the babe she bore;
And then, with a holy impulse, she sank to her knees and made
A lowly prayer in the silence there, and this was the prayer she prayed:
"Christ, who didst bear the scourging, but now dost wear the crown,
I at thy feet, O true and sweet, would lay my burden down,

Thou bad'st me love and cherish the babe thou gavest me,
And I have kept thy word, nor stepped aside from following thee;
And lo! the boy is dying, and vain is all my care,
And my burden's weight is very great! yea, greater than I can bear.
O Lord, thou know'st what peril doth threat these poor men's lives;
I, a lone woman, most weak and human, plead for their waiting wives.
Thou canst not let them perish; up, Lord, in thy strength and save
From the scorching breath of this terrible death, on the cruel winter wave.
Take thou my babe and watch it, no care is like to thine,
And let thy power, in this perilous hour, supply what lack is mine."
And so her prayer she ended, and rising to her feet,
Turned one look to the cradle nook where the child's faint pulses beat;
And then with softest footsteps retrod the chamber floor,
And noiselessly groped for the latch, and oped and crossed the cottage door.
And through the tempest bravely Jane Conquest fought her way,
By snowy deep, and slippery steep, to where her goal lay.
And she gained it, pale and breathless, and weary, and sore, and faint,
But with soul possessed with the strength, and zest, and ardour of a saint.
Silent and weird, and lonely amid its countless graves,
Stood the old gray church on its tall rock perch, secure from the flood's great waves.
Jane Conquest reached the churchyard, and stood by the old church door;
But the oak was tough, and had bolts enough, and her strength was frail and poor;

So she crept through a narrow window, and climbed the belfry stair,
And grasped the rope, sole cord of hope for the mariners in despair.
And the wild wind helped her bravely, and she wrought with an earnest will,
And the clamorous bell spake out right well to the hamlet under the hill.
And it roused the slumb'ring fishers, nor its warning task gave o'er
Till a hundred fleet and eager feet were hurrying to the shore;
And then it ceased its ringing, for the woman's work was done,
And many a boat that was now afloat showed man's work was begun.
But the ringer in the belfry lay motionless and cold,
With the cord of hope, the church-bell rope, still in her frozen hold.
How long she lay it boots not, but she woke from her swoon at last,
In her own bright room, to find the gloom and the grief of the peril past.
And they told her all the story: how a brave and gallant few
O'ercame each check, and reached the wreck, and saved the hapless crew;
And how the curious sexton had climbed the belfry stair,
And of his fright when, cold and white, he found her lying there;
And how, when they had borne her back to her home again,
The child she left with a heart bereft of hope, and wrung with pain,
Was found within its cradle in a quiet slumber laid,
With a peaceful smile on its lips the while, and the wasting sickness stayed.
And she said 'twas Christ that watched it, and brought it safely through,

And she praised his truth, and his tender ruth, who had saved her darling too.
And then there came a letter across the surging foam;
And last, the breeze that o'er the seas bore Harry Conquest home:
And they told him all the story, that still their children tell,
Of the fearful sight on that winter night, and the ringing of the bell. J. MILNE.

BECALMED.

It was as calm as calm could be; a death-still night in June: a silver sail on a silver sea, under a silver moon. No least low air the still sea stirred; but all on the dreaming deep the white ship lay, like a white sea-bird, with folded wings, asleep. For a long, long month not a breath of air—for a month not a drop of rain; and the gaunt crew watched in wild despair, with a fever in throat and brain. And they saw the shore, like a dim cloud, stand on the far horizon-sea: it was only a day's short sail to the land, and the haven where they would be.

Too faint to row—no signal brought an answer, far or nigh: Father, have mercy; leave them not alone on the deep to die. And the gaunt crew prayed on the decks above, and the women prayed below: "One drop of rain, for Heaven's great love! O Heaven, for a breeze to blow!" But never a shower from the skies would burst, and never a breeze would come: O God, to think that man can thirst, and starve, in sight of home! But out to sea with the drifting tide the vessel drifted away, till the far-off shore, like the dim cloud, died, and the wild crew ceased to pray! Like fiends they glared, with their eyes aglow, like beasts with hunger wild; but a mother prayed, in the cabin below, by the bed of her little child. It slept, and lo! in its sleep it smiled, a babe of summers three: "O Father, save my little child, whatever comes to me!"

Calm gleamed the sea, calm gleamed the sky—no cloud, no

sail in view; and they cast them lots for who should die to feed the starving crew! Like beasts they glared, with hunger wild, and their red-glazed eyes aglow; and the death-lot fell on the little child that slept in the cabin below! And the mother shrieked in wild despair: "O God, my child—my son! They will take his life—it is hard to bear, yet, Father, thy will be done!" And she waked the child from its happy sleep, and she knelt by the cradle bed: "We thirst, my child, on the lonely deep; we are dying, my child, for bread. On the lone, lone sea no sail—no breeze; not a drop of rain in the sky: we thirst—we starve—on the lonely seas, and thou, my boy, must die!"

She wept: what tears her wild soul shed not I but Heaven knows best. And the child rose up from its cradle bed, and crossed its hands on its breast. "Father," he lisped, "so good—so kind, have pity on mother's pain; for mother's sake, a little wind; Father, a little rain!" And she heard them shout for the child from the deck, and she knelt on the cabin stairs. "The child!" they cry, "the child—stand back—and a curse on your idiot prayers!" And the mother rose in her wild despair, and she bared her throat to the knife: "Strike—strike me—me; but spare, O spare my child, my dear son's life!"

Ah me! it was a ghastly sight: red eyes, like flaming brands, and a hundred belt-knives flashing bright in the clutch of skeleton hands! "Me—me—strike, ye fiends of death!"—but soft—through the ghastly air whose falling tear was that? whose breath waves through the mother's hair? A flutter of sail—a ripple of seas, a speck on the cabin-pane: thank God! it is a breeze—a breeze—and a drop of blessèd rain! And the mother rushed to the cabin below, and she wept on the babe's bright hair: "The sweet rain falls, the sweet winds blow: Father has heard thy prayer!" But the child had fallen asleep again, and lo! in its sleep it smiled. "Thank God," she cried, "for his wind and his rain; thank God for my little child!"

SAMUEL K. COWAN.

THE LADY OF PROVENCE.

The war-note of the Saracen was on the winds of France; it had stilled the harp of the troubadour, and the clash of the tourney's lance. The sounds of the sea, and the sounds of the night, and the hollow echoes of charge and flight, were around Clotilde, as she knelt to pray in a chapel where the mighty lay, on the old Provençal shore: many a Chatillon beneath, unstirred by the ringing trumpet's breath, his shroud of armour wore. But meekly the voice of the Lady rose through the trophies of their proud repose; and her fragile frame, at every blast that full of the savage war-horn passed, trembling, as trembles a bird's quick heart when it vainly strives from its cage to part—so knelt she in her woe; a weeper alone with the tearless dead!—oh, they reck not of tears o'er their quiet shed, or the dust had stirred below!

Hark!—a swift step: she hath caught its tone through the dash of the sea, through the wild wind's moan. Is her lord returned with his conquering bands?—no! a breathless vassal before her stands.

"Hast thou been on the field? art thou come from the host?"

"From the slaughter, Lady! All, all is lost! our banners are taken—our knights laid low—our spearmen chased by the Paynim foe—and thy lord"—his voice took a sadder sound— "thy lord—he is not on the bloody ground! There are those who tell that the leader's plume was seen in the flight, through the gathering gloom!"

A change o'er her mien and spirit passed: she ruled the heart which had beat so fast, she dashed the tears from her kindling eye, with a glance as of sudden royalty.

"Dost thou stand by the tombs of the glorious dead, and fear not to say that their son hath fled? Away! he is lying by lance and shield—point me the path to his battle-field!"

Silently, with lips compressed, pale hands clasped above her breast, stately brow of anguish high, deathlike cheek, but dauntless eye—silently, o'er that red plain, moved the Lady, 'midst the slain. She searched into many an unclosed eye, that looked without soul to the starry sky ; she bowed down o'er many a shattered breast, she lifted up helmet and cloven crest ;—not there, not there he lay !

" Lead where the most has been dared and done ; where the heart of the battle hath bled—lead on ! " And the vassal took the way.

He turned to a dark and lonely tree that waved o'er a fountain red : oh, swiftest there had the current free from noble veins been shed ! Thickest there the spear-heads gleamed, and the scattered plumage streamed, and the broken shields were tossed, and the shivered lances crossed—HE WAS THERE ! the leader amidst his band, where the faithful had made their last vain stand ; with the falchion yet in his cold hand grasped, and his country's flag to his bosom clasped ! She quelled in her soul the deep floods of woe—the time was not yet for their waves to flow; and a proud smile shone on her pale despair, as she turned to her followers,—

" Your lord is there ! Look on him ! know him by scarf and crest ! bear him away with his sires to rest ! "

There is no plumed head o'er the bier to bend—no brother of battle, no princely friend : by the red fountain the valiant lie —the flower of Provençal chivalry. But ONE free step, and one lofty heart, bear through that scene, to the last, their part.

" I have won thy fame from the breath of wrong ! my soul hath risen for thy glory strong ! Now call me hence by thy side to be ; the world thou leav'st has no place for me. Give me my home on thy noble heart ! well have we loved—let us both depart ! "

And pale on the breast of the dead she lay, the living cheek to the cheek of clay. The living cheek ? oh, it was not in vain that strife of the spirit to rend its chain ! She is there, at rest, in her place of pride ! in death, how queenlike !—a glorious bride! From the long heart-withering early gone: she hath lived —she hath loved—her task is done! MRS. HEMANS.

FITZ-JAMES AND RODERICK DHU.

[FROM "THE LADY OF THE LAKE."]

[NOTE.—It was the custom of King James the Fifth of Scotland to travel about the country *incognito*. In Sir Walter Scott's poem he has adopted the *nom de plume* of "Fitz-James."

Losing his way in a Highland pass, near the Trossachs, he meets a poor maniac (Blanche of Devan). While she is telling him the story of her life, and how her lover was murdered by the treachery of Roderick Dhu, an arrow from Red Murdoch's bow pierces her breast. Fitz-James swiftly avenges this dastardly deed, and returns only in time to hear poor Blanche's dying words, in which she conjures him to avenge her lover's death.

A lock of her hair he dips in blood and fixes to his cap, vowing—

> "By Him whose word is truth! I swear,
> No other favour will I wear,
> Till this sad token I imbrue
> In the best blood of Roderick Dhu!"

He then resumes his journey.]

> In dread, in danger, and alone,
> Famished and chilled, through ways unknown,
> Tangled and steep, he journeyed on;
> Till, as a rock's huge point he turned,
> A watch-fire close before him burned.
> Beside its embers red and clear,
> Basked, in his plaid, a mountaineer;
> And up he sprang with sword in hand,—
> "Thy name and purpose? Saxon, stand!"—
> "A stranger."—"What dost thou require?"—
> "Rest and a guide, and food and fire."—
> "Art thou a friend to Roderick?"—"No."—
> "Thou dar'st not call thyself a foe?"—
> "I dare! to him and all the band

He brings to aid his murderous hand."—
" Bold words !—Stranger, I am to Roderick Dhu
A clansman born, a kinsman true ;
Each word against his honour spoke,
Demands of me avenging stroke :
But not for clan nor kindred's cause
Will I depart from honour's laws ;—
To assail a wearied man were shame,
And stranger is a holy name.
Then rest thee here till dawn of day ;
Myself will guide thee on the way
As far as Coilantogle's ford ;
From thence thy warrant is thy sword."—
" I take thy courtesy, by Heaven,
As freely as 'tis nobly given ! "—
And the brave foemen, side by side,
Lay peaceful down, like brothers tried,
And slept until the dawning beam
Purpled the mountain and the stream.

*   *   *   *

So toilsome was the road to trace,
The guide, abating of his pace,
Led slowly through the pass's jaws,
And asked Fitz-James, by what strange cause
He sought these wilds, traversed by few,
Without a pass from Roderick Dhu ?
" Brave Gael, my pass in danger tried,
Hangs in my belt, and by my side ;......
But yestermorn, I knew
Nought of thy chieftain, Roderick Dhu,
Save as an outlawed, desperate man,
The head of a rebellious clan,
Who, in the Regent's court and sight,
With ruffian dagger stabbed a knight."—
" And heard'st thou why he drew his blade ?

Heard'st thou that shameful word and blow
Brought Roderick's vengeance on his foe?
What recked the Chieftain if he stood
On Highland heath, or Holy-Rood?
He rights such wrong where it is given,
If it were in the court of Heaven!"—
" Still was it outrage;......
Besides, thy Chieftain's robber life!—
Wrenching from ruined Lowland swain
His herds and harvest, reared in vain;
Methinks, a soul like thine should scorn
The spoils from such foul foray borne."—
" Saxon, from yonder mountain high,
I marked thee send delighted eye
Far to the south and east, where lay,
Extended in succession gay,
Deep waving fields and pastures green;—
These fertile plains, that softened vale,
Were once the birthright of the Gael;
The stranger came with iron hand,
And from our fathers reft the land.
Where dwell we now? See, rudely swell
Crag over crag, and fell o'er fell:
Ask we this savage hill we tread
For fattened steer, or household bread;
And well the mountain might reply,—
' To you, as to your sires of yore,
Belong the target and claymore!
I give you shelter in my breast,
Your own good blades must win the rest!'
Pent in this fortress of the north,
Think'st thou we will not sally forth
To spoil the spoiler as we may,
And from the robber rend the prey?
Ay, by my soul! While on yon plain

The Saxon rears one shock of grain;
While, of ten thousand herds, there strays
But one along yon river's maze,—
The Gael, of plain and river heir,
Shall, with strong hand, redeem his share!"—
Answered Fitz-James,—" Well, let it pass.
Enough, I am by promise tied
To match me with this man of pride;
Twice have I sought Clan-Alpine's glen
In peace; but when I come again,
I come with banner, brand, and bow,
As leader seeks his mortal foe.
For love-lorn swain, in lady's bower,
Ne'er panted for the appointed hour,
As I, until before me stand
This rebel Chieftain and his band!"

" Have, then, thy wish!"—he whistled shrill,
And he was answered from the hill;
Wild as the scream of the curlew,
From crag to crag the signal flew.
Instant, through copse and heath, arose
Bonnets, and spears, and bended bows;
On right, on left, above, below,
Sprang up at once the lurking foe;
The rushes and the willow-wand
Are bristling into axe and brand,
And every tuft of broom gives life
To plaided warrior armed for strife.

That whistle garrisoned the glen
At once with full five hundred men!
The mountaineer cast glance of pride
Along Ben-ledi's living side,
Then fixed his eye and sable brow

Full on Fitz-James—" How say'st thou now ?
These are Clan-Alpine's warriors true ;
And, Saxon—*I* am Roderick Dhu !"

Fitz-James was brave :—Though to his heart
The life-blood thrilled with sudden start,
He manned himself with dauntless air,
Returned the Chief his haughty stare ;
His back against a rock he bore,
And firmly placed his foot before :—
" Come one, come all ! this rock shall fly
From its firm base as soon as I."

Sir Roderick marked—and in his eyes
Respect was mingled with surprise,
And the stern joy which warriors feel
In foemen worthy of their steel.
Short space he stood—then waved his hand :
Down sank the disappearing band ;
Each warrior vanished where he stood,
In broom or bracken, heath or wood.
The wind's last breath had tossed in air
Pennon, and plaid, and plumage fair,—
The next but swept a lone hill-side,
Where heath and fern were waving wide.

Fitz-James looked round—yet scarce believed
The witness that his sight received ;
Sir Roderick in suspense he eyed,
And to his look the Chief replied :—
" Fear nought—nay, that I need not say—
But doubt not aught from mine array.
Thou art my guest ;—I pledged my word
As far as Coilantogle ford :
So move we on ;—I only meant

FITZ-JAMES AND RODERICK DHU.

To show the reed on which you leant,
Deeming this path you might pursue
Without a pass from Roderick Dhu."......

The Chief in silence strode before,
And reached that torrent's sounding shore,
Where Vennachar in silver breaks.
And here his course the Chieftain stayed,
Threw down his target and his plaid,
And to the Lowland warrior said :—
"Bold Saxon! to his promise just,
Vich-Alpine has discharged his trust.
This 'murderous Chief!' this 'ruthless man!'
This 'head of a rebellious clan!'
Hath led thee safe, through watch and ward,
Far past Clan-Alpine's outmost guard.
Now, man to man, and steel to steel,
A Chieftain's vengeance thou shalt feel.
See, here, all vantageless I stand,
Armed, like thyself, with single brand :
For *this* is Coilantogle ford,
And thou must keep thee with thy sword."

The Saxon paused :— " I ne'er delayed
When foeman bade me draw my blade ;
Nay, more, brave Chief, I vowed thy death ;
Yet, sure, thy fair and generous faith,
And my deep debt for life preserved,
A better meed have well deserved :
Can nought but blood our feud atone?
Are there no means?"—" No, stranger, none!
And, hear,—to fire thy flagging zeal,—
The Saxon cause rests on thy steel ;
For thus spoke Fate, by prophet bred
Between the living and the dead :

'Who spills the *foremost* foeman's life,
  His party conquers in the strife.' "

" Then, by my word," the Saxon said,
" The riddle is already read.
  Seek yonder brake beneath the cliff,—
  There lies Red Murdoch, stark and stiff.
  Thus Fate has solved her prophecy;
  Then yield to Fate, and not to me."

  Dark lightning flashed from Roderick's eye:
" Soars thy presumption, then, so high,
  Because a wretched kern ye slew,
  Homage to name to Roderick Dhu?
  He yields not, he, to man nor Fate!
  Thou add'st but fuel to my hate!
  My clansman's blood demands revenge.—
  Not yet prepared?—By heaven, I change
  My thought, and hold thy valour light
  As that of some vain carpet-knight,
  Who ill deserved my courteous care,
  And whose best boast is but to wear
  A braid of his fair lady's hair."

" I thank thee, Roderick, for the word!
  It nerves my heart, it steels my sword;
  For I have sworn this braid to stain
  In the best blood that warms thy vein.
  Now, truce, farewell! and, ruth, begone!
  Yet think not that by thee alone,
  Proud Chief! can courtesy be shown;
  Though not from copse, or heath, or cairn,
  Start at my whistle clansmen stern,
  Of this small horn one feeble blast
  Would fearful odds against thee cast.

But fear not, doubt not, which thou wilt—
We try this quarrel hilt to hilt."

Then each at once his falchion drew,
Each on the ground his scabbard threw,
Each looked to sun, and stream, and plain,
As what they ne'er might see again;
Then foot, and point, and eye opposed,
In dubious strife they darkly closed.

Ill fared it then with Roderick Dhu
That on the field his targe he threw,
Whose brazen studs and tough bull-hide
Had death so often dashed aside.......

Three times in closing strife they stood,
And thrice the Saxon blade drank blood;—
No stinted draught, no scanty tide,
The gushing flood the tartans dyed.
Fierce Roderick felt the fatal drain,
And showered his blows like wintry rain;
The foe—invulnerable still—
Foiled his wild rage by steady skill;
Till, at advantage ta'en, his brand
Forced Roderick's weapon from his hand,
And, backward borne upon the lea,
Brought the proud Chieftain to his knee.

" Now, yield thee! or by Him who made
The world, thy heart's blood dyes my blade!"—
"Thy threats, thy mercy, I defy!
Let recreant yield, who fears to die."

Like adder darting from his coil,
Like wolf that dashes through the toil,

Like mountain-cat who guards her young,
Full at Fitz-James's throat he sprung;
Received, but recked not of a wound,
And locked his arms his foeman round.—
Now, gallant Saxon, hold thine own!
No *maiden's* hand is round thee thrown!
That desperate grasp thy frame might feel
Through bars of brass and triple steel!—
They tug, they strain!—down, down they go,
The Gael above, Fitz-James below!

The Chieftain's gripe his throat compressed,
His knee was planted on his breast;
His clotted locks he backward threw,
Across his brow his hand he drew,
From blood and mist to clear his sight,
Then gleamed aloft his dagger bright!—
But—while the dagger gleamed on high,
Reeled soul and sense, reeled brain and eye.
Down came the blow! but in the heath
The erring blade found bloodless sheath.
The struggling foe may now unclasp
The fainting Chief's relaxing grasp;—
Unwounded from the dreadful close,
But breathless all, Fitz-James arose.

Sir Walter Scott.

THE RUINED COTTAGE.

None will dwell in that cottage, for they say oppression reft it from an honest man, and that a curse clings to it: hence the vine trails its green weight of leaves upon the ground; hence weeds are in that garden; hence the hedge, once sweet with honeysuckle, is half dead; and hence the gray moss on the apple tree. One once dwelt there, who had been in his youth a soldier; and when many years had passed, he sought his native village, and sat down to end his days in peace. He had one child—a little laughing thing, whose large dark eyes, he said, were like the mother's he had left buried in strangers land. And time went on in comfort and content:—and that fair girl had grown far taller than the red-rose tree her father planted on her first English birthday: and he had trained it up against an ash till it became his pride;—it was so rich in blossom and in beauty, it was called the tree of Isabel. 'Twas an appeal to all the better feelings of the heart, to mark their quiet happiness; their home—in truth a home of love; and more than all, to see them on the Sabbath, when they came among the first to church, and Isabel, with her bright colour and her clear, glad eyes, bowed down so meekly in the house of prayer; and in the hymn her sweet voice audible: her father looked so fond of her, and then from her looked up so thankfully to Heaven! And their small cottage was so very neat; their garden filled with fruits, and herbs, and flowers; and in the winter, there was no fireside so cheerful as their own.

But other days and other fortunes came—an evil power! They bore against it cheerfully, and hoped for better times; but ruin came at last, and the old soldier left his own dear home, and left it for a prison! 'Twas in June, one of June's brightest days: the bee, the bird, the butterfly, were on their lightest wing; the fruits had their first tinge of summer light; the sunny sky, the very leaves seemed glad; and the old man looked back upon his cot, and wept aloud. They hurried him away from the dear child that would not leave his side. They led him from the sight of the blue heaven, and the green trees, into a low, dark cell, the windows shutting out the blessed sun with iron grating; and for the first time he threw him on his bed, and could not hear his Isabel's good night! But the next morn she was the earliest at the prison gate, the last on whom it closed; and her sweet voice, and sweeter smile, made him forget to pine.

She brought him every morning fresh wild flowers; but

every morning could he mark her cheek grow paler, and more pale, and her low tones get fainter, and more faint, and a cold dew was on the hand he held. One day, he saw the sunshine through the grating of his cell—yet Isabel came not; at every sound, his heart-beat took away his breath—yet still she came not near him! But one sad day, he marked the dull street through the iron bars that shut him from the world; at length, he saw a coffin carried carelessly along, and he grew desperate—he forced the bars, and he stood on the street, free, and alone! He had no aim, no wish for liberty; he only felt one want, to see the corpse that had no mourners. When they set it down, ere it was lowered into the new-dug grave, a rush of passion came upon his soul, and he tore off the lid—he saw the face of Isabel, and knew he had no child! He lay down by the coffin, quietly—his heart was broken!

Mrs. Maclean.

MARY, QUEEN OF SCOTS.

I looked far back into other years, and, lo! in bright array,
I saw, as in a dream, the forms of ages passed away.
It was a stately convent, with its old and lofty walls,
And gardens with their broad green walks, where soft the footstep falls;
And o'er the antique dial-stone the creeping shadow passed,
And all around the noon-day sun a drowsy radiance cast.
No sound of busy life was heard, save, from the cloister dim,
The tinkling of the silver bell, or the sisters' holy hymn.
And there five noble maidens sat beneath the orchard trees,
In that first budding spring of youth, when all its prospects please;
And little recked they, when they sang, or knelt at vesper prayers,
That Scotland knew no prouder names—held none more dear than theirs;—

And little even the loveliest thought, before the holy shrine,
Of royal blood, and high descent from the ancient Stuart line :
Calmly her happy days flew on, uncounted in their flight;
And as they flew, they left behind a long-continuing light.

    The scene was changed. It was the court, the gay court of Bourbon,
And 'neath a thousand silver lamps a thousand courtiers throng :
And proudly kindles Henry's eye—well pleased, I ween, to see
The land assemble all its wealth of grace and chivalry :—
But fairer far than all the rest who bask on fortune's tide,
Effulgent in the light of youth, is she, the new-made bride!
The homage of a thousand hearts—the fond, deep love of one—
The hopes that dance around a life whose charms are but begun,—
They lighten up her chestnut eye, they mantle o'er her cheek,
They sparkle on her open brow, and high-souled joy bespeak :
Ah! who shall blame, if scarce that day, through all its brilliant hours,
She thought of that quiet convent's calm, its sunshine and its flowers?

    The scene was changed. It was a bark that slowly held its way,
And o'er its lee the coast of France in the light of evening lay;
And on its deck a Lady sat, who gazed with tearful eyes
Upon the fast receding hills, that dim and distant rise.
No marvel that the Lady wept,—there was no land on earth
She loved like that dear land, although she owed it not her birth;
It was her mother's land, the land of childhood and of friends,—
It was the land where she had found for all her griefs amends,—
The land where her dead husband slept—the land where she had known

The tranquil convent's hushed repose, and the splendours of a throne :
No marvel that the Lady wept—it was the land of France—
The chosen home of chivalry—the garden of romance !
The past was bright, like those dear hills so far behind her bark ;
The future, like the gathering night, was ominous and dark !
One gaze again—one long, last gaze—" Adieu, fair France, to thee ! "
The breeze comes forth—she is alone on the unconscious sea !

  The scene was changed. It was an eve of raw and surly mood,
And in a turret-chamber high of ancient Holyrood
Sat Mary, listening to the rain, and sighing with the winds,
That seemed to suit the stormy state of men's uncertain minds.
The touch of care had blanched her cheek—her smile was sadder now ;
The weight of royalty had pressed too heavy on her brow ;
And traitors to her councils came, and rebels to the field ;—
The Stuart *sceptre* well she swayed, but the *sword* she could not wield.
She thought of all her blighted hopes—the dreams of youth's brief day,
And summoned Rizzio with his lute, and bade the minstrel play
The songs she loved in early years—the songs of gay Navarre ;
The songs, perchance, that erst were sung by gallant Chatelar :
They half beguiled her of her cares, they soothed her into smiles,
They won her thoughts from bigot zeal, and fierce domestic broils :
But hark ! the tramp of armèd men ! the Douglas' battle-cry !
They come !—they come !—and, lo ! the scowl of Ruthven's hollow eye !
And swords are drawn, and daggers gleam, and tears and words are vain—

The ruffian steel is in his heart, the faithful Rizzio's slain!
Then Mary Stuart dashed aside the tears that trickling fell:
"Now for my father's arm!" she said; "my woman's heart farewell!"

The scene was changed. It was a lake, with one small lonely isle;
And there, within the prison-walls of its baronial pile,
Stern men stood menacing their Queen, till she should stoop to sign
The traitorous scroll that snatched the crown from her ancestral line.
"My lords!—my lords!" the captive said, "were I but once more free,
With ten good knights on yonder shore to aid my cause and me,
That parchment would I scatter wide to every breeze that blows,
And once more reign a Stuart Queen o'er my remorseless foes!"
A red spot burned upon her cheek—streamed her rich tresses down;
She wrote the words—she stood erect—a Queen without a crown!

The scene was changed. A royal host a royal banner bore,
And the faithful of the land stood round their smiling Queen once more.
She stayed her steed upon a hill—she saw them marching by—
She heard their shouts—she read success in every flashing eye.
The tumult of the strife begins—it roars—it dies away;
And Mary's troops and banners now, and courtiers—where are they?
Scattered and strown, and flying far, defenceless and undone;—
Alas! to think what she has lost, and all that guilt has won!—
Away! away! thy gallant steed must act no laggard's part;
Yet vain his speed—for thou dost bear the arrow in thy heart!

MARY, QUEEN OF SCOTS.

The scene was changed. Beside the block a sullen headsman stood,
And gleamed the broad axe in his hand, that soon must drip with blood.
With slow and steady step there came a Lady through the hall,
And breathless silence chained the lips, and touched the hearts of all.
I knew that queenly form again, though blighted was its bloom ;
I saw that grief had decked it out—an offering for the tomb !
I knew the eye, though faint its light, that once so brightly shone ;
I knew the voice, though feeble now, that thrilled with every tone ;
I knew the ringlets, almost gray, once threads of living gold !
I knew that bounding grace of step—that symmetry of mould !
Even now I see her far away, in that calm convent aisle,
I hear her chant her vesper-hymn, I mark her holy smile,—
Even now I see her bursting forth upon the bridal morn,
A new star in the firmament, to light and glory born !
Alas, the change !—she placed her foot upon a triple throne,
And on the scaffold now she stands—beside the block—alone !
The little dog that licks her hand, the last of all the crowd
Who sunned themselves beneath her glance, and round her footsteps bowed !
Her neck is bared—the blow is struck—the soul is passed away !
The bright, the beautiful, is now—a bleeding piece of clay !
The dog is moaning piteously ; and, as it gurgles o'er,
Laps the warm blood that trickling runs unheeded to the floor !
The blood of beauty, wealth, and power—the heart-blood of a Queen,—
The noblest of the Stuart race—the fairest earth has seen,—
Lapped by a dog ! Go think of it, in silence and alone ;
Then weigh against a grain of sand the glories of a throne !

H. G. Bell.

THE BURIAL OF MOSES.

By Nebo's lonely mountain, on this side Jordan's wave,
In a vale in the land of Moab, there lies a lonely grave:
And no man knows that sepulchre, and no man saw it e'er;
For the angels of God upturned the sod, and laid the dead man there.

That was the grandest funeral that ever passed on earth;
But no man heard the trampling, or saw the train go forth—
Noiselessly, as the daylight comes back when night is done,
And the crimson streak on ocean's cheek grows into the great sun.

Noiselessly, as the spring-time her crown of verdure weaves,
And all the trees on all the hills open their thousand leaves;
So, without sound of music, or voice of them that wept,
Silently down from the mountain's crown the great procession swept.

Perchance the bald old eagle, on gray Beth-Peor's height,
Out of his lonely eyrie, looked on the wondrous sight;
Perchance the lion stalking still shuns that hallowed spot—
For beast and bird have seen and heard that which man knoweth not!

But when the warrior dieth, his comrades in the war,
With arms reversed and muffled drum, follow his funeral car;
They show the banners taken, they tell his battles won,
And after him lead his masterless steed, while peals the minute-gun.

Amid the noblest of the land we lay the sage to rest,
And give the bard an honoured place, with costly marble drest,—

In the great minster transept, where lights like glories fall,
And the organ rings, and the sweet choir sings, along the emblazoned wall.

This was the truest warrior that ever buckled sword;
This the most gifted poet that ever breathed a word;
And never earth's philosopher traced with his golden pen,
On the deathless page, truths half so sage as he wrote down for men.

And had he not high honour? the hillside for a pall!
To lie in state, while angels wait; with stars for tapers tall!
And the dark rock-pines, like tossing plumes, over his bier to wave!
And God's own hand, in that lonely land, to lay him in the grave!

In that strange grave without a name, whence his uncoffined clay
Shall break again, O wondrous thought! before the judgment day,
And stand, with glory wrapt around, on the hills he never trod,
And speak of the strife that won our life, with the Incarnate Son of God.

O lonely grave in Moab's land! O dark Beth-Peor's hill!
Speak to these curious hearts of ours, and teach them to be still.
God hath his mysteries of grace, ways that we cannot tell;
He hides them deep, like the hidden sleep of him he loved so well!

Mrs. C. F. Alexander.

THE LEPER.

"Room for the leper! room!" And as he came, the cry passed on—"Room for the leper! room!" Sunrise was slanting on the city's gates, rosy and beautiful; and from the hills the early-risen poor were coming in, duly and cheerfully, to their toil; and up rose the sharp hammer's clink, and the far hum of moving wheels, and multitudes astir, and all that in a city-murmur swells,—unheard but by the watcher's weary ear, aching with night's dull silence; or the sick, hailing the welcome light and sounds, that chase the death-like images of the dark away.—" Room for the leper!" And aside they stood—matron, and child, and pitiless manhood,—all who met him on his way, —and let him pass. And onward through the open gate he came, a leper—with the ashes on his brow, sackcloth about his loins, and on his lip a covering,—stepping painfully and slow; and, with a difficult utterance, like one whose heart is with an iron nerve put down, crying, " Unclean! unclean!"......

'Twas now the first of the Judean autumn; and the leaves, whose shadows lay so still upon his path, had put their beauty forth beneath the eye of Judah's loftiest noble. He was young, and eminently beautiful; and life mantled in elegant fulness on his lip, and sparkled in his glance; and in his mien there was a gracious pride that every eye followed with benisons;— AND THIS WAS HE! With the soft airs of summer there had come a torpor on his frame—a drowsy sloth; day after day he lay as if in sleep; his skin grew dry and bloodless, and white scales, circled with livid purple, covered him. And Helon was a leper! He put off his costly raiment for the leper's garb, and, with the sackcloth round him, and his lip hid in a loathsome covering, stood still—waiting to hear his doom :—" Depart! depart, O child of Israel, from the temple of thy God! for he has smote thee with his chastening rod; and, to the desert wild, from all thou lov'st, away thy feet must flee, that from thy plague his people may be free. And now depart! and, when thy heart is heavy, and thine eyes are dim, lift up thy prayer beseechingly to Him who, from the tribes of men, selected thee to feel his chastening rod. Depart, O leper! and forget not God!"

And he went forth—alone! Not one of all the many whom he loved, nor she whose name was woven in the fibres of his heart breaking within him now, to come and speak comfort unto him. Yea, he went his way, sick, and heart-broken, and alone,—to die! for God had cursed the leper!......

It was noon, and Helon knelt beside a stagnant pool in the lone wilderness, and bathed his brow, hot with the burning leprosy, and touched the loathsome water to his fevered lips; praying that he might be so blest—to die! Footsteps approached; and, with no strength to flee, he drew the covering closer on his lip, crying, "Unclean! unclean!" and, in the folds of the coarse sackcloth shrouding up his face, he fell upon the earth till they should pass. Nearer the Stranger came, and, bending o'er the leper's prostrate form, pronounced his name, "Helon!" The voice was like the master-tone of a rich instrument — most strangely sweet; and the dull pulses of disease awoke, and, for a moment, beat beneath the hot and leprous scales with a restoring thrill!—"Helon, arise!" and he forgot his curse, and rose and stood before Him.

Love and awe mingled in the regard of Helon's eye, as he beheld the Stranger. He was not in costly raiment clad, nor on his brow the symbol of a princely lineage wore; no followers at his back; nor in his hand buckler, or sword, or spear;—yet, if he smiled, a kingly condescension graced his lips. His garb was simple, and his sandals worn; his stature modelled with a perfect grace; his countenance the impress of a God, touched with the opening innocence of a child; his eye was blue and calm, as is the sky in the serenest noon; his hair unshorn fell to his shoulders; and his curling beard the fulness of perfected manhood bore. He looked on Helon earnestly awhile, as if his heart were moved; and, stooping down, he took a little water in his hand, and laid it on his brow, and said, "Be clean!" And lo! the scales fell from him; and his blood coursed with delicious coolness through his veins; his dry palms grew moist, and on his brow the dewy softness of an infant's stole: his leprosy was cleansed; and he fell down prostrate at Jesus' feet and worshipped him! N. P. WILLIS.

THE FALCON OF SER FEDERIGO.

One summer morning, when the sun was hot, weary with labour in his garden-plot, on a rude bench beneath his cottage eaves, Ser Federigo sat among the leaves of a huge vine, that, with its arms outspread, hung its delicious clusters overhead. Below him, through the lovely valley, flowed the river Arno, like a winding road; and from its banks were lifted high in air the spires and roofs of Florence, called the Fair: to him a marble tomb, that rose above his wasted fortunes and his buried love. For there, in banquet and in tournament, his wealth had lavished been, his substance spent, to woo and lose, since ill his wooing sped, Monna Giovanna, who his rival wed, yet ever in his fancy reigned supreme, the ideal woman of a young man's dream.

Then he withdrew, in poverty and pain, to this small farm, the last of his domain; his only comfort and his only care to prune his vines, and plant the fig and pear; his only forester and only guest his falcon, faithful to him, when the rest, whose willing hands had found so light, of yore, the brazen knocker of his palace door, had now no strength to lift the wooden latch, that entrance gave beneath a roof of thatch. Companion of his solitary ways, purveyor of his feasts on holidays, on him this melancholy man bestowed the love with which his nature overflowed.

And so the empty-handed years went round, vacant, though voiceful with prophetic sound; and so, that summer morn, he sat and mused with folded, patient hands, as he was used, and dreamily before his half-closed sight floated the vision of his lost delight. Beside him, motionless, the drowsy bird dreamed of the chase, and in his slumber heard the sudden, scythe-like sweep of wings, that dare the headlong plunge through eddying gulfs of air; then, starting broad awake upon his perch, tinkled his bells, like mass-bells in a church, and, looking at his master, seemed to say, "Ser Federigo, shall we hunt to-day?"

Ser Federigo thought not of the chase : the tender vision of her lovely face, I will not say he seems to see—he sees in the leaf-shadows of the trellises, herself, yet not herself; a lovely child with flowing tresses, and eyes wide and wild, coming undaunted up the garden walk, and looking not at him, but at the hawk. "Beautiful falcon!" said he, "would that I might hold thee on my wrist, or see thee fly!" The voice was hers, and made strange echoes start through all the haunted chambers of his heart, as an Æolian harp through gusty doors of some old ruin its wild music pours.

"Who is thy mother, my fair boy?" he said, his hand laid softly on that shining head. "Monna Giovanna.—Will you let me stay a little while, and with your falcon play? We live there, just beyond your garden wall, in the great house behind the poplars tall."

So he spake on ; and Federigo heard as from afar each softly uttered word, and drifted onward through the golden gleams and shadows of the misty sea of dreams. Then, waking from his pleasant reveries, he took the little boy upon his knees, and told him stories of his gallant bird, till in their friendship he became a third......

Monna Giovanna, widowed in her prime, had come with friends to pass the summer time in her grand villa, halfway up the hill, o'erlooking Florence, but retired and still. Here, in seclusion, as a widow may, the lovely lady whiled the hours away, pacing in sable robes the statued hall, herself the stateliest statue among all, and seeing more and more, with secret joy, her husband risen and living in her boy. Meanwhile the boy, rejoicing in his strength, stormed down the terraces from length to length, the screaming peacock chased in hot pursuit, and climbed the garden trellises for fruit. But his chief pastime was to watch the flight of a gerfalcon, soaring into sight; and as he gazed, full often wondered he who might the master of the falcon be, until that happy morning, when he found master and falcon in the cottage ground......

And now a shadow and a terror fell on the great house, as if a passing-bell tolled from the tower, and filled each spacious room with secret awe, and preternatural gloom : the petted boy grew ill, and day by day pined with mysterious malady away. The mother's heart would not be comforted ; her darling seemed to her already dead ; and often, sitting by the sufferer's side, " What can I do to comfort thee ?" she cried. At first the silent lips made no reply, but, moved at length by her importunate cry, " Give me," he answered, with imploring tone, " Ser Federigo's falcon for my own !"

No answer could the astonished mother make : how could she ask, e'en for her darling's sake, such favour at a luckless lover's hand ? But yet, for her child's sake, she could no less than give assent, to soothe his restlessness......

Two ladies, clothed in cloak and hood, passed through the garden gate into the wood—Monna Giovanna and her bosom friend, intent upon their errand and its end. They found Ser Federigo at his toil, like banished Adam, delving in the soil. Monna Giovanna raised her stately head, and with fair words of salutation said : " Ser Federigo, we come here as friends, hoping in this to make some poor amends for past unkindness. I who ne'er before would even cross the threshold of your door ; I who in happier days such pride maintained, refused your banquets, and your gifts disdained—this morning come, a self-invited guest, to put your generous nature to the test, and breakfast with you under your own vine." To which he answered : " Poor desert of mine, not your unkindness call it, for if aught is good in me of feeling or of thought, from you it comes, and this last grace outweighs all sorrows, all regrets of other days."

And after further compliment and talk, among the dahlias in the garden walk he left his guests, and to his cottage turned ; and, as he entered, for a moment yearned for the lost splendours of the days of old—the ruby glass, the silver and the gold—and felt how piercing is the sting of pride, by want imbittered and intensified. He looked about him for some means or way to keep this unexpected holiday; searched every cupboard, and then searched again; summoned the maid, who came, but came in vain. "The signor did not hunt to-day," she said; "there's nothing in the house but wine and bread."

Then, suddenly, the drowsy falcon shook his little bells, with that sagacious look which said, as plain as language to the ear, "If anything is wanting, I am here!" Yes, everything is wanting, gallant bird! The master seized thee without further word; like thine own lure, he whirled thee round—ah me! The pomp and flutter of brave falconry; the bells, the jesses, the bright scarlet hood; the flight and the pursuit o'er field and wood—all these for evermore are ended now: no longer victor, but the victim thou!

Then on the board a snow-white cloth he spread, laid on its wooden dish the loaf of bread, brought purple grapes with autumn sunshine hot, the fragrant peach, the juicy bergamot; then in the midst a flask of wine he placed, and with autumnal flowers the banquet graced. Ser Federigo, would not these suffice, without thy falcon stuffed with cloves and spice?

When all was ready, and the courtly dame with her companion to the cottage came, upon Ser Federigo's brain there fell the wild enchantment of a magic spell: the room they entered, mean and low and small, was changed into a sumptuous banquet-hall; he ate celestial food, and a divine flavour was given to his country wine. And the poor falcon, fragrant with his spice, a peacock was, or bird of paradise!

When the repast was ended, they arose and passed again into the garden-close. Then said the lady, "Far too well I know, remembering still the days of long ago, though you betray it not, with what surprise you see me here in this familiar wise. You have no children, and you cannot guess what anguish, what unspeakable distress a mother feels, whose child is lying ill, nor how her heart anticipates his will. And yet, for this, you see me lay aside all womanly reserve and check of pride, and ask the thing most precious in your sight—your falcon, your sole comfort and delight; which if you find it in your heart to give, my poor, unhappy boy perchance may live."

Ser Federigo listens, and replies, with tears of love and pity in his eyes: "Alas, dear lady! there can be no task so sweet to me as giving, when you ask. One little hour ago, if I had known this wish of yours, it would have been my own. But, thinking in what manner I could best do honour to the presence of my guest, I deemed that nothing worthier could be than what most dear and precious was to me; and so my gallant falcon breathed his last, to furnish forth, this morning, our repast."

In mute contrition, mingled with dismay, the gentle lady turned her eyes away, grieving that he such sacrifice should make, and kill his falcon for a woman's sake; then took her leave, and passed out at the gate with footstep slow, and soul disconsolate.

Three days went by; and, lo! a passing-bell tolled from the little chapel in the dell; ten strokes Ser Federigo heard, and said, breathing a prayer, "Alas! her child is dead!"

Three months went by; and, lo! a merrier chime rang from the chapel bells at Christmas time: the cottage was deserted, and no more Ser Federigo sat beside its door; but now, with servitors to do his will, in the grand villa, halfway up the hill, sat at the Christmas feast, and at his side Monna Giovanna, his beloved bride, never so beautiful, so kind, so fair, enthroned once more in the old rustic chair, high-perched upon the back of which there stood the image of a falcon carved in wood, and underneath the inscription, with a date, "All things come round to him who will but wait."   LONGFELLOW.

KING ROBERT OF SICILY.

Robert of Sicily, brother of Pope Urbane, and Valmond, Emperor of Allemaine, apparelled in magnificent attire, with retinue of many a knight and squire, on St. John's eve, at vespers, proudly sat, and heard the priests chant the Magnificat. And, as he listened, o'er and o'er again repeated, like a burden or refrain, he caught the words, "*Deposuit potentes de sede, et exaltavit humiles;*" and slowly lifting up his kingly head, he to a learnèd clerk beside him said, "What mean these words?" The clerk made answer meet, "He has put down the mighty from their seat, and has exalted them of low degree." Thereat King Robert muttered scornfully, "'Tis well that such seditious words are sung only by priests, and in the Latin tongue; for unto priests and people be it known, there is no power can push me from my throne!" And leaning back, he yawned and fell asleep, lulled by the chant monotonous and deep.

When he awoke, it was already night; the church was empty, and there was no light, save where the lamps, that glimmered few and faint, lighted a little space before some saint. He started from his seat, and gazed around, but saw no living thing, and heard no sound. He groped towards the door, but it was locked; he cried aloud, and listened, and then knocked; and uttered awful threatenings and complaints, and imprecations upon men and saints. The sounds re-echoed from the roof and walls, as if dead priests were laughing in their stalls!

At length the sexton, hearing from without the tumult of the knocking and the shout, and thinking thieves were in the house of prayer, came with his lantern, asking, "Who is there?" Half choked with rage, King Robert fiercely said, "Open: 'tis I, the king! Art thou afraid?" The frightened sexton, muttering, with a curse, "This is some drunken vagabond, or worse!" turned the great key, and flung the portal wide: a man rushed by him at a single stride, haggard, half-naked, without hat or cloak; who neither turned, nor looked at him, nor spoke, but leaped into the blackness of the night, and vanished like a spectre from his sight.

Robert of Sicily, brother of Pope Urbane, and Valmond, Emperor of Allemaine, despoiled of his magnificent attire, bareheaded, breathless, and besprent with mire, with sense of wrong and outrage desperate, strode on and thundered at the palace gate; rushed through the court-yard, thrusting, in his rage, to right and left each seneschal and page, and hurried up the broad and sounding stair, his white face ghastly in the torches' glare. From hall to hall he passed with breathless speed; voices and cries he heard, but did not heed; until, at last, he reached the banquet-room, blazing with light, and breathing with perfume.

There, on the daïs, sat another king! wearing his robes, his crown, his signet-ring! King Robert's self in features, form, and height, but all transfigured with angelic light! It was an angel; and his presence there with a divine effulgence filled the air; an exaltation, piercing the disguise, though none the hidden angel recognize.

A moment, speechless, motionless, amazed, the throneless monarch on the angel gazed, who met his looks of anger and surprise with the divine compassion of his eyes; then said, "Who art thou? and why com'st thou here?" To which King Robert answered, with a sneer, "I am the king, and come to claim my own from an impostor, who usurps my throne!" And suddenly, at these audacious words, up sprang the angry guests, and drew their swords. The angel answered with unruffled brow, "Nay, not the king, but the king's jester! thou henceforth shalt wear the bells and scalloped cape, and for thy counsellor shalt lead an ape; thou shalt obey my servants when they call, and wait upon my henchmen in the hall!"

Deaf to King Robert's threats, and cries, and prayers, they thrust him from the hall and down the stairs; a group of tittering pages ran before, and as they opened wide the folding-door his heart failed, for he heard, with strange alarms, the boisterous laughter of the men-at-arms, and all the vaulted chamber roar and ring with the mock plaudits of "Long live the king!"

Next morning, waking with the day's first beam, he said within himself, "It was a dream!" But the straw rustled as he turned his head; there were the cap and bells beside his bed; around him rose the bare, discoloured walls; close by, the steeds were champing in their stalls; and, in the corner, a revolting shape, shivering and chattering sat the wretched ape. It was no dream: the world he loved so much had turned to dust and ashes at his touch!

Days came and went and now returned again to Sicily the old Saturnian reign; under the angel's governance benign, the happy island danced with corn and wine; and deep within the mountain's burning breast, Enceladus, the giant, was at rest.

Meanwhile, King Robert yielded to his fate, sullen, and silent, and disconsolate. Dressed in the motley garb that jesters wear; with looks bewildered and a vacant stare; close shaven above the ears, as monks are shorn; by courtiers—mocked; by pages—laughed to scorn; his only friend—the ape; his only food —what others left: he still was unsubdued. And when the angel met him on his way, and half in earnest, half in jest, would say, sternly, though tenderly, that he might feel the velvet scabbard held a sword of steel, "Art thou the king?" the passion of his woe burst from him in resistless overflow, and, lifting high his forehead, he would fling the haughty answer back, "I am—I am the king!"

Almost three years were ended, when there came ambassadors of great repute and name from Valmond, Emperor of Allemaine, unto King Robert, saying that Pope Urbane, by letter, summoned them forthwith, to come on Holy Thursday to his city of Rome. The angel with great joy received his guests, and gave them presents of embroidered vests, and velvet mantles with rich ermine lined, and rings and jewels of the rarest kind. Then he departed with them o'er the sea into the lovely land of Italy; whose loveliness was more resplendent made by the mere passing of that cavalcade—with plumes, and cloaks, and housings, and the stir of jewelled bridle and of golden spur.

And, lo! among the menials, in mock state, upon a piebald steed, with shambling gait—his cloak of foxtails flapping in the wind, the solemn ape demurely perched behind—King Robert rode, making huge merriment in all the country towns through which they went.

The Pope received them with great pomp, and blare of bannered trumpets, on Saint Peter's Square, giving his benediction and embrace, fervent, and full of apostolic grace. While with congratulations and with prayers he entertained the angel unawares, Robert, the jester, bursting through the crowd, into their presence rushed, and cried aloud, "*I* am the king! Look, and behold in me, Robert, your brother, King of Sicily! This man, who wears my semblance to your eyes, is an impostor in a king's disguise. Do you not know me? does no voice within answer my cry, and say we are akin?" The Pope, in silence, but with troubled mien, gazed at the angel's countenance serene; the emperor, laughing, said, "It is strange sport to keep a madman for thy fool at court!" and the poor, baffled jester, in disgrace, was hustled back among the populace.

In solemn state the holy week went by, and Easter Sunday gleamed upon the sky; the presence of the angel, with its light, before the sun rose, made the city bright, and with new fervour filled the hearts of men, who felt that Christ indeed had risen again. Even the jester, on his bed of straw, with haggard eyes the unwonted splendour saw: he felt, within, a power unfelt before; and, kneeling humbly on his chamber floor, he heard the rushing garments of the Lord sweep through the silent air, ascending heavenward.

And now the visit ending, and once more Valmond returning to the Danube's shore, homeward the angel journeyed, and again the land was made resplendent with his train, flashing along the towns of Italy unto Salerno, and from there by sea. And when once more within Palermo's wall, and seated on the throne in his great hall, he heard the Angelus from convent towers, as if the better world conversed with ours, he beckoned to King Robert to draw nigher, and with a gesture bade the rest retire; and when they were alone the angel said, "Art thou the king?" Then, bowing down his head, King Robert crossed both hands upon his breast, and meekly answered him: "Thou knowest best! My sins as scarlet are; let me go hence, and in some cloister's school of penitence, across those stones, that pave the way to heaven, walk barefoot, till my guilty soul is shriven!" The angel smiled, and from his radiant face a holy light illumined all the place; and through the open window, loud and clear, they heard the monks chant in the chapel near, above the stir and tumult of the street: "He has put down the mighty from their seat, and has exalted them of low degree!" and through the chant a second melody rose like the throbbing of a single string: "I am an angel, and thou art the king!"

King Robert, who was standing near the throne, lifted his eyes, and, lo! he was alone; but all apparelled as in days of old, with ermined mantle and with cloth of gold; and when his courtiers came, they found him there, kneeling upon the floor, absorbed in silent prayer! LONGFELLOW.

THE DEATH OF MARMION.

Blount and Fitz-Eustace rested still
With Lady Clare upon the hill;
On which (for far the day was spent)
The western sunbeams now were bent.
The cry they heard—its meaning knew,
Could plain their distant comrades view.
Sadly to Blount did Eustace say,
" Unworthy office here to stay,
No hope of gilded spurs to-day !"......

THE DEATH OF MARMION.

But, lo! straight up the hill there rode
  Two horsemen, drenched with gore;
And in their arms, a helpless load,
  A wounded knight they bore.
His hand still strained the broken brand;
His arms were smeared with blood and sand:
Dragged from among the horses' feet,
With dinted shield, and helmet beat—
The falcon-crest and plumage gone—
Can that be haughty Marmion?
When, doffed his casque, he felt free air,
Around 'gan Marmion wildly stare:—
"Where's Harry Blount? Fitz-Eustace where?
Linger ye here, ye hearts of hare?
Redeem my pennon—charge again!
Cry—'Marmion to the rescue!'—Vain!
Last of my race, on battle-plain
That shout shall ne'er be heard again!—
Yet my last thought is England's:—fly—
To Dacre bear my signet-ring,
Tell him his squadrons up to bring.
Fitz-Eustace, to Lord Surrey hie!
Let Stanley charge with spur of fire,
With Chester charge, and Lancashire,
Full upon Scotland's central host,
Or victory and England's lost.
Must I bid twice?—hence, varlets, fly!
Leave Marmion here alone—to die."

They parted—and alone he lay;
Clare drew her from the sight away,
Till pain wrung forth a lowly moan,
And half he murmured,—"Is there none
  Of all my halls have nursed,
Page, squire, or groom, one cup to bring

Of blessed water, from the spring,
　　To slake my dying thirst?"

O woman! in our hours of ease,
Uncertain, coy, and hard to please,
　　And variable as the shade
By the light quivering aspen made;
When pain and anguish wring the brow,
　　A ministering angel thou!—
Scarce were the piteous accents said,
When, with the Baron's casque, the maid
　　To the nigh streamlet ran:
Forgot were hatred, wrongs, and fears;
The plaintive voice alone she hears,
　　Sees but the dying man.
She stooped her by the runnel's side,
　　But in abhorrence backward drew;
For, oozing from the mountain-side,
Where raged the war, a dark red tide
　　Was curdling in the streamlet blue!
Where shall she turn?—Behold her mark
　　A little fountain cell,
Where water, clear as diamond spark,
　　In a stone basin fell.
She filled the helm, and back she hied,—
And, with surprise and joy, espied
　　A monk supporting Marmion's head;
A pious man, whom duty brought
To dubious verge of battle fought,
　　To shrive the dying, bless the dead.
Deep drank Lord Marmion of the wave,
And, as she stooped his brow to lave—
" Is it the hand of Clare," he said,
" Or injured Constance, bathes my head?"
　　Then, as remembrance rose,

THE DEATH OF MARMION.

"Speak not to me of shrift or prayer,
　　I must redress her woes!
Short space, few words, are mine to spare!—
Forgive!—and listen, gentle Clare!"
"Alas!" she said, "the while,
O think of your immortal weal!
In vain for Constance is your zeal;
　　She—died at Holy Isle!"
Lord Marmion started from the ground,
As light as though he felt no wound;
Though in the action burst the tide
In torrents from his wounded side!
"Then it was truth!" he said:—"I knew
That the dark presage must be true!
I would the Fiend, to whom belongs
The vengeance due to all her wrongs,
　　Would spare me but a day!
For, wasting fire, and dying groan,
And priests slain on the altar-stone,
　　Might bribe him for delay.
It may not be—this dizzy trance!—
Curse on yon base marauder's lance!
And doubly cursed my failing brand!—
A sinful heart makes feeble hand!"
Then, fainting, down on earth he sunk,
Supported by the trembling monk.
With fruitless labour Clara bound,
And strove to stanch, the gushing wound:
The monk, with unavailing cares,
Exhausted all the Church's prayers:
Ever, he said, that, close and near,
A lady's voice was in his ear,
And that the priest he could not hear,
　　For that she ever sung,—
"In the lost battle, borne down by the flying,

Where mingles war's rattle with groans of the dying!"
   So the notes rung.—
" Avoid thee, Fiend !—with cruel hand,
Shake not the dying sinner's sand !—
   O look, my son, upon yon sign
   Of the Redeemer's grace divine !
   O think on faith and bliss !—
By many a death-bed I have been,
And many a sinner's parting seen,
   But never aught like this !"—
The war, that for a space did fail,
Now, trebly thundering, swelled the gale,
   And—" Stanley !" was the cry :—
A light on Marmion's visage spread,
   And fired his glazing eye ;
With dying hand, above his head
He shook the fragment of his blade,
   And shouted " Victory !—
Charge ! Chester, charge ! On !—Stanley !—On !"—
Were the last words of Marmion.
                         SIR WALTER SCOTT.

"TELL" TO HIS NATIVE MOUNTAINS.

Ye crags and peaks ! I'm with you once again !
I hold to you the hands you first beheld,
To show they still are free. Methinks I hear
A spirit in your echoes answer me,
And bid your tenant welcome to his home
Again ! O sacred forms, how proud you look !
How high you lift your heads into the sky !
How huge you are, how mighty, and how free !
Ye are the things that tower, that shine ; whose smile
Makes glad—whose frown is terrible ; whose forms,
Robed or unrobed, do all the impress wear

Of awe divine! Ye guards of liberty,
I'm with you once again! I call to you
With all my voice! I hold my hands to you,
To show they still are free! I rush to you,
As though I could embrace you!

     Scaling yonder peak,
I saw an eagle wheeling near its brow,
O'er the abyss. His broad-expanded wings
Lay calm and motionless upon the air,
As if he floated there without their aid,
By the sole act of his unlorded will,
That buoyed him proudly up. Instinctively
I bent my bow; yet kept he rounding still
His airy circle, as in the delight
Of measuring the ample range beneath
And round about; absorbed, he heeded not
The death that threatened him. I could not shoot!—
'Twas liberty! I turned my bow aside,
And let him soar away!

    With what pride I used
To walk these hills, and look up to my God,
And bless him that the land was free. Yes, it was free!
From end to end, from cliff to lake, 'twas free!
Free as our torrents are that leap our rocks,
And plough our valleys, without asking leave;
Or as our peaks that wear their caps of snow,
In very presence of the regal sun.
How happy was I then! I loved
Its very storms! Yes, I have often sat
In my boat at night, when, midway o'er the lake,
The stars went out, and down the mountain gorge
The wind came roaring.—I have sat and eyed
The thunder breaking from his cloud, and smiled

To see him shake his lightnings o'er my head,
And think I had no master save his own!
On the wild jutting cliff, o'ertaken oft
By the mountain blast, I've laid me flat along,
And while gust followed gust more furiously,
As if to sweep me o'er the horrid brink,
And I have thought of other lands, whose storms
Are summer-flaws to those of mine, and just
Have wished me there—the thought that mine was free
Has checked that wish, and I have raised my head,
And cried, in thraldom to that furious wind,
Blow on—this is the land of liberty! KNOWLES.

THE SEVEN AGES.

All the world's a stage,
And all the men and women merely players:
They have their exits, and their entrances;
And one man in his time plays many parts,
His acts being seven ages.—At first the infant,
Mewling and puking in the nurse's arms.
And then the whining schoolboy, with his satchel,
And shining morning face, creeping like snail
Unwillingly to school. And then the lover,
Sighing like furnace, with a woful ballad
Made to his mistress' eyebrow. Then the soldier,
Full of strange oaths, and bearded like the pard,
Jealous in honour, sudden and quick in quarrel,
Seeking the bubble, reputation,
Even in the cannon's mouth. And then the justice,
In fair round body, with good capon lined,
With eyes severe, and beard of formal cut,
Full of wise saws and modern instances;
And so *he* plays his part. The sixth age shifts

Into the lean and slippered pantaloon,
With spectacles on nose and pouch on side;
His youthful hose, well saved, a world too wide
For his shrunk shank; and his big, manly voice,
Turning again toward childish treble, pipes
And whistles in his sound.   Last scene of all,
That ends this strange eventful history,
Is second childishness, and mere oblivion;
Sans teeth, *sans* eyes, *sans* taste, *sans* everything.
                                            SHAKESPEARE.

CATO ON THE IMMORTALITY OF THE SOUL.

It must be so!—Plato, thou reason'st well:
Else, whence this pleasing hope, this fond desire,
This longing after immortality?
Or whence this secret dread, and inward horror
Of falling into nought?   Why shrinks the soul
Back on herself, and startles at destruction?
'Tis the divinity that stirs within us;
'Tis heaven itself that points out an hereafter,
And intimates eternity to man.
Eternity! thou pleasing—dreadful thought!
Through what variety of untried being,
Through what new scenes and changes must we pass!
The wide, the unbounded prospect lies before me;
But shadows, clouds, and darkness rest upon it.
Here will I hold.   If there's a Power above us—
And that there is, all nature cries aloud
Through all her works—He must delight in virtue;
And that which He delights in, must be happy:
But when? or where?   This world—was made for Cæsar.
I'm weary of conjectures—this must end them.
                              [*Laying hand on dagger.*
Thus am I *doubly* armed.   My death and life,

My bane and antidote, are both before me,
This—in a moment brings me to an end;
But this—informs me I shall never die!
The soul, secured in her existence, smiles
At the drawn dagger, and defies its point.—
The stars shall fade away, the sun himself
Grow dim with age, and nature sink in years:
But thou shalt flourish in immortal youth,
Unhurt, amid the war of elements,
The wreck of matter, and the crash of worlds!

ADDISON.

THE WATER-MILL.

Oh! listen to the water-mill, through all the livelong day,
As the clicking of the wheels wears hour by hour away.
How languidly the autumn wind doth stir the withered leaves,
As on the field the reapers sing, while binding up the sheaves!
A solemn proverb strikes my mind, and as a spell is cast,
"The mill will never grind again with water that is past."

The summer winds revive no more leaves strown o'er earth and main;
The sickle never more will reap the yellow garnered grain;
The rippling stream flows ever on, aye tranquil, deep, and still,
But never glideth back again to busy water-mill:
The solemn proverb speaks to all, with meaning deep and vast,
"The mill will never grind again with water that is past."

Oh! clasp the proverb to thy soul, dear loving heart and true,

THE WATER-MILL.

For golden years are fleeting by, and youth is passing too :
Ah ! learn to make the most of life, nor lose one happy day,
For time will ne'er return sweet joys neglected, thrown away;
Nor leave one tender word unsaid, thy kindness sow broadcast—
" The mill will never grind again with water that is past."

Oh ! the wasted hours of life that have swiftly drifted by,
Alas ! the good we might have done, all gone without a sigh;
Love that we might once have saved by a single kindly word,
Thoughts conceived but ne'er expressed, perishing, unpenned, unheard,—
Oh ! take the lesson to thy soul, for ever clasp it fast,
" The mill will never grind again with water that is past."

Work on while yet the sun doth shine, thou man of strength and will,
The streamlet ne'er doth useless glide by clicking water-mill;
Nor wait until to-morrow's light beams brightly on thy way,
For all that thou canst call thine own lies in the phrase "to-day :"
Possessions, power, and blooming health must all be lost at last—
" The mill will never grind again with water that is past."

Oh ! love thy God and fellow man, thyself consider last,
For come it will when thou must scan dark errors of the past ;
Soon will this fight of life be o'er, and earth recede from view,
And heaven in all its glory shine where all is pure and true :
Ah ! then thou'lt see more clearly still the proverb deep and vast,
" The mill will never grind again with water that is past."

D. C. M'CALLUM.

TO-MORROW.

To-morrow, didst thou say?
Methought I heard Horatio say, To-morrow.
Go to, I will not hear of it—To-morrow!
'Tis a sharper, who stakes his penury
Against thy plenty; who takes thy ready cash,
And pays thee nought but wishes, hopes, and promises,—
The currency of idiots: injurious bankrupt,
That gulls the easy creditor!—To-morrow!
It is a period nowhere to be found
In all the hoary registers of Time,
Unless, perchance, in the fool's calendar!
Wisdom disclaims the word, nor holds society
With those who own it. No, my Horatio,
'Tis fancy's child, and folly is its father;
Wrought of such stuff as dreams are, and baseless
As the fantastic visions of the evening.
  But soft, my friend—arrest the present moments;
For, be assured, they all are arrant tell-tales,
And, though their flight be silent, and their path
Trackless as the wingèd couriers of the air,
They post to heaven, and there record thy folly;—
Because, though stationed on the important watch,
Thou, like a sleeping, faithless sentinel,
Didst let them pass unnoticed, unimproved.
And know, for that thou slumberedst on the guard,
Thou shalt be made to answer, at the bar,
For every fugitive; and when thou thus
Shalt stand impleaded at the high tribunal
Of hood-winked Justice, who shall tell thy audit?
  Then, stay the present instant, dear Horatio!
Imprint the marks of wisdom on its wings;
'Tis of more worth than kingdoms! far more precious
Than all the crimson treasures of life's fountain!—

Oh! let it not elude thy grasp; but, like
The good old patriarch upon record,
Hold the fleet angel fast, until he bless thee!
                                    COTTON.

THE OLD CLOCK ON THE STAIRS.

Somewhat back from the village street stands the old-fashioned country-seat. Across its antique portico tall poplar trees their shadows throw; and from its station in the hall, an ancient timepiece says to all, "For ever—never! never—for ever!" Half-way up the stairs it stands, and points and beckons with its hands from its case of massive oak, like a monk, who, under his cloak, crosses himself, and sighs, alas! with sorrowful voice to all who pass, "For ever—never! never—for ever!" By day its voice is low and light; but in the silent dead of night, distinct as a passing footstep's fall, it echoes along the vacant hall, along the ceiling, along the floor, and seems to say at each chamber door, "For ever—never! never—for ever!" Through days of sorrow and of mirth, through days of death and days of birth, through every swift vicissitude of changeful time, unchanged it has stood; and as if, like God, it all things saw, it calmly repeats those words of awe, "For ever—never! never—for ever!" In that mansion used to be free-hearted Hospitality. His great fires up the chimney roared, the stranger feasted at his board; but, like the skeleton at the feast, that warning timepiece never ceased—"For ever—never! never—for ever!" There groups of merry children played, there youths and maidens dreaming strayed. O precious hours! O golden prime, and affluence of love and time! Even as a miser counts his gold, those hours the ancient timepiece told—"For ever—never! never—for ever!" From that chamber, clothed in white, the bride came forth on her wedding night; there, in that silent room below, the dead lay in his shroud of snow; and in the hush that followed the prayer was heard the old clock on the stair—"For ever—never! never—for ever!" All are scattered now and fled; some are married, some are dead; and when I ask, with throbs of pain, "Ah! when shall they all meet again?" as in the days long since gone by, the ancient timepiece makes reply, "For ever—never! never—for ever!" Never here, for ever there, where all parting, pain, and care, and death, and time shall disappear—for ever there, but never here! The horologe of eternity sayeth this incessantly, "For ever—never! never—for ever!"   LONGFELLOW.

ELEGY WRITTEN IN A COUNTRY CHURCHYARD.

The curfew tolls the knell of parting day, the lowing herd winds slowly o'er the lea, the ploughman homeward plods his weary way, and leaves the world to darkness and to me. Now fades the glimmering landscape on the sight, and all the air a solemn stillness holds, save where the beetle wheels his droning flight, and drowsy tinklings lull the distant folds; save that, from yonder ivy-mantled tower, the moping owl does to the moon complain of such as, wandering near her secret bower, molest her ancient, solitary reign. Beneath those rugged elms, that yew tree's shade, where heaves the turf in many a mouldering heap—each in his narrow cell for ever laid—the rude forefathers of the hamlet sleep. The breezy call of incense-breathing morn, the swallow twittering from the straw-built shed, the cock's shrill clarion, or the echoing horn, no more shall rouse them from their lowly bed. For them no more the blazing hearth shall burn, or busy housewife ply her evening care; no children run to lisp their sire's return, or climb his knees the envied kiss to share. Oft did the harvest to their sickle yield; their furrow oft the stubborn glebe has broke. How jocund did they drive their team a-field! how bowed the woods beneath their sturdy stroke! Let not Ambition mock their useful toil, their homely joys, and destiny obscure; nor Grandeur hear with a disdainful smile the short and simple annals of the poor. The boast of heraldry, the pomp of power, and all that beauty, all that wealth e'er gave, await alike the inevitable hour: the paths of glory lead but to the grave. Nor you, ye proud, impute to these the fault, if Memory o'er their tomb no trophies raise, where, through the long-drawn aisle and fretted vault, the pealing anthem swells the note of praise. Can storied urn or animated bust back to its mansion call the fleeting breath? Can Honour's voice provoke the silent dust, or Flattery soothe the dull, cold ear of Death? Perhaps in this neglected spot is laid some heart once pregnant with celestial fire; hands that the rod of empire might have swayed, or waked to ecstasy the living lyre. But Knowledge to their eyes her ample page, rich with the spoils of time, did ne'er unroll; chill Penury repressed their noble rage, and froze the genial current of the soul. Full many a gem of purest ray serene, the dark unfathomed caves of ocean bear; full many a flower is born to blush unseen, and waste its sweetness on the desert air. Some village Hampden, that, with dauntless breast, the little tyrant of his fields withstood; some mute, inglorious Milton, here may rest; some Cromwell, guiltless of his country's blood. The applause of listening senates to command, the threats of pain and ruin to despise, to scatter plenty o'er a smiling land, and read their history in a nation's eyes, their lot forbade: nor circumscribed alone their growing virtues, but their crimes confined;—forbade to wade through slaughter to a throne, and shut the gates of mercy on mankind; the struggling pangs of conscious truth to hide; to quench the blushes of ingenuous shame; or heap the shrine of luxury and pride with incense kindled at the Muse's flame. Far from the madding crowd's ignoble strife (their sober wishes never learned to stray), along the cool, sequestered vale of life they kept the noiseless tenor of their way. Yet even these bones from insult to protect, some frail memorial still erected nigh, with uncouth rhymes and shapeless sculpture decked, implores the passing tribute of a sigh. Their names, their years, spelt by the unlettered Muse, the place of fame and elegy supply;

and many a holy text around she strews, that teach the rustic moralist to die. For who, to dumb forgetfulness a prey, this pleasing, anxious being e'er resigned; left the warm precincts of the cheerful day, nor cast one longing, lingering look behind? On some fond breast the parting soul relies, some pious drops the closing eye requires; even from the tomb the voice of Nature cries—even in our ashes live their wonted fires. For thee, who, mindful of the unhonoured dead, dost in these lines their artless tale relate,—if chance, by lonely Contemplation led, some kindred spirit shall inquire thy fate, haply some hoary-headed swain may say, "Oft have we seen him, at the peep of dawn, brushing with hasty steps the dews away, to meet the sun upon the upland lawn. There, at the foot of yonder nodding beech, that wreathes its old fantastic roots so high, his listless length at noontide would he stretch, and pore upon the brook that babbles by. Hard by yon wood, now smiling as in scorn, muttering his wayward fancies he would rove; now drooping, woful, wan, like one forlorn, or crazed with care, or crossed in hopeless love. One morn I missed him on the 'customed hill, along the heath, and near his favourite tree; another came, nor yet beside the rill, nor up the lawn, nor at the wood was he. The next, with dirges due, in sad array, slow through the church-way path we saw him borne: approach and read (for thou canst read) the lay graved on the stone beneath yon aged thorn."

THE EPITAPH.

"Here rests his head upon the lap of Earth, a youth to Fortune and to Fame unknown; fair Science frowned not on his humble birth, and Melancholy marked him for her own. Large was his bounty, and his soul sincere; Heaven did a recompense as largely send: he gave to Misery all he had—a tear; he gained from Heaven ('twas all he wished)—a friend. No further seek his merits to disclose, or draw his frailties from their dread abode (there they alike in trembling hope repose),—the bosom of his Father and his God." THOMAS GRAY.

THE BELLS.

Hear the sledges with the bells—silver bells! What a world of merriment their melody foretells! How they tinkle, tinkle, tinkle, in the icy air of night! while the stars that oversprinkle all the heavens / seem to twinkle with a crystalline delight; keeping time, time, time, in a sort of Runic rhyme, to the tintinnabulation / that so musically wells / from the jingling and the tinkling of the bells.

Hear the mellow wedding bells—golden bells! What a world of happiness their harmony foretells! Through the balmy air of night, how they ring out their delight! From the molten-golden notes, what a liquid ditty floats! what a gush of euphony voluminously wells! How it swells! how it dwells on the future! how it tells / of the rapture that impels / to the swinging and the ringing, to the rhyming and the chiming of the bells!

Hear the loud alarum bells—brazen bells! What a tale of terror, now, their turbulency tells! In the startled ear of night / how they scream out their affright / in a clamorous appealing to the mercy of the fire, in a mad expostulation with the deaf and frantic fire! What a tale their terror tells of despair! How they clang, and clash, and roar! What a horror they outpour on the bosom of the palpitating air! Yet the ear it fully knows, by the twanging and the clanging, how the danger ebbs and flows; yet the ear distinctly tells, in the jangling and the wrangling, how the danger sinks and swells, by the sinking or the swelling in the anger of the bells—in the clamour and the clangour of the bells!

Hear the tolling of the bells—iron bells! What a world of solemn thought their monody compels! In the silence of the night / how we shiver with affright / at the melancholy menace of their tone! For every sound that floats from the rust within their throats / is a groan. And the people—ah! the people—they that dwell up in the steeple, all alone, and who, tolling,

tolling, tolling, in that muffled monotone, feel a glory in so rolling on the human heart a stone—they are neither man nor woman, they are neither brute nor human—they are Ghouls! And their king it is who tolls; and he rolls, rolls, rolls a pæan from the bells; and his bosom proudly swells with the pæan of the bells! And he dances, and he yells; keeping time, time, time, in a sort of Runic rhyme, to the pæan of the bells, to the throbbing of the bells, to the sobbing of the bells, to the rolling of the bells, to the tolling of the bells, to the moaning and the groaning of the bells. EDGAR ALLAN POE.

COMING.

"It may be in the evening,
    When the work of the day is done,
And you have time to sit in the twilight
    And watch the sinking sun,
While the long, bright day dies slowly
    Over the sea,
And the hour grows quiet and holy
    With thoughts of Me;
While you hear the village children
    Passing along the street,
Among those thronging footsteps
    May come the sound of *My* feet.
Therefore I tell you: Watch
    By the light of the evening-star,
When the room is growing dusky
    As the clouds afar;
Let the door be on the latch
    In your home,
For it may be through the gloaming
    I will come.

COMING.

"It may be when the midnight
    Is heavy upon the land,
And the black waves lying dumbly
    Along the sand;
When the moonless night draws close,
And the lights are out in the house;
When the fires burn low and red,
And the watch is ticking loudly
    Beside the bed.
Though you sleep, tired out, on your couch,
Still your heart must wake and watch
    In the dark room;
For it may be that at midnight
    I will come.

"It may be at the cock-crow,
When the night is dying slowly
    In the sky,
And the sea looks calm and holy,
    Waiting for the dawn
    Of the golden sun
    Which draweth nigh;
When the mists are on the valleys, shading
    The rivers chill,
And the morning-star is fading, fading
    Over the hill:
Behold I say unto you: Watch!
Let the door be on the latch
    In your home;
In the chill before the dawning,
Between the night and morning,
    I may come.

"It may be in the morning,
    When the sun is bright and strong,

And the dew is glittering sharply
    Over the lawn;
When the waves are laughing loudly
    Along the shore,
And the little birds are singing sweetly
    About the door;
With the long day's work before you,
    You rise up with the sun,
And the neighbours come in to talk a little
    Of all that must be done:
But remember that *I* may be the next
    To come in at the door,
To call you from all your busy work
    For evermore.
As you work your heart must watch;
For the door is on the latch
    In your room,
And it may be in the morning
    I will come."

So He passed down my cottage garden,
    By the path that leads to the sea,
Till He came to the turn of the little road
    Where the birch and laburnum tree
Lean over and arch the way;
There I saw Him a moment stay,
    And turn once more to me,
    As I wept at the cottage door,
And lift up His hands in blessing—
    Then I saw His face no more.

And I stood still in the doorway,
    Leaning against the wall,
Not heeding the fair white roses,
    Though I crushed them and let them fall;

COMING.

Only looking down the pathway,
    And looking toward the sea,
And wondering, and wondering
    When He would come back for me;
Till I was aware of an angel
    Who was going swiftly by,
With the gladness of one who goeth
    In the light of God Most High.

He passed the end of the cottage
    Toward the garden gate—
(I suppose he was come down
At the setting of the sun,
To comfort some one in the village
    Whose dwelling was desolate)—
And he paused before the door
    Beside my place,
And the likeness of a smile
    Was on his face:
"Weep not," he said, "for unto you is given
    To watch for the coming of His feet
Who is the glory of our blessed heaven;
The work and watching will be very sweet,
    Even in an earthly home;
And in such an hour as you think not,
    He will come."

So I am watching quietly
    Every day.
Whenever the sun shines brightly,
    I rise and say:
"Surely it is the shining of His face!"
And look unto the gates of His high place
    Beyond the sea;
For I know He is coming shortly
    To summon me.

COMING.

And when a shadow falls across the window
    Of my room,
Where I am working my appointed task,
I lift my head to watch the door, and ask
    If He is come;
And the angel answers sweetly
    In my home:
"Only a few more shadows
    And He will come."

B. M.

DIALOGUES.

CANUTE AND HIS COURTIERS.

Canute. Is it true, my friends, as you have often told me, that I am the greatest of monarchs?

1st. Courtier. It is true, my liege; you are the most powerful of all kings.

2nd. Cour. We are all your slaves; we kiss the dust of your feet.

1st. Cour. Not only we, but even the elements, are your slaves. The land obeys you from shore to shore, and the sea obeys you.

Can. Does the sea, with its loud, boisterous waves, obey me? Will that terrible element be still at my bidding?

2nd. Cour. Yes, the sea is yours; it was made to bear your ships upon its bosom, and to pour the treasures of the world at your royal feet. It is boisterous to your enemies, but it knows you to be its sovereign.

Can. Is not the tide coming up?

1st. Cour. Yes, my liege; you may perceive the swell already.

Can. Bring me a chair then; set it here upon the sands.

2nd. Cour. Where the tide is coming up, my gracious lord?

Can. Yes, set it just here.

1st. Cour. [*Aside*] I wonder what he is going to do!

2nd. Cour. [*Aside*] Surely he is not so silly as to believe us!

Can. O mighty ocean, thou art my subject! My courtiers tell me so, and it is thy duty to obey me. Thus, then, I stretch my sceptre over thee, and command thee to retire. Roll back thy swelling waves, nor let them presume to wet the feet of me, thy royal master.

1st. Cour. [*Aside*] I believe the sea will pay very little regard to his royal commands.

2nd. Cour. [*Aside*] Regard! nay, see how fast the tide is rising!

1st. Cour. The next wave will come up to the chair. It is folly to stay; we shall be covered with salt water.

Can. Well, does the sea obey my commands? If it be my subject, it is a very rebellious subject. See how it swells and dashes the angry foam and salt spray over my sacred person! Sycophants, did you think that I believed your abject flatteries? Know there is but one Being whom the sea will obey. He is Sovereign of heaven and earth, King of kings, and Lord of lords. It is only He who can say to the ocean, "Thus far shalt thou go, but no farther; and here shall thy proud waves be stayed." A king is but a man, and a man is but a worm. Shall a worm assume the power of the great God, and think the elements will obey him? May kings learn to be humble from my example, and courtiers learn truth from your disgrace.   BARBAULD.

THE TWO ROBBERS.

Alexander. What, art thou the Egyptian robber of whose exploits I have heard so much?

Robber. I am an Egyptian, and a soldier.

Alex. A soldier!—a thief, a plunderer, an assassin; the pest of the country!

Rob. What have I done of which you can complain?

Alex. Hast thou not set at defiance my authority, violated the public peace, and passed thy life in injuring the persons and properties of thy fellow subjects?

THE TWO ROBBERS.

Rob. Alexander, I am your captive; I must hear what you please to say, and endure what you please to inflict. But my soul is unconquered; and if I reply at all to your reproaches, I will reply like a free man.

Alex. Speak freely.

Rob. I must then answer your question by another: How have you passed your life?

Alex. Like a hero. Ask Fame, and she will tell you. Among the brave, I have been the bravest; among sovereigns, the noblest; among conquerors, the mightiest.

Rob. And does not fame speak of me too? Was there ever a bolder captain of a more valiant band? Was there ever?—but I scorn to boast. You yourself know that I have not been easily subdued.

Alex. Still, what are you but a robber—a base, dishonest robber?

Rob. And what is a conqueror? Have not you, too, gone about the earth like an evil genius, blasting the fair fruits of peace and industry; plundering, ravaging, killing, without law, without justice, merely to gratify an insatiable lust for dominion? All that I have done to a single district with a hundred followers, you have done to whole nations with a hundred thousand. If I have stripped individuals, you have ruined kings and princes. If I have burned a few hamlets, you have desolated the most flourishing kingdoms and cities of the earth. What is the difference, but that as you were born a king, and I a private man, you have been able to become a mightier robber than I?

Alex. But if I have taken like a king, I have given like a king. If I have subverted empires, I have founded greater. I have cherished arts, commerce, and philosophy.

Rob. I, too, have freely given to the poor what I took from the rich. I have established order and discipline among the most ferocious of mankind. I have stretched out my protecting arm over the oppressed. I know little of the philosophy you talk of, but I believe neither you nor I shall ever repay to the world the mischiefs we have done it.

Alex. Leave me. [*Exit Robber.*] Are we then so much alike? Alexander a robber! Let me reflect. [*Exit.*]   BARBAULD.

FROM "WILLIAM TELL."

TELL, ALBERT (his Son), GESLER, and SARNEM.

Sar. [*To Tell*] Behold the governor. Down, slave, upon thy knees, and beg for mercy.

Ges. Does he hear?

Sar. He does, but braves thy power. —Down, slave, and ask for life.

Ges. [*To Tell*] Why speak'st thou not?

Tell. For wonder! Yes, for wonder—that thou seem'st a man.

Ges. What should I seem?

Tell. A monster.

Ges. Ha! beware!—think on thy chains.

Tell. Think on my chains! How came they on me?

Ges. Dar'st thou question me? Beware my vengeance.

Tell. Can it more than kill?

Ges. Enough; it may do that.

Tell. No, not enough. It cannot take away the grace of life—the comeliness of look that virtue gives—its port erect, with consciousness of truth—its rich attire of honourable deeds—its fair report that's rife on good men's tongues;—it cannot lay its hand on these, no more than it can pluck his brightness from the sun, or with polluted finger tarnish it.

Ges. But it may make thee writhe.

Tell. It may; and I may say, "Go on!" though it should make me groan again.

Ges Whence comest thou?

Tell. From the mountains; there they watch no more the avalanche.

Ges. Why so?

Tell. Because they look for thee. The hurricane comes unawares upon them; from its bed the torrent breaks and finds them in its track—

Ges. What then?

Tell. They thank kind Providence it is not thou! Thou hast perverted nature in them. The earth presents her fruits to them, and is not thanked. There's not a blessing Heaven vouchsafes them, but the thought of thee doth wither to a curse —as something they must lose, and had far better lack.

Ges. 'Tis well. I'd have them as their hills—that never smile, though wanton summer tempt them e'er so much.

Tell. But they do sometimes smile.

Ges. Ah!—when is that?

Tell. When they do talk of vengeance! and the true hands are lifted up to Heaven on every hill for justice on thee!

Ges. [*To Sarnem*] Lead in his son. [*Aside*] Now will I take exquisite vengeance. [*Enter Sarnem and Albert.*] [*To Tell*] I would see thee make a trial of thy skill with that same bow. 'Tis said thy arrows never miss.

Tell. What is the trial?

Ges. Thou look'st upon thy boy as though instinctively thou guessest it.

Tell. Look upon my boy! What mean you? Look upon my boy as though I guessed it!—guessed at the trial thou wouldst have me make!—guessed it—instinctively! Thou dost not mean—no—no. Thou wouldst not have me make a trial of my skill upon my child? Impossible! I do not guess thy meaning.

Ges. I'd see thee hit an apple on his head a hundred paces off.

Tell. Great Heaven!

Ges. On this condition I will spare his life and thine.

Tell. Make a father murder his own child!—'Tis beyond horror! 'tis too much for flesh and blood to bear!

FROM "WILLIAM TELL."

Ges. Dost thou consent?

Tell. My hands are free from blood. I'll not murder my boy for Gesler.

Boy. You will not hit me, father. You'll be sure to hit the apple; will you not save me, father?

Tell. Lead me forth; I'll make the trial.

Boy. Father—

Tell. Speak not to me—let me not hear thy voice; thou must be dumb, and so should all things be—earth should be dumb, and heaven, unless its thunder muttered at the deed, and sent a bolt to stop it.—Give me my bow and quiver.

Ges. When all is ready.—Sarnem, measure hence the distance —three hundred paces.

Tell. Will he do it fairly?

Ges. What is't to thee, fairly or not?

Tell. Oh, nothing! a little thing—a very little thing! I only shoot at my child! [*Sarnem prepares to measure.*] Stop! you measure 'gainst the sun.

Ges. And what of that? What matter whether to or from the sun?

Tell. I'd have it at my back. The sun should shine upon the mark, not on him that shoots. I will not shoot against the sun.

Ges. Give him his way. [*Sarnem measures paces and goes out.*

Tell. I should like to see the apple I must hit.

Ges. There, take that.

Tell. You've picked the smallest one.

Ges. I know I have. Thy skill will be the greater if thou hittest it.

Tell. True! true!—I did not think of that. I wonder I did not think of that. A larger one had given me a chance to save my boy.—Give me my bow and quiver.

Ges. [*To an attendant*] Give him a single arrow.

Tell. [*Looks at it, and breaks it*] Let me see my quiver. It is not one arrow in a dozen I would use to shoot with at a dove, much less a dove like that.

Ges. Show him the quiver.

[*Sarnem takes the apple, and leads out the boy to place them; meanwhile Tell conceals an arrow under his garment. He then selects another arrow.*]

Tell. Is the boy ready? Keep silence now for Heaven's sake, and be my witnesses that, if his life's in peril from my hand, 'tis only for the chance of saving it. For mercy's sake, keep motionless and silent!

[*He aims and shoots in the direction of the boy. Albert enters with the apple on the arrow's point.*]

Tell. Thank Heaven!

[*As he raises his arms the concealed arrow falls.*]

Ges. Unequalled archer!—Ha! why this concealed?

Tell. To kill THEE, tyrant, had I slain my boy.

KNOWLES.

A GAOL MOUSE.

(*By permission of the Author.*)

JUDGE, WARDER, and PRISONER.

Scene: A Court of Justice.

Warder. My name is John White. I am a warder in the gaol in which the prisoner was confined for embezzlement. He was convicted fourteen months ago. Since his conviction, his behaviour has been marked "exceptionally good." I know the prosecutor, William Hinde; he also is a warder in the gaol. Yes, I remember the night you mention; it was the first of May, about nine o'clock. I heard a scuffle in the cell of number fifty-six, the prisoner. I heard some one cry, "You hound!" and then I saw Hinde running out, blood oozing from his mouth. "What's the matter, Hinde?" I asked. "That brute in there," he said, "has hit me on the mouth." "Whatever made him do it, Hinde? he's not the fighting sort." Hinde replied, "I tried to kill his precious mouse." That's my evidence, my lord.

A GAOL MOUSE.

Judge. Prisoner at the bar, since you are not defended by learned counsel, it rests with you to plead your own defence. You have heard the evidence against you. Now is your time to speak.

Prisoner. Fourteen months ago I was convicted of a crime of which I am innocent. This misfortune nearly broke me down. I had lost all—wife, children, friends, home, my own good name. One night, when I was served my prison fare, a little mouse crept out upon the floor, and eyed, askance, the dreaded human form. I threw some food; but, scared, it scampered off. By-and-by, out it crept again; and this time shared my meal. A welcome guest! So every night it came, until, at last, it grew so tame, I fed it from my hand; it slept with me, and nestled in my sleeve.

I had no friends; I grew to love this mouse, as these dumb animals are often loved by those who find all others cold and false.

One night, the warder, Hinde, came into my cell when my little pet was sporting on my hand.

"They talk about that mouse of yours," he said; "let's see if it's as tame White says it is. Will it feed from my hand? Let's see."

Suspecting nothing, into his hand I gave my little pet; the cruel hand closed on it, and he laughed. "Come, bid your friend good-bye; I'm going to crush it!" "You hound!" I cried, and struck him in the face with all my might; he dropped the mouse, which ran, and found a shelter e'en from whence it came.

This is my crime, and I am in your hands.

Judge. This tale is touching, and, I doubt not, true; but, gentlemen of the jury, you are here to deal with facts, not sentiments. It now rests with you to give your verdict.

Foreman of the Jury. We are agreed, my lord. We find the prisoner guilty, but we recommend him strongly to the mercy of the court.

Judge. Prisoner at the bar, you stand convicted of an assault upon your warder, William Hinde, for which the sentence of the court receive :—That you be imprisoned for one day, to run concurrently with the sentence you are undergoing. Furthermore, I have here—now, can you bear good news ?—I have here a packet from the Home Office, commanding your release. Another has confessed the crime for which you have already suffered wrongfully. You are a free man !

One moment more. John White, the warder, has for you, outside, a little friend of yours—your pet <u>mouse</u>.

If I may say so, I think I should have done to Hinde exactly as you did. I wish you well. JOHN COX.

FROM "THE HEART OF MIDLOTHIAN."

I.—JEANIE DEANS AND THE LAIRD OF DUMBIEDYKES.

Scene: The Courtyard of Dumbiedykes House.

Dum. Jeanie woman, come in by, an' rest ye.

Jeanie. Na, Laird, I hae a lang day's journey afore me. I maun be twenty mile the nicht, if feet will carry me.

Dum. Twenty mile ! twenty mile on your feet ! Hoot, toot ! ye maun never think o' that ; come in by.

Jeanie. What I hae tae say tae ye, Laird, I can say here : I'm gaun a lang journey, Laird, oot o' my faither's kennin'.

Dum. Oot o' his kennin', Jeanie? That's no richt. Ye maun think on't again.

Jeanie. Ay, Laird, I'm gaun tae Lunnon tae speak tae the Queen, for my puir Effie's life.

Dum. Lunnon ! The Queen ! Effie's life ! The lassie's demented !

Jeanie. Sink or swim, I'm determined tae gang ; though I suld beg my way frae door tae door. An' sae I maun, unless ye wad lend <u>me</u> a sma' sum tae pay my expenses—little wad dae't —an' ye ken, Laird, my faither's a man o' means, an' wad let nae man—far less you, Laird—come tae loss by me. I see ye're no for helpin' me, Laird, sae fare-ye-weel! Gang an' see my faither as often as you can—he'll be lanely eneugh noo.

Dum. Whaur's the silly bairn gaun? Come in by, Jeanie woman! come in by! [*Takes her into the parlour.*] That's my bank, Jeanie lass! Nane o' yer goldsmiths' bills for me—they bring folk to ruin. Jeanie! I'll mak' ye Leddy Dumbiedykes afore the sun sets, an' ye can ride to Lunnon in your ain coach, if ye like.

Jeanie. Na, Laird, that can never be,—my faither's grief—my sister's situation—the shame tae you!

Dum. That's *my* business, Jeanie lass; if ye werena jist a fule, ye wad ne'er say a word aboot that; an' yet—I like ye the better for't.

Jeanie. Ay, Laird, but—I like anither man better than you.

Dum. Like anither man better than me, Jeanie? it's no possible—ye hae kenned me sae lang.

Jeanie. Ay, Laird, but I—hae kenned him langer.

Dum. Langer! it canna be, Jeanie! Ye were born on the land! Eh, Jeanie woman! look at the siller! it's a' gowd! a' gowd! an' then, there's bonds for siller lent! an' the rental-book! clear three hunder sterlin.' There they're a'—look at them! Ye're no lookin'! look at them, Jeanie woman! An' then, there's my mither's wardrobe up the stair; an' my gran'-mither's forby! Silk gowns, wad stand on their ends—an' rings—an' ear-rings—an'—eh, Jeanie woman! Just gang up the stair an' look at them.

Jeanie. It canna be, Laird. I canna break my word till him, though ye suld gie me the haill Barony o' Dalkeith, an' Lugton into the bargain.

Dum. Yer word tae *him!* ay, but wha is he? I haena heard his name yet. Come noo, Jeanie, ye're just queerin' me—it's a blaw i' my lug. Wha is he, Jeanie? Wha is he?

Jeanie. Weel, Laird, it's just—Reuben Butler—the schule-maister.

Dum. Reuben Butler! Reuben Butler, the dominie! Reuben! the son o' my cottar! Verra weel, lass! verra weel! A wilfu' woman will hae her way. But it doesna signify—it doesna— Reuben Butler!—as for wastin' my substance on ither folk's Joes!

Jeanie. I was beggin' nane frae yer honour! Least o' a', on sic a score as that! Fare-ye-weel, Laird—ye hae been kind tae my faither, an' it isna in my heart tae think but kindly o' you.

Dum. Ye maunna gang this wilfu' gate, sillerless—come o't what like. Tak' this bit purse wi' ye—tut, tut! there's only five-an'-twenty guineas in't—an' gang whaur ye like, dae what ye like—marry a' the Butlers in the cuintry if ye like, an' sae —guid mornin' tae ye, Jeanie.

Jeanie. An' God bless you, Laird, wi' mony a guid mornin', an' the Lord's peace be wi' ye, if I suld never see ye again.

[*Exit Jeanie.*

Dum. Eh! Jeanie woman!—[*Exit Dum.*]

II.—JEANIE DEANS AND THE DUKE OF ARGYLL.

Scene: The Duke's Study in London.

Duke. Well, my bonnie lass, do you wish to speak to the Duchess, or myself?

Jeanie. It was wi' yer Honour—I beg yer Lordship's pardon —I mean yer Grace—that I wanted tae speak. Yer Honour—I beg yer Lordship's pardon—I mean yer Grace.

Duke. Never mind my Grace, lassie, speak out a plain tale, and show you have a Scotch tongue in your head.

Jeanie. Oh, sir, I'm muckle obleeged. Sir, I'm the sister o' that puir unfortunate lassie, Effie Deans, lyin' under sentence at Edinburgh, an' I hae come up frae the North tae see what could be dune for her, in the way o' gettin' a reprieve, or a pardon, or the like o' that.

Duke. My poor girl! you have taken a long and a sad journey to very little purpose. Your sister is condemned to death.

Jeanie. Ay, sir; but I'm gi'en tae understaun' there's a law for reprievin' her—if it be the King's pleesure.

Duke. Certainly there is. But that lies only in the King's power. What friends have you at Court?

Jeanie. Nane! exceptin' God—an' yer Grace.

Duke. Alas! my good girl, I have no means of averting your sister's fate. Whoever made you come to me?

Jeanie. It was yoursell, sir.

Duke. Myself! Why, you have never seen me before.

Jeanie. No, sir; but a' the warld kens the Duke o' Argyll is Scotland's frien'. Ye speak for the richt, an' ye fecht for the richt! An' if ye wadna help tae save an innocent cuintrywoman o' your ain frae a shamefu' death, what can we expect frae Sootheners an' strangers.

Duke. Innocent! Yes, yes, but how can you think your sister innocent?

Jeanie. Because, sir, she has never been proved guilty—as ye may see for yourself, if ye'll only read thae papers.

Duke. [*after having read papers*] Young woman! your poor sister's case is a very hard one—it has not been proved that the murder was ever committed.

Jeanie. God bless ye, sir! God bless ye for that word!

Duke. And now, leave these papers with me, and come again—let me see—yes, the day after to-morrow; and be sure to be dressed just as you are.

Jeanie. I wad hae putten on a cap, but I thocht yer Honour's heart wad warm tae the tartan.

Duke. And you thought quite right, my good girl. MacCallum-More's heart will be as cold as death can make it, when it does *not* warm to the tartan.

III.—QUEEN CAROLINE, DUKE OF ARGYLL, and JEANIE DEANS.

Scene: The Duke's Study.

Duke. You are punctual, my good lass. I have asked an

audience of a lady whose influence with the King is very high. You shall speak to her yourself.

Jeanie. I wad like tae ken what tae ca' her—whether yer Honour, or yer Leddyship—for I hear that leddies are fully mair parteek'ler aboot their titles o' honour than gentlemen.

Duke. Call her simply Madam. Tell your story plainly and boldly, as you did to me.

Scene: The Queen's Garden at Richmond.

Queen. And now, your Grace, what of that young woman? She is some thirtieth cousin, I suppose?

Duke. No, Madam! but I should be proud of any relation with half her worth, honesty, and affection.

Queen. Ah! her name must be Campbell, at least?

Duke. No, Madam! her name, if I may be allowed to say so, is not so distinguished.

Queen. Well, then, she comes from Inveraray, or Argyllshire?

Duke. No, Madam! she has never been farther north than Edinburgh. Her sister, Effie Deans, is the first, and *I* think, Madam, unjust victim of a severe law.

Queen. Effie Deans! Yes, I myself have read the case, and doubt the justice of it.

Duke. Will your Highness be pleased to hear my poor countrywoman?

Queen. Surely, your Grace! [*Duke beckons to Jeanie.*

Queen. Tell me, young woman, how you travelled up to London.

Jeanie. Maistly on my feet, Madam!

Queen. All that immense way on foot! How far can you travel in a day?

Jeanie. Five-an'-twenty miles an' a bittock, Madam.

Queen. And a what, your Grace?

Duke. And about five miles more, Madam.

Queen. Dear me! I thought I was a good walker, but this

shames me sadly. And have you walked all this way for your sister's sake?

Jeanie. Ay, Madam! an' I wad walk tae the warld's end tae save my puir Effie. It isna when we sleep saft, an' wauken happy, that we think on ither folks' sufferin's; but when the hour o' trouble comes—seldom may it come tae yer Leddyship! —an' when the hour o' death comes—that comes tae high and low; lang an' late may it be yours—then, my Leddy, it isna what we hae dune for oorsells, but what we hae dune for ithers that we think on maist pleesantly; an' the thocht that ye hae intervened tae save the puir thing's life, will be sweeter in that hour—come when it may—than if a word o' yer mouth could hang the haill Porteous mob at the end o' ae tow.

Queen. THIS IS ELOQUENCE! *I* cannot grant a pardon to your sister, but you shall not lack my warm intercession with his Majesty. Take this small token! It will remind you that you have had an interview with Queen Caroline.

SIR WALTER SCOTT.

KING JAMES AND GEORGE HERIOT.

[Adapted from "The Fortunes of Nigel."]

KING JAMES, GEORGE HERIOT, and MAXWELL.

Scene: The King's Private Chamber.

Maxwell. Master Heriot waits without, so please your Majesty.

King James. Admit him, instanter, Maxill; hae ye hair-boured sae lang at Court, an' not yet learned that gold an' silver is ever welcome? Admit him, instanter!

[*Exit Maxwell, and re-enter showing in George Heriot.*

K. James. Weel, Jinglin' Geordie! an' what hae ye brocht wi' ye noo, tae cheat yer lawfu' king and sov'reign liege?

George Heriot. Heaven forbid! I have but brought your Majesty a piece of antique plate for your royal inspection.

K. James. Body o' me, man, let's see't, Herrit! Bring't intae oor praisence, Maxill! [*Exit Maxwell.*] An' whaur gat ye't, Geordie?

G. Heriot. From Italy, sire. [*Enter Maxwell.*

K. James. Etaly, Etaly! Pit it doon, Maxill; pit it doon. Ay, it's a curious piece; an', as I think, fit for a king's chaumer—the subject verra adequate an' beseemin'; bein', as I see, "The Jidgment o' Solomon"—a prince in whose pauths it weel becomes a' leevin' monarchs tae walk wi' emulation.

Max. But whose footsteps, sire, only one hath ever been able to overtake.

K. James. Haud yer tongue, Maxill! Look at the bonnie piece o' warkmanship, an' haud yer claverin' tongue!—An' wha's handywark may it be, Geordie?

G. Heriot. It was wrought, sire, by the famous Florentine artist, Cellini; and was designed for Francis the First of France.

K. James. Francis o' France! Send Solomon, King o' the Jews, tae Francis o' France! I tell ye, sir, he was a fechtin' fule—a mere fechtin' fule! If they could hae sent him Solomon's wit, an' love o' peace an' godliness! but "Solomon's Jidgment" suld sit in ither company than Francis o' France.

G. Heriot. I hope it will find a fitter master, your Majesty.

K. James. It is a curious an' verra artificial sculptur', but yet, methinks, the executioner there is brandishin' his gully ower near the king's face! What think ye, Geordie?

G. Heriot. Only in appearance, your Majesty, the perspective being allowed for.

K. James. The prospecteeve! There canna be a waur prospecteeve, man, for a lawfu' king wha wishes tae reign in love, an' dee in peace an' honour, than tae hae naked swurds flashin' afore his een; but, a'thegither, it is a brave piece. An' what's the price o't, Geordie?

G. Heriot. A hundred and fifty pounds sterling, your Majesty.

K. James. A hunder an' fifty punds sterlin'! My sang,

Jinglin' Geordie, but ye're determined your purse sall jingle tae a bonny tune! Hoo am I tae tell doon a hunder an' fifty punds, when ye ken my verra hoosehold servitors are sax months in arrear?

G. Heriot. I shall be happy to wait your convenience, my liege; the money lying at the usual interest.

K. James. Spoken like an honest an' raisonable dealer! Awa' wi' it, Maxill—awa' wi' it. [*Exit Maxwell.*] An', noo, my guid auld frien' Geordie—noo that we are secret, I opine that oor cuintrymen hae a' gane daft! frantic, man—clean brain-crazed! Yesterday, nae faurer gane, a ragged rascal—every dud upon his back biddin' guid-day tae the ither—wi' a coat an' hat wad hae served a pease-bogle, thrusts intae oor royal haun' some supplicawtion aboot debts awin' by oor gracious mither, an' sic-like nonsense. Whaurat oor horse spangs on end; an' but for oor admirable sittin'—whaurin we hae been thocht tae excel maist sov'reign princes (no tae speak o' subjects) in Europe—we wad been laid end-lang on the causey! I tell ye, sir, there's no a loon amang them can deleever a supplicawtion as it suld be, in the face o' Mâjesty!

G. Heriot. I would I knew the most fitting mode to do so, were it but to instruct our poor countrymen in better manners, my liege.

K. James. By my halidome! but ye're a ceevileezed fallah, an' I care na if I fling awa' as muckle time as may teach ye. Gang faurer that wiy, Geordie; faurer that wiy. An' first, then, see ye, sir, ye sall approach the praisence o' Mâjesty thus,—shadin' yer een wi' yer haun'—so— Verra weel, Geordie! verra weel! Then, see ye, sir; ye sall come nearer — nearer, Geordie, nearer! Then, sir, ye sall kneel. Get doon, Geordie, get doon! Noo, then, sir, ye sall mak' tae kiss the hem o' oor garment, the latch o' oor shoe, or sic like. Verra weel enackit, Geordie; verra weel enackit! We then motion tae ye tae rise —thus— Gudesake, man, dinna rise yet! Havin' a boon tae ask, as yet, ye obey not, but slippin' yer haun' intae yer pooch

—that wiy, Geordie, that wiy—ye bring forth yer supplicawtion, an' place it reverentially in oor royal pâlm.

[*At this point of the ceremonial George Heriot places in the king's hand a bona-fide supplication on behalf of his young friend, Lord Nigel.*]

K. James. What means this, ye fause loon?

G. Heriot. Pardon my boldness, my most gracious Majesty, on behalf of a friend.

K. James. A frien'! Sae muckle the waur! sae muckle the waur, I tell ye, sir! Had it been for yersell, noo, ye wadna hae askit twice; for ye are oor auld an' faithfu' servant, Geordie. On my word, Jingler, when I look back on auld times, I'm no sure but we were happier in auld Holyrood than we are in St. James's here. Nae supplicawtions then, Geordie! It was ower weel kent we had naething tae gie.

G. Heriot. Does my liege remember the awful task we had to collect gold and silver work to make some show before the Spanish ambassador?

K. James. Brawly, I mind, Geordie, brawly! But I remember not the name o' that richt leal lord wha helpit us wi' every unce o' gold he had in his hoose.

G. Heriot. If you will cast your eye over that paper, my liege, I think you will remember his name.

K. James. Say ye sae, Geordie? say ye sae? "Lord Glenvaurloch." That was his name, indeed! But this supplicawtor maun be his son, for Lord Randal has lang gane whaur king an' lord maun gang, as weel as puir folk like you, Geordie. Ay, he was a leal an' lovin' subject, was Lord Randal; an' lent us siller mair than aince.

G. Heriot. Of which loan, sire, his son now begs payment.

K. James. Body o' me, man! I mind the thing! That suld be *quantum sufficit* atween prince an' subject!

G. Heriot. Pardon me, my liege, but Lord Nigel is on the point of losing his estate, by virtue of an unredeemed warrant.

K. James. Gude sake, man, we maun suspend the diligence!

G. Heriot. That may hardly be, sire ; your learnèd counsel of the law say it must be paid at once.

K. James. Ay ; that's what thae fallahs aye say ! Weel, weel ! just it is we suld piy oor debts that the young man may piy his. And he must be piyed, an' *in verbo regis* he shall be piyed ! But hoo tae cum by the siller, man ; hoo tae cum by the siller is a deeficult chapter ! Ye maun try the ceety, Geordie !

G. Heriot. Ah, sire, the city's funds are—

K. James. Dinna tell me, sir, what the ceety's funds are ! Oor ain exchequer's as dry as Dean Giles's discoorses on the Penetentiary Psâlms ! The ceety, Herrit ! ye maun try the ceety ! Dinna haggle aboot terms ! Only get me the loan ; an' on the word o' a king, I'll piy the puir lad ! Noo, awa' wi' ye, Jingler ; awa' wi' ye. An' atween you an' me, Geordie —atween you an' me, we will redeem the brave auld estate o' Glenvaurloch !
Sir Walter Scott.

FROM "THE OLD LIEUTENANT AND HIS SON."

(By permission of Messrs. Wm. Isbister and Co.*)*

[Edward Fleming was an old, half-pay lieutenant of the navy. One day he said to his only son :—]

Old Lieut. Neddy, my boy, did you ever think what profession you would like to follow ?

Ned. Yes, father ; the sea, with your permission.

Old L. The sea, my boy ! I needn't tell you, Ned, that I honour the sea ; all the honours your old father ever gained were gained on the sea. Ned, I'd give my right hand to see you in the navy, if we had the old ships, the old men, the old officers, and the old wars. But these, all these, are gone !

Ned. Well, I must do something, father. I can't hang on you and mother much longer ; and I won't.

Old L. Bless you, my boy ! I like your spirit. Well, well, we'll think about it. I'll have a talk with old Freeman ; he's a man of sound/common sense. Any man who was boatswain in the *Arethusa* must have the right stuff/in him. Yes; I'll have a talk with old Freeman.

[One evening Mrs. Fleming said to the Old Lieutenant:—]

Mrs. F. Edward dear, what think you of the Church for Neddy? I do so fear the temptations and dangers of the sea.

Old L. Mary, my love, do you think a parson has no temptations, or the pulpit no dangers. I have known parsons firing broadsides, and showing bunting on Sundays, but all the week silent, and without a signal. Don't tell me a parson has no temptations.

Mrs. F. A doctor, then, Edward?

Old L. Well, you see, Mary, neither Neddy nor I ever took medicine ourselves, and we wouldn't like to give it to other people.

Mrs. F. Any profession, Edward, any profession to keep Neddy at home.

Old L. Well, well, we'll see about it. One thing I'm resolved on—and that is, that our Neddy shan't enter one of the idle professions. Look at some of our young swells—these fellows talk big English, swagger along the streets, and flirt with the girls. They ape at being gentlemen, without work to soil their fingers, or thoughts to shake up their brains—if they have any. I tell you, Mary, I'd rather see our Neddy a tailor, sewing his own clothes, than see him parade the streets, an idle fool, in clothes he might have worked for, but wouldn't.

[One day the old Bo'sun, Freeman, called on the Old Lieutenant.]

Old L. We've been thinking, Freeman, we've been thinking what to make of Neddy. His mother thinks the sea dangerous.

Freeman. Cap'n, I've often remarked that men drown boats oftener than boats drown men.

Old L. You're quite correct, Freeman, you're quite correct—

the seaman makes the vessel. His mother would like him to be a parson.

Freeman. No, no, Cap'n.

Old L. You're quite correct, Freeman, you're quite correct; Ned has ballast, but not bunting for a parson.—A doctor, Freeman, eh?

Freeman. A doctor, Cap'n! Give me a man who will lose his own legs on deck, fighting for queen and country, and not waste his time, sawing off the legs of other men, in the cock-pit.

Old L. You're quite correct, Freeman, you're quite correct; pills and plasters won't do for Ned.—A lawyer, Freeman, eh?

Freeman. A lawyer, Cap'n! No, no, a lawyer's rig won't do.

Old L. You're quite correct, Freeman, you're quite correct; I don't understand these lawyer fellows a bit.

Freeman. No, nor nobody else, Cap'n. The sea, the old sea's the thing for Ned! Blow, breezes, blow; it's in the lad, Cap'n, it's in the lad!

"A life on the ocean-wave,
A home on the rolling deep!"

The old sea's the thing for Ned!

Old L. You're quite correct, Freeman, you're quite correct.

[One day Mrs. Fleming said to her old and faithful servant:—]

Mrs. F. Well, Babby, we have at last resolved to let Ned go to sea.

Babby. Oor Neddy gaun tae the sea! Never tell *me* he's gaun tae the sea!—a nesty, jumblin' pairt o' creation. Can ye no mak' him a shopkeeper or—somethin' at hame?

Mrs. F. No, no, Babby! That would never do for our Neddy.

Babby. Maybe no; he's ower prood for that. Eh, sirs, the day! it's a wunnerfu' thing this pride! Ye'll no let yer laddie hannle tea, but ye think taur's nicer for his hauns. Ye objec' tae saft sugar, but no tae saut water. There's ae thing—if he was a shopkeeper he wad never be drooned; an' he micht be a bailie, or the provost, maybe, an' merry a fine, winsome lass. An'—noo, Mistress Fleemin', ye needna lauch at me, for I'm positeeve I'm richt—for my sake, for a' oor sakes, keep my bonnie laddie in his auld nest!

[Ned's last night in the dear, old home had arrived.]

Babby. Noo, Maister Ned, ye'll no put on thae fine socks, unless ye be askit oot tae yer denner.

Ned. Asked out to dinner, Babby! Who's to ask me? a mermaid, eh?

Babby. I'm no heedin' wha asks ye. A merrmaid, as ye ca' her, is just as guid as onybody else, if she's a nice bit lassie. When it's cauld ye'll put on the comforter I made ye; an' if ye're wyse, ye'll tak' yer umbrella wi' ye, tae keep the saut water aff yer new pilot jaicket. What are ye lauchin' at, ye silly laddie?

[It was now about midnight, and Ned's mother entered the room.]

Mrs. F. Darling Ned, you and I shall have no sad farewells; but promise me, that you will read a little of this Bible, every day, and that you will never neglect your prayers to God.

Ned. I do promise, mother, with heart, soul, and strength.

[At that moment the Old Lieutenant entered.]

Old L. You'll go and kill yourself with this packing business! Leave us, Mary; I want to speak to Ned. [*Ned's mother slowly left the room.*]—Ned, you know, *I* have no present to give you.

Ned. Present, father! You!

Old L. No, my boy, no; but, for all that, I mean to give you my dearest treasure on earth—look at that signature.

Ned. Nelson! an order from him to you, father—to make certain signals.

Old L. Ay, lad, an order from him to me, your father. Ned, I give *that* to you as *my* parting gift, that, as you look at it, in storm or sunshine, at home or abroad, you may remember that "England expects every man to do his duty," and that you may never disgrace your old father by neglecting yours.

Ned. Thank you, father. Whatever happens to me, I'll never part with it; and I hope I won't disgrace you.

Old L. My own boy! I'm sure you never will. Ned, I never had much learning, never could tell you what was passing here; can't do it now; a heavy sea swamps me when I want to sail a-head. Ned, you must be a better man than your old father; for I never saw my father at all, and hardly ever my poor mother. Ned, you must do what your good mother has taught you; though God knows how I love you, Ned!

Ned. Dear father, don't speak in that way, as if you weren't the best father in the world! What did I ever see in you but good? what did I ever get from you but good?

Old L. Do you say so, Ned? do you believe that? I tell you, Ned, to hear that from your own lips—I tell you—I—I—God bless you! God bless and keep you, my own boy!

Dr. Norman Macleod.

FROM "THE SCHOOL FOR SCANDAL."
Sir Peter and Lady Teazle.

Sir P. When an old bachelor marries a young wife, what is he to expect? 'Tis now above six months since my Lady Teazle made me "the happiest of men," and I have been the most miserable dog ever since! We tifted a little going to church, and fairly quarrelled before the bells were done ringing. I was more than once nearly choked with gall during the honeymoon, and had lost every satisfaction in life before my friends had done wishing me joy. And, yet, I chose with caution a girl bred wholly in the country, who had never known luxury beyond one silk gown, or dissipation beyond the annual gala of a race-ball. Yet, now, she plays her part in all the extravagant fopperies of the town, with as good a grace as if she had never seen a bush or a grass-plot out of Grosvenor Square. I am sneered at by all my acquaintance—paragraphed in the newspapers; she dissipates my fortune, and contradicts all my humours. And yet, the worst of it is, I doubt I love her, or I should never bear all this; but I am determined never to let her know it.—No, no, no! Oh, here she comes. [*Enter Lady T.*] Lady Teazle, Lady Teazle, I won't bear it!

Lady T. Very well, Sir Peter, you may bear it or not, just as you please; but I know I ought to have my own way in everything, and, what's more, I will.

Sir P. What, madam! is there no respect due to the authority of a husband?

Lady T. Why, don't I know that no woman of fashion does as she is bid after her marriage? Though I was bred in the country, I'm no stranger to that. If you wanted me to be obedient, you should have adopted me, not married me—I'm sure you're old enough."

Sir P. Ay, there it is! Madam, what right have you to run into all this extravagance?

Lady T. I'm sure I'm not more extravagant than a woman of quality ought to be.

Sir P. Madam, I'll have no more sums squandered away upon such unmeaning luxuries: you have as many flowers in your dressing-room as would turn the Pantheon into a greenhouse.

Lady T. O Sir Peter! how can you be angry at my little elegant expenses?

Sir P. Had you any of those little elegant expenses when you married me?

Lady T. O Sir Peter! you would not have me be out of the fashion? I should think you would like to have your wife thought a woman of taste.

Sir P. Madam, you had no taste when you married me!

Lady T. Very true, indeed; and, after having married you, I should never pretend to taste again.

Sir P. Very well, very well, madam; you have entirely forgot what your situation was when I first saw you.

Lady T. No, no; I have not—a very disagreeable situation it was, or I'm sure I never would have married you.

Sir P. You forget the humble state I took you from—the daughter of a poor country squire. When I came to your father's I found you sitting at your tambour, in a linen gown, a bunch of keys at your side, and your hair combed smoothly over a roll.

Lady T. Yes, I remember very well;—my daily occupations were to overlook the dairy, superintend the poultry, make extracts from the Family Receipt-Book, and comb my aunt Deborah's lap-dog.

Sir P. Oh, I am glad to find you have so good a recollection!

Lady T. My evening employments were to draw patterns for ruffles—which I had not material to make up;—play at Pope Joan with the curate; read a sermon to my aunt Deborah, or, perhaps, be stuck up at an old spinet to thrum my father to sleep after a fox-chase.

Sir P. Then you were glad to take a ride out behind the butler upon the old docked coach-horse.

Lady T. No, no; I deny the butler and the coach-horse.

Sir P. I say you did. This *was* your situation.—Now, madam, you must have your coach, viz-a-viz, and three powdered footmen to walk before your chair, and in summer two white cats, to draw you to Kensington Gardens; and, instead of your living in that hole in the country, I have brought you home here, made a woman of fortune of you, a woman of quality—in short, I have made you my wife.

Lady T. Well! and there is but one thing more you can now add to the obligation, and that is—

Sir P. To make you my widow, I suppose.

Lady T. Hem!—

Sir P. Very well, madam, very well; I am much obliged to you for the hint.

Lady T. Why, then, will you force me to say shocking things of you? But now we have finished our morning conversation, I want you to be in a monstrous good humour; come, do be good-humoured, and let me have two hundred pounds.

Sir P. What! can't I be in good humour without paying for it?—But look always thus, and you shall want for nothing. You shall have the money.

Lady T. You can't think, Sir Peter, how good humour becomes you; now you look just as you did before I married you.

Sir P. Do I, indeed?

Lady T. Don't you remember when you used to walk with me under the elms, and tell me stories of what a gallant you were in your youth, and asked me if I could like an old fellow who would deny me nothing?

Sir P. Ay; and you were so attentive and obliging to me then!

Lady T. To be sure I was, and used to take your part against all my acquaintance; and when my cousin Sophy used to laugh at me for thinking of marrying a man old enough to be my father, and called you an ugly, stiff, formal, old bachelor, I contradicted her, and said I did not think you so ugly by any means, and that I dared say you would make a very good sort of a husband.

Sir P. That was very kind of you. Well, and you were not mistaken; you have found it so, have you not? But shall we always live thus happy?

Lady T. With all my heart. I don't care how soon we leave off quarrelling, provided you will own you are tired first.

Sir P. With all *my* heart.

Lady T. Then we shall be as happy as the day is long, and never, never, never quarrel more.

Sir P. Never—never—never—never! and let our future contest be who shall be most obliging.

Lady T. Ay!

Sir P. But, my dear Lady Teazle!—my love!—indeed you must keep a strict watch over your temper; for, you know, my dear, that in all our disputes and quarrels you always begin first.

Lady T. No, no, Sir Peter, my dear, 'tis always you that begin.

Sir P. No, no; no such thing!

Lady T. Have a care! this is not the way to live happy, if you fly out thus.

Sir P. Madam, I say 'tis you!

Lady T. I never saw such a man in my life—just what my cousin Sophy told me!

Sir P. Your cousin Sophy is a forward, saucy, impertinent minx!

Lady T. You are a very great bear, I am sure, to abuse my relations.

Sir P. But I am very well served for marrying you—a pert, forward, rural coquette, who had refused half the honest squires in the county.

Lady T. I am sure I was a great fool for marrying you—a stiff, cross, dangling, old bachelor, who was unmarried at fifty because nobody would have him.

Sir P. You were very glad to have me; you never had such an offer.

Lady T. Oh yes, I had—there was Sir Tivey Terrier, who everybody said would be a better match; for his estate was full as good as yours—and he has broke his neck since we were married.

Sir P. Very well, very well, madam! You are an ungrateful woman; and may plagues light on me if I ever try to be friends with you again—you shall have a separate maintenance.

Lady T. By all means, a separate maintenance.

Sir P. Very well, madam! oh, very well! Ay, madam, and I'll have a divorce, madam! I'll make an example of myself for the benefit of all old bachelors.

Lady T. Well, Sir Peter, I see you are going to be in a passion, so I'll leave you; and when you are come properly to your temper, we shall be the happiest couple in the world, and never, never, never quarrel more! Ha, ha, ha! Sir Peter!

[*Exit Lady T.*

Sir P. So! I have got much by my intended expostulation. —What a charming air she has! and how pleasingly she shows her contempt for my authority! Well, though I can't make her love me, 'tis some pleasure to tease her a little; and I think she never appears to such advantage, as when she is doing everything to vex and plague me. SHERIDAN.

FROM "THE SCHOOL FOR SCANDAL."

CHARLES SURFACE, SIR OLIVER SURFACE as MR. PREMIUM, MOSES, and CARELESS.

Scene: Picture-room at Charles Surface's House.

Charles. Walk in, gentlemen; pray walk in: here they are, the family of the Surfaces, up to the Conquest.

Sir O. And, in my opinion, a goodly collection.

Charles. Ay, ay, these are done in the true spirit of portrait-painting. Not like the works of your modern Raphaels, who give you the strongest resemblance, yet contrive to make your portrait independent of you, so that you may sink the original, and not hurt the picture. No, no; the merit of these is the inveterate likeness: all stiff and awkward as the originals, and like nothing in human nature besides.

Sir O. Ah! we shall never see such figures of men again.

Charles. I hope not. Well, you see, Master Premium, what a domestic character I am: here I sit of an evening surrounded by my family. But, come, get to your pulpit, Mr. Auctioneer; here's an old gouty chair of my grandfather's will answer the purpose.

Care. Ay, ay; this will do. But, Charles, I have not a hammer; and what's an auctioneer without his hammer?

Charles. That's true. (*Taking pedigree down*) what parchment have we here? Oh! our genealogy in full. Here, Careless, you shall have no common bit of mahogany; here's the family tree for you! this shall be your hammer. And now you may knock down my ancestors with their own pedigree.

Sir O. [*Aside*] What an unnatural rogue! an *ex post facto* parricide!

Care. Charles, this is the most convenient thing you could have found for the business, for 'twill not only serve as a hammer, but a catalogue into the bargain. Come, begin: going! going! going!

Charles. Bravo, Careless! Well, here's my great uncle, Sir Richard Raveline, a marvellous good general in his day, I assure you. He served in all the Duke of Marlborough's wars, and got that cut over his eye at the battle of Malplaquet. What say you, Mr. Premium? look at him: there's a hero, not cut out of his feathers, as your modern clipped captains are, but enveloped in wig and regimentals, as a general should be. What do you bid?

Sir O. [*Apart to* MOSES] Bid him speak.

Moses. Mr. Premium would have you speak.

Charles. Why, then, he shall have him for ten pounds; and I'm sure that's not dear for a staff-officer.

Sir O. [*Aside*] His famous uncle Richard for ten pounds! —Very well, sir, I take him at that.

Charles. Careless, knock down my uncle Richard. Here, now, is a maiden sister of his, my great-aunt Deborah; done by Kneller in his best manner, and esteemed a very formidable likeness. There she is, you see, a shepherdess feeding her flock. You shall have her for five pounds ten: the sheep are worth the money.

Sir O. [*Aside*] Ah! poor Deborah! a woman who set such a value on herself!—Five pounds ten! she's mine.

Charles. Knock down my aunt Deborah, Careless! This, now, is a grandfather of my mother's, a learnèd judge, well known on the western circuit. What do you rate him at, Moses?

Moses. Four guineas.

Charles. Four guineas! You don't bid me the price of his wig.—Mr. Premium, you have more respect for the woolsack; do let us knock his lordship down at fifteen.

Sir O. By all means.

Care. Gone!

Charles. And there are two brothers of his, William and Walter Blunt, Esquires, both members of parliament, and noted speakers; and what's very extraordinary, I believe this is the first time they were ever bought or sold.

Sir O. That is very extraordinary indeed; I'll take them at your own price, for the honour of parliament.

Care. Well said, little Premium! I'll knock them down at forty.

Charles. Here's a jolly fellow—I don't know what relation, but he was mayor of Norwich: take him at eight pounds.

Sir O. No, no; six will do for the mayor.

Charles. Come, make it guineas, and I'll throw the two aldermen there into the bargain.

Sir O. They're mine.

Charles. Careless, knock down the mayor and aldermen. But we shall be all day retailing in this manner: do let us deal wholesale: what say you, little Premium? Give me three hundred pounds, and take all that remains on each side, in a lump.

Care. Ay, ay, that will be the best way.

Sir O. Well, well; anything to accommodate you; they are mine. But there is one portrait which you have always passed over.

Care. What, that ill-looking little fellow over the settee?

Sir O. Yes, sir, I mean that; though I don't think him so ill-looking a little fellow, by any means.

Charles. What! that? Oh! that's my uncle Oliver; 'twas done before he went to India.

Care. Your uncle Oliver! Then you'll never be friends, Charles. That, now, to me, is as stern a looking rogue as ever I saw; an unforgiving eye, and a disinheriting countenance! an inveterate knave, depend on't. Don't you think so, little Premium? [*Slapping him on the shoulder.*]

Sir O. Sir, I do not; I think it as honest a looking face as any in the room, dead or alive; but I suppose Uncle Oliver goes with the rest of the lumber?

Charles. No! I'll not part with poor Noll. The old fellow has been very good to me, and I'll keep his picture while I've a room to put it in.

Sir O. [*Aside*] The rogue's my nephew after all.—But, sir, I have somehow taken a fancy to that picture.

Charles. I am sorry for it, for you certainly will not have it. Haven't you got enough of them?

Sir O. [*Aside*] I forgive him everything.—But, sir, when I take a whim in my head I don't value money. I'll give you as much for that as for all the rest.

Charles. Don't tease me, master broker; I tell you, I'll not part with it, and there's an end of it.

Sir O. [*Aside*] How like his father the rascal is!—Well, well, I have done. Here is a cheque for your sum.

Charles. Why, 'tis for eight hundred pounds!

Sir O. You will not let Sir Oliver go?

Charles. No.

Sir O. Then never mind the difference; we'll balance that another time; but give me your hand on the bargain. You are an honest fellow, Charles—I beg pardon, sir, for being so free. —Come, Moses.

Charles. This is a whimsical old fellow! But, harkye! Premium, you'll prepare lodgings for these gentlemen?

Sir O. Yes, yes; I'll send for them in a day or two.

Charles. But, hold! do now send a genteel conveyance for

them; for I assure you, they were most of them used to ride in their own carriages.

Sir O. I will, I will—for all but Oliver.

Charles. Ay, all but the little nabob.

Sir O. You're fixed on that?

Charles. Peremptorily.

Sir O. [*Aside*] A dear extravagant rogue!— Good-day! —Come, Moses.   SHERIDAN.

FROM "THE RIVALS."

MRS. MALAPROP, SIR ANTHONY ABSOLUTE, and LYDIA LANGUISH.

Mrs. M. There, Sir Anthony! there sits the deliberate simpleton, who wants to disgrace her family, and lavish herself on a fellow not worth a shilling.

Lyd. Madam, I thought you once—

Mrs. M. You thought, miss! I don't know any business you have to think at all; thought does not become a young woman. But the point we would request of you is, that you will promise to forget this fellow; to illiterate him, I say, from your memory.

Lyd. Ah! madam, our memories are independent of our wills; it is not so easy to forget.

Mrs. M. But I say it *is*, miss; there is nothing so easy as to forget, if a person chooses to set about it. I'm sure I have as much forgot your poor, dear uncle as if he had never existed; and I thought it my duty so to do. And, let me tell you, Lydia, these violent memories don't become a young woman.

Sir Anth. Why, sure, she won't pretend to remember what she's ordered not! Ay, this comes of her reading!

Lyd. What crime, madam, have I committed, to be treated thus?

Mrs. M. Now, don't attempt to extirpate yourself from the matter; you know I have proof controvertible of it. But, tell me, will you promise to do as you're bid? Will you take a husband of your friends' choosing?

Lyd. Madam, I must tell you plainly that, had I no preference for any one else, the choice you have made would be my aversion.

Mrs. M. What business have you, miss, with preference and aversion? They don't become a young woman; and you ought to know that, as both always wear off, 'tis safest in matrimony to begin with a little aversion. I am sure I hated your poor, dear uncle before marriage, as if he'd been a blackamoor; and yet, miss, you are sensible what a wife I made, and, when it pleased Heaven to release me from him, 'tis unknown what tears I shed! But, suppose we were going to give you another choice, will you promise to give up this Beverley?

Lyd. Could I belie my thoughts so far as to give that promise, my actions would certainly as far belie my words.

Mrs. M. Take yourself to your room, miss. You are fit company for nothing but your own ill humours.

Lyd. Willingly, madam; I cannot change for the worse.

[*Exit Lydia.*

Mrs. M. There's a little intricate vixen for you.

Sir Anth. It is not to be wondered at, ma'am; all that is the natural consequence of teaching girls to read. On my way hither, Mrs. Malaprop, I observed your niece's maid coming forth from a circulating library. She had a book in each hand; they were half-bound volumes with yellow covers: from that moment I guessed how full of duty I should find her mistress. But, Mrs. Malaprop, in moderation, now, what would you have a young woman know?

Mrs. M. Observe me, Sir Anthony: I would by no means wish a daughter of mine to be a progeny of learning; I don't think so much learning becomes a young woman. For instance, I would never let her meddle with Greek, or Hebrew, or algebra, or simony, or paradoxes, or such inflammatory branches of learning; nor would it be necessary for her to handle any of your mathematical, astronomical, diabolical instruments; but, Sir Anthony, I would send her, at nine years old, to a boarding school, in order to learn a little ingenuity and artifice. Then, sir, she should have a supercilious knowledge in accounts; and, as she grew up, I would have her instructed in geometry, that she might know something of the contagious countries. This, Sir Anthony, is what I would have a young woman know; and I don't think there is a superstitious article in it.

Sir Anth. Well, well, Mrs. Malaprop, I will dispute the point no further with you; though I must confess that you are a truly moderate and polite arguer, for almost every third word you say is on my side of the question. But, Mrs. Malaprop, to the more important point in the debate: you say you have no objection to my proposal?

Mrs. M. None, I assure you. I am under no positive engagement with Mr. Acres; and, as Lydia is so obstinate against him, perhaps your son may have better success.

Sir Anth. Well, madam, I will write for the boy directly. He knows not a syllable of this yet, though I have, for some time, had the proposal in my head. He is at present with his regiment.

Mrs. M. We have never seen your son, Sir Anthony; but I hope no objection on his side.

Sir Anth. Objection! let him object if he dare! No, no, Mrs. Malaprop; Jack knows that the least demur puts me into a frenzy directly. My process was always very simple: in his younger days, 'twas "Jack, do this;" if he demurred, I knocked him down! if he grumbled at that, I always sent him out of the room!

Mrs. M. Ay, and the properest way! nothing is so conciliating to young people as severity. Well, Sir Anthony, I shall give Mr. Acres his discharge, and prepare Lydia to receive your son's invocations; and I hope you will represent her to the captain as an object not altogether illegible.

Sir Anth. Madam, I will handle the subject prudently. Well, I must leave you; and, let me beg you, Mrs. Malaprop, to enforce this matter roundly to the girl: take my advice, keep a tight hand; if she reject this proposal, clap her under lock and key; and if you were just to let the servant forget to bring her dinner for three or four days, you can't conceive how she'd come about. Good-morning, Mrs. Malaprop.

SHERIDAN.

FROM "KING JOHN."

Scene: A Room in a Castle.

HUBERT, ARTHUR, and two Attendants.

Hub. Heat me these irons hot; and look thou stand
Within the arras: when I strike my foot
Upon the bosom of the ground, rush forth,
And bind the boy which you shall find with me
Fast to the chair: be heedful.—
Young lad, come forth; I have to say with you.

Enter ARTHUR.

Arth. Good-morrow, Hubert.
Hub.   Good-morrow, little prince.
Arth. You are sad, Hubert.
Hub. Indeed, I have been merrier.
Arth. Methinks nobody should be sad but I:
Yet, I remember, when I was in France,
Young gentlemen would be as sad as night,
Only for wantonness. By my christendom,
So I were out of prison and kept sheep,
I should be as merry as the day is long;
And so I would be here, but that I doubt
My uncle practises more harm to me.
He is afraid of me, and I of him:
Is it my fault that I was Geoffrey's son?

No, indeed, is't not; and I would to heaven
I were your son, so you would love me, Hubert.
   Hub. [*Aside*] If I talk to him, with his innocent prate
He will awake my mercy, which lies dead :
Therefore I will be sudden, and despatch.
   Arth. Are you sick, Hubert? you look pale to-day :
In sooth, I would you were a little sick,
That I might sit all night and watch with you :
I warrant I love you more than you do me.
   Hub. [*Aside*] His words do take possession of my bosom.
Read here, young Arthur.   [*Showing a paper.*
[*Aside*] I must be brief, lest resolution drop
Out at mine eyes in tender womanish tears.—
Can you not read it? is it not fair writ?
   Arth. Too fairly, Hubert, for so foul effect :
Must you with hot irons burn out both mine eyes?
   Hub. I must.
   Arth.   And will you?
Have you the heart? When your head did but ache,
I knit my handkercher about your brows,—
The best I had, a princess wrought it me,—
And I did never ask it you again ;
And with my hand at midnight held your head ;
And like the watchful minutes to the hour,
Still and anon cheered up the heavy time,
Saying, "What lack you?" and "Where lies your grief?"
Many a poor man's son would have lain still,
And ne'er have spoke a loving word to you ;
But you at your sick service had a prince.
Nay, you may think my love was crafty love,
And call it cunning : do, an if you will :
If heaven be pleased that you must use me ill,
Why then you must.—Will you put out mine eyes?
These eyes that never did, nor never shall,
So much as frown on you.

Hub. I have sworn to do it;
And with hot irons must I burn them out.
   Arth. If an angel should have come to me
And told me, Hubert should put out mine eyes,
I would not have believed him—no tongue but Hubert's.
   Hub. Come forth!   [*Enter two Attendants*
Do as I bid you do.
   Arth. Oh, save me, Hubert, save me! my eyes are out
Even with the fierce looks of these murderous men.
   Hub. Give me the iron, I say, and bind him here.
   Arth. Alas, what need you be so boisterous-rough?
I will not struggle, I will stand stone-still.
For heaven's sake, Hubert, let me not be bound!
Nay, hear me, Hubert! drive these men away,
And I will sit as quiet as a lamb;
I will not stir, nor wince, nor speak a word,
Nor look upon the iron angerly:
Send but these men away, and I'll forgive you,
Whatever torment you do put me to.
   Hub. Go, stand within; let me alone with him.—
                 [*Exeunt Attendants.*
Come, boy, prepare yourself.
   Arth. Is there no remedy?
   Hub. None, but to lose your eyes.
   Arth. Oh, that there were but a mote in yours,
A grain, a dust, a gnat, a wandering hair,
Any annoyance in that precious sense!
Then feeling what small things are boisterous there,
Your vile intent must needs seem horrible.
   Hub. Is this your promise? go to, hold your tongue.
   Arth. Hubert, the utterance of a brace of tongues
Must needs want pleading for a pair of eyes:
Let me not hold my tongue, let me not, Hubert;
Or, Hubert, if you will, cut out my tongue,
So I may keep mine eyes: oh, spare mine eyes,

FROM "KING JOHN."

Though to no use but still to look on you!
Look! the instrument is cold,
And would not harm me.
    Hub.   I can heat it, boy.
    Arth. No; the fire is dead with grief:
                              See for yourself;
There is no malice in this burning coal;
The breath of heaven has blown his spirit out,
And strewed repentant ashes on his head.
    Hub. But with my breath I can revive it, boy.
    Arth. An if you do, you will but make it blush
And glow with shame of your proceedings, Hubert:
Nay, it perchance will sparkle in your eyes;
And like a dog that is compelled to fight,
Snatch at his master that doth spur him on.
All things that you would use to do me wrong
Deny their office: only *you* do lack
That mercy which fierce fire and iron extends.
    Hub. I will not touch thine eyes
For all the treasure that thine uncle owes:
Yet am I sworn, and I did purpose, boy,
With this same very iron to burn them out.
    Arth. Now you look like Hubert! all this while
You were disguised.
    Hub.   Peace; no more. Adieu!
Your uncle must not know but you are dead;
I'll fill these doggèd spies with false reports:
And, pretty child, sleep doubtless and secure,
That Hubert, for the wealth of all the world,
Will not offend thee.
    Arth.   O heaven! I thank you, Hubert.
    Hub. Silence; no more:
Much danger do I undergo for thee.
                                              SHAKESPEARE.

FROM "ROMEO AND JULIET."
The Balcony Scene.
ROMEO, JULIET, and NURSE.

Rom. He jests at scars that never felt a wound.—
                                          [*Juliet appears at window.*
But, soft! what light through yonder window breaks?
It is the east, and Juliet is the sun!
Arise, fair sun, and kill the envious moon,
Who is already sick and pale with grief,
That thou her maid art far more fair than she.
   Jul. Ah me!
   Rom.   She speaks!—
Oh, speak again, bright angel! for thou art
As glorious to this night, being o'er my head,
As is a wingèd messenger of heaven
Unto the white upturnèd wondering eyes
Of mortals, that fall back to gaze on him
When he bestrides the lazy-pacing clouds,
And sails upon the bosom of the air.
   Jul. O Romeo, Romeo! wherefore art thou Romeo?
Deny thy father, and refuse thy name;
Or, if thou wilt not, be but sworn my love,
And I'll no longer be a Capulet.
   Rom. [*Aside*] Shall I hear more, or shall I speak at this?
   Jul. 'Tis but thy name that is my enemy;
What's in a name? that which we call a rose
By any other name would smell as sweet;
What's Montague?—Romeo, doff thy name,
And for that name, which is no part of thee,
Take all myself.
   Rom.   I take thee at thy word!
Henceforth I never will be Romeo.
   Jul. What man art thou that, thus bescreened in night,
So stumblest on my counsel?

Rom.   By a name
I know not how to tell thee who I am.
My name is hateful to myself,
Because it is an enemy to thee.
    Jul. Art thou not Romeo, and a Montague?
    Rom. Neither—if either thee dislike.
    Jul. How camest thou hither?
The orchard walls are high, and hard to climb,
And the place, death, considering who thou art,
If any of my kinsmen find thee here.
    Rom. With love's light wings did I o'erperch these walls.
And what love can do, *that* does love attempt;
Therefore thy kinsmen are no let* to me.
    Jul. If they do see thee, they will murder thee!
    Rom. There lies more peril in thine eye
Than twenty of their swords.
    Jul. I would not for the world they saw thee here.
    Rom. I have night's cloak to hide me from their eyes;
And but thou love me, let them find me here;
My life were better ended by their hate,
Than death proroguèd, wanting of thy love.
    Jul. By whose direction found'st thou out this place?
    Rom. By love, who first did prompt me to inquire.
I am no pilot; yet, wert thou as far
As that vast shore washed with the farthest sea,
I would adventure for such merchandise.
    Jul. Thou know'st the mask of night is on my face,
Else would a maiden blush bepaint my cheek
For that which thou hast heard me speak to-night.
But trust me, gentleman, I'll prove more true
Than those that have more cunning to be strange.
    Rom. Lady, by yonder blessed moon, I swear,
That tips with silver all these fruit-tree tops—

* Hindrance.

Jul. Oh, swear not by the moon, the inconstant moon,
That monthly changes in her circled orb.
　Rom. What shall I swear by?
　Jul.　　　　　　　　Do not swear at all;
Or, if thou wilt, swear by thy gracious self,
And I'll believe thee.
　Rom.　　　　　　If my heart's dear love—
　Jul. Well, do not swear; although I joy in thee,
I have no joy in this contráct to-night:
It is too rash, too unadvised, too sudden;
Too like the lightning, which doth cease to be
Ere one can say, "It lightens." Good-night,
Good-night! as sweet repose and rest
Come to thy heart, as that within my breast.
　Nurse. [*Within*] Juliet!
　Jul.　　　　　　Anon, good nurse!—
Stay but a little, I will come again.　　　[*Exit Juliet.*
　Rom. O blessed, blessed night! I am afeard,
Being in night, all this is but a dream,
Too flattering-sweet to be substantial.

　　　　　　　Re-enter JULIET.

　Jul. Three words, dear Romeo, and good-night indeed.
　Nurse. [*Within*] Madam!
　Jul.　　　　　　I come, good nurse.—
A thousand times good-night!　　　　　[*Exit Juliet.*
　Rom. Love goes toward love, as schoolboys from their books,
But love from love, toward school with heavy looks.
　　　　　　　　　　　　　　　　[*Romeo retiring.*

　　　　　　　Re-enter JULIET.

　Jul. Hist! Romeo, hist!—Oh, for a falconer's voice
To lure this tassle-gentle back again!
Bondage is hoarse, and may not speak aloud.—Romeo!
　Rom. How silver-sweet sound lovers' tongues by night,
Like softest music to attending ears!

Jul. Romeo!
Rom. My dear?
Jul. I have forgot why I did call thee back.
Rom. Let me stand here till thou remember it.
Jul. I shall forget, to have thee still stand there.
Rom. And I'll still stay, to have thee still forget.
Jul. 'Tis almost morning; good-night, good-night!
Parting is such sweet sorrow,
That I shall say good-night till it be morrow. [*Exit Juliet.*
Rom. Sleep dwell upon thine eyes, peace in thy breast!
Would I were sleep and peace, so sweet to rest!

SHAKESPEARE.

THE COURTSHIP OF HENRY V.

KING HENRY and PRINCESS KATHERINE of France.

Henry. Fair Katherine, wilt thou vouchsafe to teach a soldier terms that will enter at a lady's ear, and plead his love-suit to her gentle heart?

Kath. Your Majestee sall mock at me; I cannot speak your England.

Henry. If you will love me soundly with your French heart, I will be glad to hear you confess it, brokenly, with your English tongue! Do you like me, Kate?

Kath. Pardonnez-moi, I cannot tell vat is "like me."

Henry. An angel is like you, Kate, and you are like an angel.

Kath. Ah, de tongues of de mans is be full of deceits.

Henry. I' faith, Kate, I am glad thou canst speak no better English; for, if thou couldst, thou wouldst find me such a plain king, that thou wouldst think I had sold my farm to buy my crown. If I could win a lady at leap-frog, or by vaulting into my saddle with my armour on my back (under the correction of bragging be it spoken), I should quickly leap into a wife. Or if I might buffet for my love, I could lay on like a butcher. I speak to thee plain soldier: if thou canst love me for this, Kate, take me; if not, to say that I shall die, is true; but for thy love—by Saint Denis! No! Yet I love thee too; and while thou livest, dear Kate, take a fellow of plain and uncoined constancy. What! a speaker is but a prater; a rhyme is but a ballad; a straight back will stoop; a black beard will turn white; a curled pate will grow bald; a fair face will wither; a full eye will wax hollow: but a good heart, Kate, is like the sun, for *it* shines bright, and never changes. If thou would have such a one, take me; and take me, take a soldier; take a soldier, take a king. What sayest thou, then, fair Kate, to my love?

Kath. Is it possible dat I sould love de enemy of France?

Henry. No; it is not possible that you should love the enemy of France, Kate: but, in loving me, you should love the friend of France; for I love France so well I will not part with a village of it; I will have it all mine; and, Kate, when France is mine, and I am yours, then yours is France, and you are mine.

Kath. I cannot tell vat is dat.

Henry. No, Kate? Then I will tell thee in French—*Quand j'ai la possession de France, et quand vous avez la possession de moi* (let me see—what then? Saint Denis be my speed!) *donc votre est France et vous êtes mienne.* I tell thee, Kate, it is as easy to conquer the kingdom as to speak so much more French. Dost thou understand *thus* much English—CANST THOU LOVE ME?

Kath. I cannot tell.

Henry. Can any of your neighbours tell, Kate? I'll ask *them.* Put off your maiden blushes; take me by the hand, and say, "Harry of England, I am thine." With that word bless mine ear, and I will tell thee aloud, "England is thine, Ireland is thine, France is thine, and Henry Plantagenet is thine;" who, though I speak it before his face, if he be not fellow with the best king, thou shalt find the best king of good fellows.

Come, your answer in broken music—for thy voice is music, and thy English broken; therefore, break thy mind to me in broken English—Wilt thou have me?

Kath. Dat is as it sall please de *roi mon père.*

Henry. Nay, it will please him well, Kate; it shall please him, Kate.

Kath. Den it sall also content me.

Henry. Then I will kiss your lips, Kate.

Kath. Non, non; it is not de fashion for *les demoiselles* in France to—vat is de England for *baiser?*

Henry. To kiss.

Kath. Oui, to kiss *devant leur nōces.*

Henry. It is not the fashion for the maids in France to kiss before they are married, would you say?

Kath. Oui, vraiment.

Henry. Dear Kate, you and I cannot be confined within the weak list of a country's fashion: we are the makers of manners, Kate; and the liberty that follows, stops the mouths of all findfaults;—as I will do yours, for upholding the nice fashion of your country, in denying me a kiss.—You have witchcraft in your lips, Kate: there is more eloquence in a touch of them than in the tongues of the French council; and they should sooner persuade Harry of England than a general petition of monarchs. May God, the best maker of all marriages, combine our hearts in one, our realms in one, that the contending kingdoms of France and England, whose very shores look pale with envy of each other's happiness, may cease their hatred; that never war advance his bleeding sword 'twixt England and fair France.   SHAKESPEARE.

CLARENCE'S DREAM.

SIR ROBERT BRACKENBURY and DUKE OF CLARENCE.

Brak. Why looks your Grace so heavily to-day?
Clar. Oh, I have passed a miserable night!

So full of ugly sights, of ghastly dreams,
That, as I am a Christian faithful man,
I would not spend another such a night,
Though 'twere to buy a world of happy days;
So full of dismal terror was the time.

 Brak. What was your dream, my lord? I pray you
  tell me.

 Clar. Methought that I had broken from the Tower,
And was embarked to cross to Burgundy;
And, in my company, my brother Glöster,
Who, from my cabin, tempted me to walk
Upon the hatches: thence we looked toward England,
And cited up a thousand heavy times,
During the wars of York and Lancaster,
That had befall'n us. As we paced along
Upon the giddy footing of the hatches,
Methought that Glöster stumbled, and, in falling,
Struck me (that thought to stay him) overboard,
Into the tumbling billows of the main.
O Lord! methought what pain it was to drown!
What dreadful noise of waters in mine ears!
What ugly sights of death within mine eyes!
Methought I saw a thousand fearful wrecks;
A thousand men that fishes gnawed upon;
Wedges of gold, great anchors, heaps of pearl,
Inestimable stones, unvalued jewels,
All scattered in the bottom of the sea.
Some lay in dead men's skulls; and, in those holes
Where eyes did once inhabit, there were crept,
As 'twere in scorn of eyes, reflecting gems,
That wooed the slimy bottom of the deep,
And mocked the dead bones that lay scattered by.

 Brak. Had you such leisure in the time of death
To gaze upon these secrets of the deep?

 Clar. Methought I had; and often did I strive

To yield the ghost: but still the envious flood
Stopped in my soul, and would not let it forth
To find the empty, vast, and wandering air;
But smothered it within my panting bulk,
Which almost burst to belch it in the sea.
 Brak. Awaked you not in this sore agony?
 Clar. Ah, no, my dream was lengthened after
  life.—
Oh, then began the tempest of my soul!
I passed, methought, the melancholy flood
With that grim ferryman (which poets write of),
Unto the kingdom of perpetual night.
The first that there did greet my stranger soul
Was my great father-in-law, renownèd Warwick,
Who cried aloud—"What scourge for perjury
Can this dark monarchy afford false Clarence?"
And so he vanished: then came wandering by
A shadow like an angel, with bright hair
Dabbled in blood; and he shrieked out aloud—
"Clarence is come; false, fleeting, perjured Clarence,
That stabbed me in the field by Tewksbury;—
Seize on him, Furies, take him to your torments!"
With that, methought, a legion of foul fiends
Environed me, and howlèd in mine ears
Such hideous cries, that, with the very noise,
I trembling waked, and, for a season after,
Could not believe but that I was in hell,—
Such terrible impression made my dream.
       SHAKESPEARE.

FROM "HENRY VIII."

WOLSEY AND HIS SECRETARY.

 Wol. Farewell, a long farewell, to all my greatness!
This is the state of man: to-day he puts forth

FROM "HENRY VIII."

The tender leaves of hope; to-morrow blossoms,
And bears his blushing honours thick upon him;
The third day comes a frost, a killing frost,
And,—when he thinks, good easy man, full surely
His greatness is a-ripening,—nips his root,
And then he falls, as I do. I have ventured,
Like little wanton boys that swim on bladders,
This many summers in a sea of glory,
But far beyond my depth: my high-blown pride
At length broke under me; and now has left me,
Weary, and old with service, to the mercy
Of a rude stream, that must for ever hide me.
Vain pomp and glory of this world, I hate ye:
I feel my heart new opened. Oh, how wretched
Is that poor man that hangs on princes' favours!
There is, betwixt that smile we would aspire to,
That sweet aspéct of princes, and their ruin,
More pangs and fears than wars or women have:
And when he falls, he falls like Lucifer,
Never to hope again.

Enter CROMWELL.

       Why, how now, Cromwell!
 Crom. I have no power to speak, sir.
 Wol.   What! amazed
At my misfortunes? Speechless! Nay, an you weep,
I am fall'n indeed.
 Crom. How does your grace?
 Wol.   Why, well;
Never so truly happy, my good Cromwell.
I know myself now; and I feel, within me,
A peace above all earthly dignities,
A still and quiet conscience. The king has cured me—
I humbly thank his grace;—and from these shoulders,
These ruined pillars, out of pity, taken

A load would sink a navy,—too much honour:
Oh, 'tis a burden, Cromwell, 'tis a burden
Too heavy for a man that hopes for heaven!
   Crom. I am glad your grace has made that right use
of it.
   Wol. I hope I have: I am able now, methinks,
(Out of a fortitude of soul I feel,)
To endure more miseries, and greater far,
Than my weak-hearted enemies dare offer.—
What news abroad?
   Crom.   The heaviest, and the worst,
Is your displeasure with the king.
   Wol.   God bless him!
   Crom. The next is, that Sir Thomas More is chosen
Lord Chancellor in your place.
   Wol.   That's somewhat sudden:
But he's a learnèd man. May he continue
Long in his highness' favour, and do justice
For truth's sake, and his conscience; that his bones,
When he has run his course, and sleeps in blessings,
May have a tomb of orphans' tears wept on them!—
What more?
   Crom. That Cranmer is returned with welcome,
Installed Lord Archbishop of Canterbury.
   Wol. That's news indeed!
   Crom.   Last, that the Lady Anne,
Whom the king hath in secrecy long married,
This day was viewed in open as his queen,
Going to chapel; and the voice is now
Only about her coronation.
   Wol. There was the weight that pulled me down. O
       Cromwell,
The king has gone beyond me,—all my glories
In that one woman I have lost for ever:
No sun shall ever usher forth mine honours,

Or gild again the noble troops that waited
Upon my smiles. Go, get thee from me, Cromwell;
I am a poor, fall'n man, unworthy now
To be thy lord and master. Seek the king:
(That sun, I pray, may never set!) I have told him
What, and how true thou art; he will advance thee;
Some little memory of me will stir him
(I know his noble nature) not to let
Thy hopeful service perish too: good Cromwell,
Neglect him not; make use now, and provide
For thine own future safety.
 Crom.   O my lord,
Must I then leave you? must I needs forego
So good, so noble, and so true a master?
Bear witness, all that have not hearts of iron,
With what a sorrow Cromwell leaves his lord.—
The king shall have my service; but my prayers
For ever, and for ever, shall be yours.
 Wol. Cromwell, I did not think to shed a tear
In all my miseries; but thou hast forced me,
Out of thy honest truth, to play the woman.
Let's dry our eyes; and thus far hear me, Cromwell;
And,—when I am forgotten, as I shall be,
And sleep in dull cold marble, where no mention
Of me more must be heard of,—say, I taught thee;
Say, Wolsey,—that once trod the ways of glory,
And sounded all the depths and shoals of honour,—
Found thee a way, out of his wreck, to rise in;
A sure and safe one, though thy master missed it.
Mark but my fall, and that that ruined me.
Cromwell, I charge thee, fling away ambition;
By that sin fell the angels: how can man, then,
The image of his Maker, hope to win by't?
Love thyself last; cherish those hearts that hate thee;
Corruption wins not more than honesty.

Still in thy right hand carry gentle peace,
To silence envious tongues. Be just, and fear not;
Let all the ends thou aim'st at be thy country's,
Thy God's, and truth's; then if thou fall'st, O Cromwell,
Thou fall'st a blessed martyr. Serve the king;
And,—pr'ythee, lead me in :—
There, take an inventory of all I have,
To the last penny; 'tis the king's : my robe,
And my integrity to Heaven, is all
I dare now call mine own. O Cromwell, Cromwell,
Had I but served my God with half the zeal
I served my king, He would not in mine age
Have left me naked to mine enemies.
 Crom. Good sir, have patience.
 Wol.   So I have. Farewell
The hopes of court! my hopes in heaven do dwell.
SHAKESPEARE.

FROM "HAMLET."

HAMLET, HORATIO, MARCELLUS, and BERNARDO.

 Hor. Hail to your lordship!
 Ham.   I am glad to see you well:
Horatio—or I do forget myself.
 Hor. The same, my lord, and your poor servant ever.
 Ham. Sir, my good friend; I'll change that name with
  you.
And what make you from Wittenberg, Horatio?—
Marcellus?
 Mar. My good lord—
 Ham. I am very glad to see you; good even, sir [*to Bernardo*].
But what, in faith, make you from Wittenberg?
 Hor. A truant disposition, good my lord.
 Ham. I would not hear your enemy say so;
Nor shall you do mine ear that violence,

To make it truster of your own report
Against yourself. I know you are *no* truant.
But what is your affair in Elsinore?
We'll teach you to drink deep ere you depart.
 Hor. My lord, I came to see your father's funeral.
 Ham. I pray thee, do not mock me, fellow-student;
I think it was to see my mother's wedding.
 Hor. Indeed, my lord, it followed hard upon.
 Ham. Thrift, thrift, Horatio! the funeral-baked meats
Did coldly furnish forth the marriage tables.
Would I had met my dearest foe in heaven
Or ever I had seen that day, Horatio!
My father!—methinks I see my father.
 Hor. Where, my lord?
 Ham.   In my mind's eye, Horatio.
 Hor. I saw him once; he was a goodly king.
 Ham. He was a man, take him for all in all,
I shall not look upon his like again.
 Hor. My lord, I think I saw him yesternight.
 Ham. Saw? who?
 Hor. My lord, the king your father.
 Ham. The king my father!
 Hor. Season your admiration for a while
With an attent ear, till I may deliver,
Upon the witness of these gentlemen,
This marvel to you.
 Ham.   For God's love, let me hear.
 Hor. Two nights together had these gentlemen,
Marcellus and Bernardo, on their watch,
In the dead vast and middle of the night,
Been thus encountered. A figure like your father,
Armèd at point, exactly, cap-à-pié,
Appears before them, and with solemn march
Goes slow and stately by them; thrice he walked
By their oppressed and fear-surprisèd eyes,

Within his truncheon's length ; whilst they, distilled
Almost to a jelly with the act of fear,
Stand dumb, and speak not to him. This to me
In dreadful secrecy impart they did;
And I, with them, the third night kept the watch:
Where, as they had delivered, both in time,
Form of the thing, each word made true and good,
The apparition comes. I knew your father;
These hands are not more like.
   Ham.   But where was this?
   Hor. Upon the platform where we watched.
   Ham. Did you not speak to it?
   Hor.   My lord, I did;
But answer made it none: yet once, methought,
It lifted up its head, and did address
Itself to motion, like as it would speak;
But, even then, the morning cock crew loud,
And at the sound it shrunk in haste away,
And vanished from our sight.
   Ham.   'Tis very strange.
   Hor. As I do live, my honoured lord, 'tis true:
And we did think it writ down in our duty
To let you know of it.
   Ham. Indeed, indeed, sirs, but this troubles me.
Hold you the watch to-night?
   All. We do, my lord.
   Ham. Armed, say you?
   All. Armed, my lord.
   Ham. From top to toe?
   All. My lord, from head to foot.
   Ham. Then saw you not his face?
   Hor. Oh yes, my lord; he wore his beaver up.
   Ham. What looked he? frowningly?
   Hor. A countenance more in sorrow than in anger.
   Ham. Pale, or red?

Hor. Nay, very pale.
Ham. And fixed his eyes upon you?
Hor. Most constantly.
Ham. I would, I had been there.
Hor. It would have much amazed you.
Ham. Very like, very like. Stayed it long?
Hor. While one with moderate haste might tell a hundred.
Mar. Ber. Longer, longer.
Hor. Not when I saw it.
Ham. His beard was grizzled? No?
Hor. It was, as I have seen it in his life,
A sable silvered.
Ham. I will watch to-night;
Perchance 'twill walk again.
Hor. I warrant it will.
Ham. If it assume my noble father's person,
I'll speak to it, though hell itself should gape,
And bid me hold my peace. I pray you all,
If you have hitherto concealed this sight,
Let it be tenable in your silence still;
And whatsoever else shall hap to-night,
Give it an understanding, but no tongue;
I will requite your loves. So, fare you well.
Upon the platform, 'twixt eleven and twelve,
I'll visit you.
All. Our duty to your honour.
Ham. Your loves, as mine to you. Farewell.
[*Exeunt Horatio, Marcellus, and Bernardo.*
My father's spirit in arms! all is not well;
I doubt some foul play: would the night were come!
Till then sit still, my soul: foul deeds will rise,
Though all the earth o'erwhelm them, to men's eyes.

SHAKESPEARE.

FROM "THE MERCHANT OF VENICE."
The Bond Scene.
SHYLOCK, BASSANIO, and ANTONIO.

Shy. Three thousand ducats,—well?

Bass. Ay, sir, for three months.

Shy. For three months,—well?

Bass. For the which, as I told you, Antonio shall be bound.

Shy. Antonio shall become bound,—well?

Bass. May you stead me? will you pleasure me? shall I know your answer?

Shy. Three thousand ducats, for three months, and Antonio bound.

Bass. Your answer to that.

Shy. Antonio is a good man.

Bass. Have you heard any imputation to the contrary?

Shy. Ho, no, no, no, no. My meaning, in saying he is a good man, is, to have you understand me, that he is sufficient. Yet his means are in supposition. He hath an argosy bound to Tripolis, another to the Indies; I understand, moreover, upon the Rialto, he hath a third at Mexico, a fourth for England; and other ventures he hath, squandered abroad. But ships are but boards; sailors but men. There be land-rats and water-rats, land-thieves and water-thieves — I mean pirates; and then there is the peril of waters, winds, and rocks. The man is, notwithstanding, sufficient. Three thousand ducats?—I think I may take his bond.

Bass. Be assured you may.

Shy. I will be assured I may; and, that I may be assured, I will bethink me.—May I speak with Antonio?

Bass. If it please you to dine with us.

Shy. Yes, to smell pork; to eat of the habitation which your prophet, the Nazarite, conjured the devil into. I will buy with you, sell with you, talk with you, walk with you, and so following; but I will not eat with you, drink with you, nor pray with you.—What news on the Rialto?—Who is he comes here?

Enter ANTONIO.

Bass. This is Signior Antonio.

Shy. [*Aside*] How like a fawning publican he looks!
I hate him, for he is a Christian;
But more, for that in low simplicity
He lends out money gratis, and brings down
The rate of usance here with us in Venice.
If I can catch him once upon the hip,
I will feed fat the ancient grudge I bear him.
He hates our sacred nation; and he rails,
Even there where merchants most do congregate,
On me, my bargains, and my well-won thrift,
Which he calls interest. Cursèd be my tribe,
If I forgive him!

Bass.   Shylock, do you hear?

Shy. I am debating of my present store;
And, by the near guess of my memory,
I cannot instantly raise up the gross
Of full three thousand ducats: what of that?
Tubal, a wealthy Hebrew of my tribe,
Will furnish me.—But, soft! how many months
Do you desire?—[*To Ant.*] Rest you fair, good signior;
Your worship was the last man in our mouths.

Ant. Shylock, albeit I neither lend nor borrow,
By taking nor by giving of excess,
Yet to supply the ripe wants of my friend,
I'll break a custom. Is he yet possessed
How much you would?

Shy. Ay, ay, three thousand ducats.

Ant. And for three months.

Shy. I had forgot,—three months, you told me so.
Well then, your bond; and, let me see.—But hear you:

Methought you said you neither lend nor borrow
Upon advantage.
  Ant.   I do never use it.
  Shy. Three thousand ducats!—'tis a good round sum.
Three months from twelve : then, let me see ; the rate—
  Ant. Well, Shylock, shall we be beholden to you?
  Shy. Signior Antonio, many a time and oft,
On the Rialto, you have rated me
About my moneys and my usances :
Still have I borne it with a patient shrug ;
For sufferance is the badge of all our tribe.
You call me misbeliever, cut-throat dog,
And spit upon my Jewish gabardine ;
And all for use of that which is mine own.
Well, then, it now appears you need my help :
Go to, then ; you come to me, and you say,
"Shylock, we would have moneys:" you say so ;
You, that did void your rheum upon my beard,
And foot me, as you spurn a stranger cur
Over your threshold : moneys is your suit.
What should I say to you? Should I not say,
"Hath a dog money? Is it possible
A cur can lend three thousand ducats?" Or,
Shall I bend low, and, in a bondman's key,
With bated breath, and whispering humbleness
Say this :—
"Fair sir, you spit on me on Wednesday last ;
You spurned me such a day ; another time
You called me dog ; and, for these courtesies,
I'll lend you this much moneys?"
  Ant. I am as like to call thee so again,
To spit on thee again, to spurn thee too.
If thou wilt lend this money, lend it not
As to thy friends—for when did friendship take
A breed for barren metal of his friend?

But lend it rather to thine enemy;
Who, if he break, thou mayst with better face
Exact the penalty.

Shy. Why, look you, how you storm!
I would be friends with you, and have your love;
Forget the shames that you have stained me with;
Supply your present wants, and take no doit
Of usance for my moneys; and you'll not hear me.
This is kind I offer.

Ant. This were kindness.

Shy. This kindness will I show:—
Go with me to a notary, seal me there
Your single bond; and, in a merry sport,
If you repay me not on such a day,
In such a place, such sum or sums as are
Expressed in the condition, let the forfeit
Be nominated for an equal pound
Of your fair flesh, to be cut off and taken
In what part of your body pleaseth me.

Ant. Content, in faith; I'll seal to such a bond,
And say there is much kindness in the Jew.

Bass. You shall not seal to such a bond for me;
I'd rather dwell in my necessity.

Ant. Why, fear not, man; I will not forfeit it:
Within these two months, that's a month before
This bond expires, I do expect return
Of thrice three times the value of this bond.

Shy. O father Abraham! what these Christians are,
Whose own hard dealings teaches them suspect
The thoughts of others!—Pray you, tell me this:
If he should break his day, what should I gain
By the exaction of the forfeiture?
A pound of man's flesh, taken from a man,
Is not so estimable, profitable neither,
As flesh of muttons, beefs, or goats. I say,

To buy his favour, I extend this friendship:
If he will take it, so; if not, adieu:
And, for my love, I pray you, wrong me not.
  Ant. Yes, Shylock, I will seal unto this bond.
  Shy. Then meet me forthwith at the notary's;
Give him direction for this merry bond,
And I will go and purse the ducats straight;
See to my house, left in the fearful guard
Of an unthrifty knave; and presently
I will be with you.
  Ant. Hie thee, gentle Jew.— [*Exit Shylock.*
This Hebrew will turn Christian; he grows kind.
  Bass. I like not fair terms and a villain's mind.
  Ant. Come on: in this there can be no dismay;
My ships come home a month before the day.
                                        SHAKESPEARE.

FROM "THE MERCHANT OF VENICE."

The Trial Scene.

THE DUKE OF VENICE, ANTONIO, BASSANIO, GRATIANO, SHYLOCK, and PORTIA (disguised as a Doctor of Laws).

  Duke. What! is Antonio here?
  Ant. Ready, so please your grace.
  Duke. I am sorry for thee: thou art come to answer a stony adversary, an inhuman wretch incapable of pity, void and empty from any dram of mercy.
  Ant. I have heard your grace hath ta'en great pains to qualify his rigorous course; but, since he stands obdúrate, and that no lawful means can carry me out of his envy's reach, I do oppose my patience to his fury; and am armed to suffer, with a quietness of spirit, the very tyranny and rage of his.
  Duke. Go one, and call the Jew into the court.
  Gra. He's ready at the door: he comes, my lord.
  Duke. Make room, and let him stand before our face. [*Enter*

FROM "THE MERCHANT OF VENICE."

Shylock.] Shylock, the world thinks, and I think so too, that thou but lead'st this fashion of thy malice to the last hour of act; and then, 'tis thought thou'lt show thy mercy and remorse more strange than is thy strange apparent cruelty; and, where thou now exact'st the penalty (which is a pound of this poor merchant's flesh), thou wilt not only loose the forfeiture, but, touched with human gentleness and love, forgive a moiety of the principal; glancing an eye of pity on his losses, that have of late so huddled on his back, enough to press a royal merchant down. We all expect a gentle answer, Jew.

Shy. I have possessed your grace of what I purpose; and by our holy Sabbath have I sworn to have the due and forfeit of my bond! If you deny it, let the danger light upon your charter and your city's freedom. You'll ask me, why I rather choose to have a weight of carrion flesh, than to receive three thousand ducats? I'll not answer that; but say, it is my humour: is it answered? What if my house be troubled with a rat, and I be pleased to give ten thousand ducats to have it baned? what, are you answered yet? Some men there are love not a gaping pig; some, that are mad if they behold a cat. Now for your answer: as there is no firm reason to be rendered, why he cannot abide a gaping pig; why he, a harmless necessary cat; so can I give no reason, nor I will not,—more than a lodged hate, and a certain loathing, I bear Antonio, that I follow thus a losing suit against him. Are you answered?

Bass. This is no answer, thou unfeeling man, to excuse the current of thy cruelty.

Shy. I am not bound to please thee with my answer.

Bass. Do all men kill the things they do not love?

Shy. Hates any man the thing he would not kill?

Bass. Every offence is not a hate at first.

Shy. What! would'st thou have a serpent sting thee twice?

Ant. I pray you, think you question with the Jew? you may as well go stand upon the beach, and bid the main flood bate his usual height; you may as well use question with the wolf, why he hath made the ewe bleat for the lamb; you may as well forbid the mountain pines to wag their high tops, and to make no noise, when they are fretted with the gusts of heaven; you may as well do anything most hard, as seek to soften that (than which what's harder?) his Jewish heart:—therefore, I do beseech you, make no more offers, use no further means; but, with all brief and plain conveniency, let me have judgment, and the Jew his will.

Bass. For thy three thousand ducats here are six.

Shy. If every ducat, in six thousand ducats, were in six parts, and every part a ducat, I would not draw them—I would have my bond!

Duke. How shalt thou hope for mercy, rendering none?

Shy. What judgment shall I dread, doing no wrong? The pound of flesh, which I demand of him, is dearly bought—is mine, and I will have it! If you deny me, fie upon your law! There is no force in the decrees of Venice! I stand for judgment: answer, shall I have it?

Duke. Upon my power, I may dismiss this court, unless Bellario, a learnèd doctor, whom I have sent for to determine this, come here to-day.

Bass. Good cheer, Antonio! What, man, courage yet! the Jew shall have my flesh, blood, bones, and all, ere thou shalt lose for me one drop of blood.

Ant. I am a tainted wether of the flock, meetest for death; the weakest kind of fruit drops earliest to the ground, and so let me. You cannot better be employed, Bassanio, than to live still, and write mine epitaph. [*Shylock kneels and whets his knife.*

Bass. Why dost thou whet thy knife so earnestly?

Shy. To cut the forfeit from that bankrupt there.

Gra. Can no prayers pierce thee?

Shy. No, none that thou hast wit enough to make.

Gra. Oh, be thou foiled, inexorable dog! and for thy life let justice be accused. Thou almost mak'st me waver in my faith, to hold opinion with Pythagoras, that souls of animals infuse themselves into the trunks of men; for thy desires are wolfish, bloody, starved, and ravenous!

Shy. Till thou canst rail the seal from off my bond, thou but offend'st thy lungs to speak so loud: repair thy wit, good youth, or it will fall to cureless ruin!—I stand here for law.

Duke. O here, I take it, is the doctor come. [*Enter Portia.*] You are welcome: take your place. Are you acquainted with the difference that holds this present question in the court?

Por. I am informèd throughly of the cause. Which is the merchant here, and which the Jew?

Duke. Antonio, and old Shylock, both stand forth.

Por. Is your name Shylock?

Shy. Shylock is my name.

Por. Of a strange nature is the suit you follow; yet, in such rule, that the Venetian law cannot impugn you as you do proceed.—You stand within his danger, do you not?

Ant. Ay, so he says.

Por. Do you confess the bond?

Ant. I do.

Por. Then must the Jew be merciful.

Shy. On what compulsion must I? tell me that.

Por. The quality of mercy is not strained; it droppeth, as the gentle rain from heaven, upon the place beneath: it is twice bless'd; it blesseth him that gives, and him that takes: 'tis mightiest in the mightiest: it becomes the thronèd monarch better than his crown; his sceptre shows the force of temporal power, the attribute to awe and majesty, wherein doth sit the dread and fear of kings; but mercy is above this sceptred sway: it is enthronèd in the hearts of kings; it is an attribute to God himself; and earthly power doth then show likest God's when mercy seasons justice. Therefore, Jew, though justice be thy plea, consider this—that, in the course of justice, none of us should see salvation: we do pray for mercy; and that same prayer doth teach us all to render the deeds of mercy.—I have spoke thus much to mitigate the justice of thy plea; which if thou follow, this strict court of Venice must needs give sentence 'gainst the merchant there.

Shy. My deeds upon my head! I crave the law—the penalty and forfeit of my bond.

Por. Is he not able to discharge the money?

Bass. Yes, here I tender it for him in the court; yea, thrice the sum: if that will not suffice, I will be bound to pay it ten times o'er, on forfeit of my hands, my head, my heart: if this will not suffice, it must appear that malice bears down truth. And I beseech you, wrest once the law to your authority: to do a great right, do a little wrong, and curb this cruel devil of his will.

Por. It must not be; there is no power in Venice can alter a decree establishèd: 'twill be recorded for a precedent, and many an error, by the same example, will rush into the state: it cannot be.

Shy. A Daniel come to judgment! yea, a Daniel!—O wise young judge, how do I honour thee!

Por. I pray you, let me look upon the bond.

Shy. Here 'tis, most reverend doctor, here it is.

Por. Shylock, there's thrice thy money offered thee.

Shy. An oath, an oath; I have an oath in heaven. Shall I lay perjury upon my soul? no, not for Venice!

Por. Why, this bond is forfeit; and lawfully by this the Jew may claim a pound of flesh, to be by him cut off nearest the merchant's heart.—Be merciful: take thrice thy money; bid me tear the bond.

Shy. When it is paid according to the tenor. It doth appear you are a worthy judge; you know the law—your exposition hath been most sound: I charge you by the law, whereof you are a well-deserving pillar, proceed to judgment. By my soul I swear there is no power in the tongue of man to alter me: I stay here on my bond.

Ant. Most heartily I do beseech the court to give the judgment.

Por. Why, then, thus it is:—you must prepare your bosom for his knife.

Shy. O noble judge! O excellent young man!

Por. For the intent and purpose of the law hath full relation to the penalty, which here appeareth due upon the bond.

Shy. 'Tis very true, O wise and upright judge! how much more elder art thou than thy looks!

Por. Therefore, lay bare your bosom.

Shy. Ay, his breast: so says the bond;—doth it not, noble judge? "Nearest his heart!" these are the very words.

Por. It is so. Are there balance here to weigh the flesh?

Shy. I have them ready.

Por. Have by some surgeon, Shylock, on your charge, to stop his wounds, lest he do bleed to death.

Shy. Is it so nominated in the bond?

Por. It is not so expressed; but what of that? 'twere good you do so much for charity.

Shy. I cannot find it; 'tis not in the bond.

Por. Come, merchant, have you anything to say?

Ant. But little: I am armed, and well prepared.—Give me your hand, Bassanio: fare you well! Grieve not that I am fallen to this for you; for herein Fortune shows herself more kind than is her custom. It is still her use to let the wretched man outlive his wealth; to view, with hollow eye and wrinkled brow, an age of poverty: from which lingering penance of such a misery doth she cut me off. Repent not you that you shall lose your friend, and he repents not that he pays your debt; for, if the Jew do cut but deep enough, I'll pay it instantly—with all my heart.

Shy. We trifle time: I pray thee, pursue sentence.

Por. A pound of that same merchant's flesh is thine: the court awards it, and the law doth give it.

Shy. Most rightful judge!

Por. And you must cut this flesh from off his breast: the law allows it, and the court awards it.

Shy. Most learnèd judge!—A sentence! Come, prepare!

Por. Tarry a little; there is something else. This bond doth give thee here no jot of blood,—the words expressly are, "a pound of flesh:" take then thy bond—take thou thy pound of flesh; but, in the cutting it, if thou dost shed one drop of Christian blood, thy lands and goods are, by the laws of Venice, confiscate unto the state of Venice.

Gra. O upright judge! Mark, Jew;—a learnèd judge!

Shy. Is that the law?

Por. Thyself shalt see the act; for, as thou urgest justice, be assured thou shalt have justice, more than thou desir'st.

Gra. O learnèd judge! Mark, Jew;—a learnèd judge!

Shy. I take this offer, then:—pay the bond thrice, and let the Christian go.

Bass. Here is the money.

Por. Soft! the Jew shall have all justice;—soft! no haste; he shall have nothing but the penalty.

Gra. O Jew! an upright judge! a learnèd judge!

Por. Therefore, prepare thee to cut off the flesh. Shed thou no blood; nor cut thou less, nor more, but just "a pound" of flesh: if thou tak'st more or less than a just pound,—be it but so much as makes it light or heavy in the substance, or the division of the twentieth part of one poor scruple, nay, if the scale do turn but in the estimation of a hair,—thou diest, and all thy goods are confiscate.

Gra. A second Daniel! a Daniel, Jew!

Por. Why doth the Jew pause? take thy forfeiture.

Shy. Give me my principal, and let me go.

Bass. I have it ready for thee; here it is.

Por. He hath refused it in the open court; he shall have merely justice, and his bond.

Gra. A Daniel, still say I; a second Daniel!—I thank thee, Jew, for teaching me that word.

Shy. Shall I not barely have my principal?

Por. Thou shalt have nothing but the forfeiture, to be so taken at thy peril, Jew.

Shy. Why, then, I'll stay no longer question.

Por. Tarry, Jew: the law hath yet another hold on you. It is enacted in the laws of Venice,—If it be proved against an alien that, by direct or indirect attempts, he seek the life of any citizen, the party 'gainst the which he doth contrive shall seize one-half his goods; the other half comes to the privy coffer of the state; and the offender's life lies in the mercy of the Duke only, 'gainst all other voice. In which predicament, I say, thou stand'st; for it appears, by manifest proceeding, that, indirectly, and directly too, thou hast contrived against the very life of the defendant; and thou hast incurred the danger formally by me rehearsed. Down, therefore, and beg mercy of the Duke.

Gra. Beg that thou may'st have leave to hang thyself!—and yet, thy wealth being forfeit to the state, thou hast not left the value of a cord; therefore thou must be hanged at the state's charge.

Duke. That thou shalt see the difference of our spirits, I pardon thee thy life before thou ask it. For half thy wealth, it is Antonio's; the other half comes to the general state, which humbleness may drive unto a fine.

Shy. Nay, take my life and all; pardon not that. You take my house, when you do take the prop that doth sustain my house; you take my life, when you do take the means whereby I live.

Por. What mercy can you render him, Antonio?

Gra. A halter gratis! nothing else, I pray you.

Ant. So please my lord the Duke, and all the court, to quit the fine for one-half of his goods, I am content; so he will let me have the other half in use,—to render it, upon his death, unto the gentleman that lately stole his daughter. Two things provided more: that, for this favour, he presently become a Christian; the other, that he do record a gift, here in the court, of all he dies possessed, unto his son Lorenzo, and his daughter.

Duke. He shall do this, or else I do recant the pardon that I late pronouncèd here.

Por. Art thou contented, Jew? what dost thou say?

Shy. I am content. I pray you, give me leave to go from hence; I am not well: send the deed after me, and I will sign it.

Duke. Get thee gone, but do it.

Gra. In christening, thou shalt have two godfathers; had I been judge, thou shouldst have had ten more—to bring thee to the gallows, not the font! SHAKESPEARE.

SELECTIONS FROM "AS YOU LIKE IT."

Scene: Oliver's Orchard.

Enter ORLANDO *and* ADAM.

Orlan. As I remember, Adam, it was in this fashion bequeathed me: By will, but a poor thousand crowns; and, as thou sayest, charged my brother, on his blessing, to breed me well: and there begins my sadness. My brother Jaques he keeps at school, and report speaks goldenly of his profit: for my part, he keeps me rustically at home, or, to speak more properly, stays me here at home unkept; for call you that keeping, for a gentleman of my birth, that differs not from the stalling of an ox? His horses are bred better; he lets me feed with his hinds, and bars me the place of a brother. This is it, Adam, that grieves me; and the spirit of my father, which I think is within me, begins to mutiny against this servitude: I will no longer endure it, though yet I know no wise remedy how to avoid it.

Adam. Yonder comes my master, your brother.

Orlan. Go apart, Adam, and thou shalt hear how he will shake me up. [*Adam retires.*

Enter OLIVER.

Oliver. Now, sir! what make you here?

Orlan. Nothing; I am not taught to make anything.

Oliver. What mar you then, sir?

Orlan. Marry, sir, I am helping you to mar that which Heaven made—a poor unworthy brother of yours—with idleness.

Oliver. Marry, sir, be better employed.

Orlan. Shall I keep your hogs, and eat husks with them? What prodigal portion have I spent, that I should come to such penury?

Oliver. Know you where you are, sir?

Orlan. Oh, sir, very well: here, in your orchard.

Oliver. Know you before whom, sir?

Orlan. Ay, better than him I am before knows me. I know you are my eldest brother; and, in the gentle condition of blood, you should so know me. The courtesy of nations allows you my better, in that you are the first-born; but the same tradition takes not away my blood, were there twenty brothers betwixt us. I have as much of my father in me as you; albeit, I confess, your coming before me is nearer to his reverence.

Oliver. What, boy! [*Attempts to strike Orlando.*

Orlan. Come, come, elder brother, you are too young in this.

Oliver. Wilt thou lay hands on me, villain?

Orlan. I am no villain; I am the youngest son of Sir Rowland de Bois. Wert thou not my brother, I would not take this hand from thy throat till this other hand had pulled out thy tongue for saying so: thou hast railed on thyself.

Adam. [Comes forward] Sweet masters, be patient; for your father's remembrance, be at accord.

Oliver. Let me go, I say!

Orlan. I will not, till I please; you shall hear me! My father charged you, in his will, to give me good education: you have trained me up like a peasant, obscuring and hiding from me all gentleman-like qualities. The spirit of my father grows strong in me, and I will no longer endure it: therefore, allow me such exercises as may become a gentleman, or give me the poor allottery my father left me by testament; with that I will go buy my fortunes.

Oliver. And what wilt thou do—beg, when that is spent? Well, sir, get you in: I will not long be troubled with you; you shall have some part of your will: I pray you, leave me.

Orlan. I will no further offend you than becomes me for my good. [*Exit Orlando.*

Oliver. Get you with him, you old dog!

Adam. Is "old dog" my reward? Most true, I have lost my teeth in your service. Heaven be with my old master! he would not have spoke such a word. [*Exit Adam.*

Oliver. Is it even so? begin you to grow upon me? I will physic your rankness, and yet give you no thousand crowns neither. [*Exit.*

Scene: *A Room in the Duke's Palace.*

Enter ROSALIND *and* CELIA.

Celia. Why, cousin! why, Rosalind! not a word?

Ros. Not one word to throw at a dog.

Celia. No, thy words are too precious to be cast away upon curs; throw some of them at me.

Ros. Oh, how full of briers is this working-day world!

Celia. They are but burrs, cousin, thrown upon thee in holiday foolery.

Ros. I could shake them off my coat: these burrs are in my heart.—Look! here comes the Duke.

Celia. With his eyes full of anger.

Enter DUKE FREDERICK.

Duke. Mistress, despatch you with your safest haste.
And get you from our court!

Ros. Me, uncle?

Duke.   You, niece:—
Within these ten days, if that thou be'st found
So near our public court as twenty miles,
Thou diest for it!

Ros.   Dear uncle,
Never so much as in a thought unborn
Did I offend your highness.
   Duke.   Thus say all traitors:
Let it suffice thee, that I trust thee not.
   Ros. Yet your mistrust cannot make me a traitor.
Tell me, whereon the likelihood depends.
   Duke. Thou art thy father's daughter; there's enough.
   Ros. So was I when your highness took his dukedom;
So was I when your highness banished him.
Treason is not inherited, my lord;
Or, if we did derive it from our friends,
What's that to me? my father was no traitor:
Then, good my liege, mistake me not so much,
To think my poverty is treacherous.
   Celia. Dear father, hear me speak.
   Duke. Ay, Celia; we but stayed her for your sake,
Else had she with her father ranged along.
   Celia. I did not then entreat to have her stay,—
I was too young that time to value her;
But now I know her: if she be a traitor,
Why, so am I; we still have slept together,
Rose at an instant, learned and played together;
And wheresoe'er we went, like Juno's swans,
Still we went coupled, and inseparable.
   Duke. She is too subtle for thee; and her smoothness,
Her very silence, and her patience,
Speak to the people, and they pity her.
She robs thee of thy name;
And thou wilt show more bright, and seem more virtuous,
When she is gone. Then open not thy lips:
Firm, and irrevocable, is the doom
Which I have passed upon her—she is banished.
   Celia. Pronounce that sentence then on me, my liege;
I cannot live out of her company.

Duke. You are a fool!—*You*, niece, provide yourself:
If you outstay the time, upon mine honour,
And in the greatness of my word, you die! [*Exit Duke.*
　Celia. O my poor Rosalind! whither wilt thou go?
Wilt thou change fathers?—I will give thee mine.
I charge thee, be not more grieved than I am.
　Ros. I have more cause.
　Celia. 　　　　　　Thou hast not, cousin;
Pr'ythee, be cheerful: know'st thou not the Duke
Hath banished me, his daughter?
　Ros. 　　　　　　That he hath not.
　Celia. No! hath not? Rosalind lacks then the love
Which teacheth me that thou and I am one.
Shall we be sundered? shall we part, sweet girl?
No! let my father seek another heir.
Therefore devise with me how we may fly,
Whither to go, and what to bear with us;
For, by this heaven, now at our sorrows pale,
Say what thou canst, I'll go along with thee!
　Ros. Why, whither shall we go?
　Celia. To seek my uncle, in the forest of Arden.
　Ros. Alas, what danger will it be to us,
Maids as we are, to travel forth so far!
　Celia. I'll put myself in poor and mean attire;
The like do you: so shall we pass along,
And never stir assailants.
　Ros. 　　　　　　Were it not better,
Because that I am more than common tall,
That I did suit me all points like a man?
A gallant curtle-axe upon my side,
A boar-spear in my hand; and—in my heart
Lie there what hidden woman's fear there will—
We'll have a swashing and a martial outside,
As many other mannish cowards have
That do outface it with their semblances.

Celia. What shall I call thee when thou art a man?

Ros. I'll have no worse a name than Jove's own page,
And, therefore, look you, call me Ganymede.
But what will you be called?

Celia. Something that hath a reference to my state;
No longer Celia, but Aliena.

Ros. But, cousin, what if we assayed to steal
The clownish fool out of your father's court?
Would he not be a comfort to our travel?

Celia. He'll go along o'er the wide world with me:
Leave me alone to woo him. Let's away,
And get our jewels and our wealth together;
Devise the fittest time and safest way
To hide us from pursuit that will be made
After my flight. Now go we in content
To liberty, and not to banishment. [*Exeunt.*

Scene: Before Oliver's House.

Enter ORLANDO *and* ADAM.

Adam. O my young master! O you memory
Of old Sir Rowland! what make you here?
Why are you virtuous? why do people love you?
And wherefore are you gentle, strong, and valiant?

Orlan. Why, Adam, what's the matter?

Adam. Come not within these doors:
Your brother this night means
To burn the lodging where you use to lie,
And you within it. I overheard him.
This is no place—this house is but a butchery;
Abhor it, fear it, do not enter it.

Orlan. Why, whither, Adam, wouldst thou have me go?

Adam. No matter whither, so you come not here.

Orlan. Why, wouldst thou have me go and beg my food?
Or, with a base and boisterous sword, enforce

A thievish living on the common road?
This I must do, or know not what to do:
Yet this I will not do, do how I can.
   Adam. But do not so: I have five hundred crowns—
The thrifty hire I saved under your father.
Take that; and He that doth the ravens feed,
Yea, providently caters for the sparrow,
Be comfort to my age!
Let me be your servant:
Though I look old, yet I am strong and lusty;
My age is as a lusty winter,
Frosty, but kindly;—let me go with you;
I'll do the service of a younger man
In all your business and necessities.
   Orlan. O good old man! how well in thee appears
The constant service of the antique world.
Thou art not for the fashion of these times,
Where none will sweat but for promotion;
It is not so with thee.
Come thy ways; we'll go along together,
And light upon some settled low content.
   Adam. Master, go on; and I will follow thee
To the last gasp, with truth and loyalty.   [*Exeunt.*

Scene: The Forest of Arden.

Enter ROSALIND, CELIA, *and* TOUCHSTONE.

Ros. Oh, how weary are my spirits! I could find in my heart to cry like a woman: but I must comfort the weaker vessel. Courage, good Aliena!

Celia. I pray you, bear with me; I can go no further.

Touch. For my part, I had rather bear with you than bear you.

Ros. Well, this is the Forest of Arden.

Touch. Ay, now I am in Arden: the more fool I; when I

was at home, I was in a better place: but travellers must be content.

Ros. Ay, be so, good Touchstone. Look you, who comes here?

Enter SHEPHERD.

Celia. I pray you, question yon man,
If he for gold will give us any food;
I faint almost to death.
 Touch.   Holloa, you clown!
 Ros. Peace, fool! he's not thy kinsman.
 Shep. Who calls?
 Touch.   Your betters, sir.
 Shep. Else they are very wretched.
 Ros. Peace, I say.—Good-even to you, friend.
 Shep. And to you, and to you all.
 Ros. I pr'ythee, shepherd, if that love, or gold,
Can in this desert place buy entertainment,
Bring us where we may rest ourselves, and feed.
Here's a young maid, with travel much oppressed,
And faints for succour.
 Shep.   I pity her;
And wish, for her sake more than for mine own,
My fortunes were more able to relieve:
But I am shepherd to another man.
My master is of churlish disposition,
And little recks to find the way to heaven
By doing deeds of hospitality.
His cote and flocks are now on sale:
By reason of his absence, there is nothing
That you will feed on; but what is, come see,
Most welcome shall you be.
 Ros. Buy thou the cottage, pasture, and the flock,
And thou shalt have the pay of them from us;
And we will mend thy wages: I like this place,
And willingly could waste my time in it.

Shep. Assuredly the thing is to be sold:
Go with me; if you like upon report
The soil, the profit, and this kind of life,
I will your very faithful shepherd be,
And buy it with your gold right suddenly.   [*Exeunt.*

Scene: Road leading to the Forest.
Enter ORLANDO *and* ADAM.

Adam. Dear master, I can go no further: oh, I die for food! Here lie I down, and measure out my grave. Farewell, kind master!

Orlan. Why, how now, Adam! no greater heart in thee? Comfort a little; cheer thyself a little. If this uncouth forest yield anything savage, I will either be food for it, or bring it for food to thee. For my sake, be comfortable; hold death awhile at the arm's end: I will be here with thee presently; and if I bring thee not something to eat, I'll give thee leave to die: but if thou diest before I come, thou art a mocker of my labour. Well said! thou lookest cheerily; and I'll be with thee quickly. Yet thou art in the bleak air: come, I will bear thee to some shelter; and thou shalt not die for lack of a dinner, if there live anything in this desert. Cheerily, good Adam! cheerily! cheerily!   [*Exeunt.*

Scene: The Forest.
Enter THE EXILED DUKE *and* JAQUES.

Duke. Why, how now, monsieur! what a life is this,
That your poor friends must woo your company?
What, you look merrily!

Jaques. A fool, a fool!—I met a fool i' the forest,
A motley fool!—a miserable world!—
As I do live by food, I met a fool;
Who laid him down, and basked him in the sun,
And railed on Lady Fortune in good terms,
In good set terms—and yet a motley fool.

"Good-morrow, fool," quoth I. "No, sir," quoth he,
"Call me not a fool, till heaven hath sent me fortune:"
And then he drew a dial from his poke,
And, looking on it with lack-lustre eye,
Says, very wisely, "It is ten o'clock.
Thus may we see," quoth he, "how the world wags:
'Tis but an hour ago since it was nine;
And after one hour more 'twill be eleven;
And so, from hour to hour, we ripe and ripe,
And then, from hour to hour, we rot and rot;
And thereby hangs a tale." When I did hear
The motley fool thus moral on the time,
My lungs began to crow like chanticleer,
That fools should be so deep contemplative;
And I did laugh, sans intermission,
An hour by his dial.—O noble fool!
A worthy fool! Motley's the only wear.

Enter ORLANDO.

Orlan. Forbear, and eat no more.
Jaques. Why, I have eat none yet.
Orlan. Nor shalt not, till necessity be served.
Duke. Art thou thus boldened, man, by thy distress?
Or else a rude despiser of good manners,
That in civility thou seem'st so empty?
What would you have? Your gentleness shall force,
More than your force move us to gentleness.
Orlan. I almost die for food; and let me have it.
Duke. Sit down, and welcome to our table.
Orlan. Speak you so gently? Pardon me, I pray you:
I thought that all things had been savage here;
And therefore put I on the countenance
Of stern commandment.
If ever you have looked on better days:
If ever been where bells have knolled to church;

If ever sat at any good man's feast;
If ever from your eyelids wiped a tear,
And know what 'tis to pity and be pitied,
Let gentleness my strong enforcement be:
In the which hope I blush, and hide my sword.

Duke. True is it, that we have seen better days,
And have with holy bell been knolled to church;
And sat at good men's feasts; and wiped our eyes
Of drops that sacred pity had engendered:
And therefore sit you down in gentleness.

Orlan. Then but forbear your food a little while.
There is an old poor man,
Who after me hath many a weary step
Limped in pure love: till he be first sufficed—
Oppressed with two weak evils, age and hunger—
I will not touch a bit.

Duke.   Go find him out,
And we will nothing waste till you return.

Orlan. I thank ye; and be blest for your good comfort!
          [*Exit Orlando.*

Duke. Thou seest, we are not all alone unhappy:
This wide and universal theatre
Presents more woful pageants than the scene
Wherein we play in.

Jaques.   All the world's a stage,
And all the men and women merely players:
They have their exits, and their entrances;
And one man, in his time, plays many parts,
His acts being seven ages. At first the infant,
Mewling and puking in the nurse's arms.
And then the whining school-boy, with his satchel,
And shining morning face, creeping like snail,
Unwillingly to school. And then the lover,
Sighing like furnace, with a woful ballad
Made to his mistress' eyebrow. Then the soldier,

Full of strange oaths, and bearded like the pard,
Jealous in honour, sudden and quick in quarrel,
Seeking the bubble, reputation,
Even in the cannon's mouth. And then the justice,
In fair round body with good capon lined,
With eyes severe, and beard of formal cut,
Full of wise saws and modern instances ;
And so he plays his part. The sixth age shifts
Into the lean and slippered pantaloon,
With spectacles on nose and pouch on side ;
His youthful hose, well saved, a world too wide
For his shrunk shank ; and his big, manly voice,
Turning again toward childish treble, pipes
And whistles in his sound. Last scene of all,
That ends this strange eventful history,
Is second childishness, and mere oblivion ;
Sans teeth, sans eyes, sans taste, sans everything.

Re-enter ORLANDO, *with* ADAM.

Duke. Welcome ! Set down your venerable burden,
And let him eat.

Orlan. I thank you most for him.

Adam. So had you need ;
I scarce can speak to thank you for myself.

Duke. Welcome ! fall to : I will not trouble you
As yet, to question you about your fortunes.—
Give us some music ; and, good cousin, sing.

SONG.

Blow, blow, thou winter wind,
Thou art not so unkind
  As man's ingratitude !
Thy tooth is not so keen,
Because thou art not seen,
  Although thy breath be rude.

Freeze, freeze, thou bitter sky,
Thou dost not bite so nigh
  As benefits forgot ;

> Though thou the waters warp,
> Thy sting is not so sharp
> As friend remembered not.

Duke. If that you are the good Sir Rowland's son,
As you have whispered faithfully you are,
Be truly welcome hither: I am the Duke
That loved your father. The residue of your fortune,
Go to my cave and tell me.—Good old man,
Thou art right welcome, as thy master is.—
Support him by the arm.—Give me your hand,
And let me all your fortunes understand. [*Exeunt.*

Enter TOUCHSTONE *and* SHEPHERD.

Shep. And how like you this shepherd's life, Master Touchstone?

Touch. Truly, shepherd, in respect of itself, it is a good life; but in respect that it is a shepherd's life, it is naught. In respect that it is solitary, I like it very well; but in respect that it is private, it is a very vile life. Now, in respect it is in the fields, it pleaseth me well; but in respect it is not in the court, it is tedious. Hast any philosophy in thee, shepherd?

Shep. No more but that I know the more one sickens, the worse at ease he is; and that he that wants money, means, and content, is without three good friends: that the property of rain is to wet, and fire to burn: that good pasture makes fat sheep: and that a great cause of the night is lack of the sun.

Touch. Such a one is a natural philosopher. Wast ever at court, shepherd?

Shep. No, truly: I earn that I eat, get that I wear, owe no man hate, envy no man's happiness, am glad of other men's good, content with my harm. Give you good-day, Master Touchstone. [*Exit Shepherd.*

Enter ROSALIND (*reading*).

> "From the east to western Ind,
> No jewel is like Rosalind.
> Her worth, being mounted on the wind,

Through all the world bears Rosalind.
All the pictures fairest lined,
Are but black to Rosalind.
Let no fair be kept in mind
But the fair of Rosalind."

Touch. I'll rhyme you so eight years together, dinners, and suppers, and sleeping-hours excepted.

Ros. Out, fool!

Touch. For a taste :—

If a hart do lack a hind,
Let him seek out Rosalind.
If the cat will after kind,
So, be sure, will Rosalind.
They that reap must sheaf and bind,
Then to cart with Rosalind.
Sweetest nut hath sourest rind,
Such a nut is Rosalind.
He that sweetest rose will find,
Ti tum—ti tum—Rosalind.

Ros. Peace, you dull fool! I found them on a tree.

Touch. Truly, the tree yields bad fruit.

Ros. Peace!

Here comes my sister, reading. Stand aside!

Enter CELIA *(reading).*

" Why should this a desert be ?
For it is unpeopled ? No ;
Tongues I'll hang on every tree,
That shall civil sayings show.
Some of violated vows
'Twixt the souls of friend and friend ;
But upon the fairest boughs,
Or at every sentence end,
Will I Rosalinda write ;
Teaching all that read, to know

The quintessence of every sprite
Heaven would in little show.
Helen's cheek, but not her heart;
Cleopatra's majesty;
Atalanta's better part;
Sad Lucretia's modesty.
Heaven would that she these gifts should have,
And I to live and die her slave!"

Ros. O most gentle pulpiter! what tedious homily of love have you wearied your parishioners withal, and never cried, "Have patience, good people!"

Celia. Didst thou hear these verses?

Ros. Oh yes, I heard them all, and more too; for some of them had in them more feet than the verses would bear.

Celia. But didst thou hear, without wondering, how thy name should be hanged and carved upon these trees?

Ros. I was seven of the nine days out of the wonder, before you came; for look here what I found on a palm-tree.

Celia. Trow you who hath done this?

Ros. I pr'ythee, who?

Celia. Is it possible—

Ros. Nay, I pr'ythee now, with most petitionary vehemence, tell me who it is?

Celia. Oh, wonderful, wonderful! and most wonderful, wonderful! and, yet again, wonderful!

Ros. I pr'ythee, tell me who it is? quickly and apace.

Celia. It is young Orlando.

Ros. Orlando?

Celia. Orlando.

Ros. What did he when thou sawest him? What said he? How looked he? What makes he here? Did he ask for me? Where remains he? How parted he with thee? and when shalt thou see him again? Answer me in one word.

Celia. To say "ay," and "no," to these particulars, is more than to answer in a catechism.

Ros. Doth he know that I am in this forest? Looks he as freshly as he did the day he wrestled?

Celia. It is as easy to count atomies as to resolve the propositions of a lover. I found him under an oak tree; there lay he, stretched along, like a wounded knight. He was furnished like a hunter.

Ros. Oh, ominous! he comes to kill my heart.

Celia. I would sing my song without a burden: thou bringest me out of tune. Soft, comes he not here?

Ros. 'Tis he: slink by, and note him. [*They retire.*

Enter ORLANDO *and* JAQUES.

Jaques. I thank you for your company; but, good faith, I had as lief have been myself alone.

Orlan. And so had I; but yet, for fashion sake, I thank you too for your society.

Jaques. Heaven be with you! let's meet as little as we can.

Orlan. I do desire we may be better strangers.

Jaques. I pray you, mar no more trees with writing love-songs on their barks.

Orlan. I pray you, mar no more of my verses with reading them ill-favouredly.

Jaques. Rosalind is your love's name?

Orlan. Yes, just.

Jaques. I do not like her name.

Orlan. There was no thought of pleasing you when she was christened.

Jaques. What stature is she of?

Orlan. Just as high as my heart.

Jaques. You are full of pretty answers. Will you sit down with me? and we two will rail against the world and all our misery.

Orlan. I will chide no breather in the world but myself, against whom I know most faults.

Jaques. The worst fault you have is to be in love.

Orlan. 'Tis a fault I would not change for your best virtue. I am weary of you.

Jaques. I was seeking for a fool, when I found you.

Orlan. He is drowned in the brook: look but in, and you shall see him.

Jaques. There I shall see mine own figure.

Orlan. Which I take to be either a fool or a cypher.

Jaques. I'll tarry no longer with you: farewell, good Signior Love. [*Exit Jaques.*

Orlan. I'm glad of your departure; adieu, good Monsieur Melancholy!

Ros. I will speak to him like a saucy lackey, and under that habit play the knave with him.—Do you hear, forester?

Orlan. Very well; what would you?

Ros. I pray you, what is't o'clock?

Orlan. You should ask me what time o' day; there's no clock in the forest.

Ros. Then there is no true lover in the forest; else sighing every minute, and groaning every hour, would detect the lazy foot of Time as well as a clock.

Orlan. And why not the swift foot of Time? had not that been as proper?

Ros. By no means, sir: Time travels in divers paces with divers persons. I'll tell you who Time ambles withal, who Time trots withal, who Time gallops withal, and who he stands still withal.

Orlan. I pr'ythee, who doth he trot withal?

Ros. Marry, he trots hard with a young maid between the contract of her marriage and the day it is solemnized: if the interim be but a se'nnight, Time's pace is so hard that it seems the length of seven years.

Orlan. Who ambles Time withal?

Ros. With a priest that lacks Latin, and a rich man that hath not the gout; for the one sleeps easily because he cannot study, and the other lives merrily because he feels no pain. These Time ambles withal.

Orlan. Who doth he gallop withal?

Ros. With a thief to the gallows; for, though he go as softly as foot can fall, he thinks himself too soon there.

Orlan. Who stays he still withal?

Ros. With lawyers in the vacation; for they sleep between term and term, and then they perceive not how Time moves.

Orlan. Where dwell you, pretty youth?

Ros. With yon shepherdess, my sister; here, in the skirts of the forest, like fringe upon a petticoat.

Orlan. Your accent is somewhat finer than you could purchase in so removed a dwelling.

Ros. I have been told so of many; but, indeed, an old religious uncle of mine taught me to speak, who was, in his youth, an inland man; one that knew courtship too well, for there he fell in love. I have heard him read many lectures against it; and I thank heaven I am not a woman, to be touched with so many giddy offences as he hath generally taxed their whole sex withal.

Orlan. Can you remember any of the principal evils that he laid to the charge of women?

Ros. They were none principal; they were all like one another, as half-pence are; every one fault seeming monstrous till his fellow-fault came to match it.

Orlan. I pr'ythee, recount some of them.

Ros. No; I will not cast away my physic, but on those that are sick. There is a man haunts the forest, that abuses our young plants with carving Rosalind on their barks; hangs odes upon hawthorns and elegies on brambles; all, forsooth, deifying the name of Rosalind. If I could meet that fancy-monger, I would give him some good counsel, for he seems to have the quotidian of love upon him.

Orlan. I am he that is so love-shaked; I pray you, tell me your remedy.

Ros. There is none of my uncle's marks upon you: he

taught me how to know a man in love; in which cage of rushes I am sure you are not prisoner.

Orlan. What were his marks?

Ros. A lean cheek, which you have not; a blue eye, and sunken, which you have not; an unquestionable spirit, which you have not; a beard neglected, which you have not: but I pardon you for that; for, simply your having in beard is a younger brother's revenue. Then your hose should be ungartered, your bonnet unbanded, your sleeve unbuttoned, your shoe untied, and everything about you demonstrating a careless desolation. But you are no such man; you are rather point-device in your accoutrements—as loving yourself, than seeming the lover of any other.

Orlan. Fair youth, I would I could make thee believe I love!

Ros. Me believe it! you may as soon make her that you love believe it; which, I warrant, she is apter to do than confess she does. But, in good sooth, are you he that hangs the verses on the trees, wherein Rosalind is so admired.

Orlan. I swear to thee, youth, by the white hand of Rosalind, I am that he, that unfortunate he.

Ros. But are you so much in love as your rhymes speak?

Orlan. Neither rhyme nor reason can express how much.

Ros. Love is merely a madness; and, I tell you, deserves as well a dark house and a whip as madmen do: and the reason why they are not so punished and cured is, that the lunacy is so ordinary, the whippers are in love too. Yet I profess curing it by counsel.

Orlan. Did you ever cure any so?

Ros. Yes, one; and in this manner. He was to imagine me his love, his mistress; and I set him every day to woo me: at which time would I, being but a moonish youth, grieve—be effeminate—changeable—longing, and liking; proud, fantastical—apish, shallow, inconstant—full of tears—full of smiles; for every passion something, and for no passion truly anything, as boys and women are, for the most part, cattle of this colour:

would now like him, now loathe him; then entertain him, then forswear him; now weep for him, then spit at him; that I drave my suitor from his mad humour of love to a living humour of madness; which was, to forswear the full stream of the world, and live in a nook merely monastic. And thus I cured him; and this way will I take upon me to cure you.

Orlan. I would not be cured, youth.

Ros. I would cure you, if you would but call me Rosalind, and come every day to my cote and woo me.

Orlan. Now, by the faith of my love, I will! Tell me where it is.

Ros. Go with me to it, and I'll show it you; and, by the way, you shall tell me where in the forest you live. Will you go?

Orlan. With all my heart, good youth.

Ros. Nay, you must call me Rosalind. [*Exeunt.*

Enter ROSALIND *and* CELIA, *meeting* OLIVER.

Oliver. Good-morrow! pray you, if you know,
Where, in the purlieus of this forest, stands
A sheep-cote, fenced about with olive trees?

Celia. West of this place, by the murmuring stream.
But, at this hour, the house doth keep itself,—
There's none within.

Oliver. If that an eye may profit by a tongue,
Then should I know you by description:
                              Are not you
The owner of the house I did inquire for?

Celia. It is no boast, being asked, to say we are.

Oliver. Orlando doth commend him to you both;
And to you he calls his Rosalind
He sends this kerchief. Are you he?

Ros. I am. What must we understand by this?

Oliver. Some of my shame: if you will know of me
What man I am, and how, and why, and where
This handkerchief was stained.

Celia. I pray you, tell it.
Oliver. When last the young Orlando parted from you,
He left a promise to return again
Within an hour, and pacing through the forest,
Chewing the food of sweet and bitter fancy,
Lo, what befell! he threw his eye aside,
And, mark, what object did present itself!
Under an oak, whose boughs were mossed with age,
A wretched man lay sleeping.
About his neck a green and gilded snake had wreathed itself;
But suddenly, seeing Orlando, it unlinked itself,
And, with indented glides, did slip away
Into a bush: under which bush's shade
A lioness lay couching, head on ground, with cat-like watch,
When that the sleeping man should stir; for 'tis
The royal disposition of that beast
To prey on nothing that doth seem as dead:
This seen, Orlando did approach the man,
And found it was his brother, his elder brother.
Ros. I have heard him speak of that same brother;
And he did render him the most unnatural
That lived 'mongst men.
Oliver. And well he might so do,
For well I know he was unnatural.
Ros. But to Orlando:—did he leave him there,
Food to the hungry lioness?
Oliver. Twice did he turn his back, and purposed so:
But kindness, nobler ever than revenge,
Made him give battle to the lioness,
Who quickly fell before him; then
From miserable slumber I awaked.
Celia. Are you his brother?
Ros. Was it you he rescued?
Celia. Was't you that did so oft contrive to kill him?
Oliver. 'Twas I, but 'tis not I. I do not shame

To tell you what I was, since my conversion
So sweetly tastes, being the thing I am.
   Ros. But, the handkerchief?
   Oliver.   By-and-by.—Here upon his arm
The lioness had torn some flesh away,
Which all this while had bled : then he fainted,
And cried, in fainting, upon Rosalind.
Brief, I recovered him ; bound up his wound ;
And, after some small space,
He sent me hither, stranger as I am,
To tell this story, that you might excuse
His broken promise ; and to give this kerchief,
Dyed in his blood, unto the shepherd youth
That he in sport doth call his Rosalind.   [*Rosalind faints.*
   Celia. Why, how now, Ganymede! sweet Ganymede!
   Oliver. Many will swoon when they do look on blood.
   Celia. There is more in it.—Cousin!—Ganymede!
   Ros. I would I were at home!
   Oliver. Be of good cheer, youth.—You a man!
You lack a man's heart.

   Ros. I do so, I confess it. Ah, sir, a body would think this was well counterfeited. I pray you, tell your brother how well I counterfeited. Heigh-ho!

   Oliver. This was not counterfeit : there is too great testimony in your complexion that it was a passion of earnest.

   Ros. Counterfeit, I assure you.

   Oliver. Well, then, take a good heart, and counterfeit to be a man.

   Ros. So I do : but, i' faith, I should have been a woman by right.

   Celia. Come, you look paler and paler ; pray you, draw homewards.—Good sir, go with us.

   Oliver. That will I ; for I must bear answer back how you excuse my brother.

   Ros. I shall devise something : but, I pray you, commend my counterfeiting to him.   [*Exeunt.*

Enter TOUCHSTONE *and* AUDREY.

Touch. Audrey, there is a youth here in the forest lays claim to you.

Aud. Ay, I know who 'tis; he hath no interest in me in the world: here comes the man you mean.

Touch. It is meat and drink to me to see a clown.

Enter WILLIAM.

Wil. Good-even, Audrey.

Aud. Give ye good-even, William.

Wil. And good-even to you, sir.

Touch. Good-even, gentle friend. Cover thy head, cover thy head; nay, pr'ythee, be covered. How old are you, friend?

Wil. Five-and-twenty, sir.

Touch. A ripe age. Is thy name William?

Wil. William, sir.

Touch. A fair name. Wast born i' the forest here?

Wil. Ay, sir, I thank heaven!

Touch. "Thank heaven!" a good answer. Art rich?

Wil. 'Faith, sir, so so.

Touch. "So so" is good; very good; very excellent good—and yet it is not; it is but so so. Art thou wise?

Wil. Ay, sir, I have a pretty wit.

Touch. Why, thou sayest well. I do now remember a saying: "The fool doth think he is wise, but the wise man knows himself to be a fool." The heathen philosopher, when he had a desire to eat a grape, would open his lips when he put it into his mouth; meaning thereby, that grapes were made to eat, and lips to open. You do love this maid?

Wil. I do, sir.

Touch. Give me your hand. Art thou learnèd?

Wil. No, sir.

Touch. Then learn this of me:—to have is to have; for it is a figure in rhetoric that drink, being poured out of a cup into a glass, by filling the one doth empty the other; for all your writers do consent that *ipse* is he: now, you are not *ipse*, for I am he.

Wil. Which he, sir?

Touch. He, sir, that must marry this woman. Therefore, you clown—abandon—which is in the vulgar, leave—the society—which in the boorish is, company—of this female—which in the common is, woman; which together is, abandon the society of this female, or, clown, thou perishest; or, to thy better understanding, diest; or, to wit, I kill thee, make thee away, translate thy life unto death, thy liberty into bondage: I will deal in poison with thee, or in bastinado, or in steel; I will bandy with thee in faction; I will o'errun thee with policy; I will kill thee a hundred and fifty ways: therefore tremble, and depart. [*Exit William.*

Touch. Trip, Audrey! trip! [*Exeunt.*

Enter ORLANDO *and* OLIVER.

Orlan. Is't possible, that on so little acquaintance you should like her? that, but seeing, you should love her? and loving, woo? and wooing, she should grant?

Oliver. Neither call the giddiness of it in question, the small acquaintance, my sudden wooing, nor her sudden consenting; but say with me, I love Aliena; say with her, that she loves me; consent with both: it shall be to your good; for my father's house, and all the revenue that was old Sir Rowland's, will I estate upon you, and here live and die a shepherd.

Orlan. Let your wedding be to-morrow: thither will I invite the Duke and all his followers. Go you, and prepare Aliena; for, look you, here comes my Rosalind!

Enter ROSALIND.

Ros. Heaven save you, brother!

Oliver. And you, fair sister. [*Exit Oliver.*

Ros. O my dear Orlando! how it grieves me to see thee wear thy heart in a scarf!

Orlan. It is my arm.

Ros. I thought thy heart had been wounded with the claws of a lion.

Orlan. Wounded it is, but with the eyes of a lady.

Ros. Did your brother tell you how I counterfeited to swoon when he showed me your handkerchief?

Orlan. Ay, and greater wonders than that.

Ros. Oh, I know where you are. Nay, 'tis true: there was never anything so sudden.

Orlan. They shall be married to-morrow, and I will bid the Duke to the nuptial. But oh, how bitter a thing it is to look into happiness through another man's eyes! By so much the more shall I, to-morrow, be at the height of heart-heaviness; by how much I shall think my brother happy in having what he wishes for.

Ros. Why, then, to-morrow I cannot serve your turn for Rosalind?

Orlan. I can live no longer by thinking.

Ros. I will weary you, then, no longer with idle talking. Know of me, then (for now I speak to some purpose), that I can do strange things: I have, since I was three years old, conversed with a magician, most profound in art. If you do love Rosalind so near the heart as your gesture cries it out, when your brother marries Aliena, shall you marry her: I know into what straits of fortune she is driven; and it is not impossible to me, if it appear not inconvenient to you, to set her before your eyes, human as she is, and without any danger.

Orlan. Speakest thou in sober meanings?

Ros. By my life, I do! Therefore, put you in your best array; bid your friends; for, if you will be married to-morrow, you shall, and to Rosalind, if you will. So fare you well.

[*Exeunt.*

Enter DUKE *and* ORLANDO.

Duke. Dost thou believe, Orlando, that the boy
Can do all this that he hath promisèd?

Orlan. I sometimes do believe, and sometimes do not;

As those that fear they hope, and know they fear.
 Duke. I do remember in this shepherd boy
Some lively touches of my daughter's favour.
 Orlan. My lord, the first time that I ever saw him
Methought he was a brother to your daughter.

Enter JAQUES.

Jaques. There is, sure, another flood toward, and these couples are coming to the ark.

Enter TOUCHSTONE *and* AUDREY.

Touch. Salutation and greeting to you all.

Jaques. Good, my lord, bid him welcome. This is the motley-minded gentleman that I have so often met in the forest: he hath been a courtier, he swears.

Touch. I have trod a measure; I have flattered a lady; I have been politic with my friend, smooth with mine enemy; I have undone three tailors; I have had four quarrels, and like to have fought one.

Jaques. And how was that ta'en up?

Touch. 'Faith, we met, and found the quarrel was upon the seventh cause.

Jaques. How did you find the quarrel on the seventh cause?

Touch. Upon a lie seven times removed :—bear your body more seeming, Audrey :—as thus, sir. I did dislike the cut of a certain courtier's beard; he sent me word, if I said his beard was not cut well, he was in the mind it was: this is called the Retort Courteous. If I sent him word again, "it was not well cut;" he would send me word, he cut it to please himself: this is called the Quip Modest. If again, "it was not well cut," he disabled my judgment: this is called the Reply Churlish. If again, "it was not well cut," he would answer, I spake not true: this is called the Reproof Valiant. If again, "it was not well cut," he would say, I lied. This is called the Countercheck quarrelsome; and, so, to the Lie Circumstantial, and the Lie Direct.

Jaques. And how oft did you say his beard was not well cut?

Touch. I durst go no further than the Lie Circumstantial, nor he durst not give me the Lie Direct; and so we measured swords, and parted.

Jaques. Can you nominate in order now the degrees of the lie?

Touch. Oh, sir, we quarrel in print, by the book; as you have books for good manners. I will name you the degrees. The first, the Retort Courteous; the second, the Quip Modest; the third, the Reply Churlish; the fourth, the Reproof Valiant; the fifth, the Countercheck Quarrelsome; the sixth, the Lie with Circumstance; the seventh, the Lie Direct. All these you may avoid, but the Lie Direct; and you may avoid that, too, with an "If." I knew when seven justices could not take up a quarrel; but when the parties were met themselves, one of them thought but of an "If," as—"If you said so, then I said so;" and they shook hands, and swore brothers. Your "If" is the only peacemaker; much virtue in "If."

Jaques. Is not this a rare fellow, my lord? he's good at anything, and yet a fool!

Duke. He uses his folly like a stalking-horse, and under the presentation of that he shoots his wit.

Enter JAQUES DE BOIS.

Jaq. de B. Let me have audience for a word or two.
I am the second son of old Sir Rowland,
That bring these tidings to this fair assembly:—
Duke Frederick, hearing how that every day
Men of great worth resorted to this forest,
Addressed a mighty power, which were on foot,
In his own conduct, purposely to take
His brother here, and put him to the sword:
And to the skirts of this wild wood he came;
Where, meeting with an old religious man,
After some question with him, was converted
Both from his enterprise and from the world:
His crown bequeathing to his banished brother,

And all their lands restored to them again
That were with him exiled:—This to be true,
I do engage my life!
 Duke.   Welcome, young man!
Thou offer'st fairly to thy brother's wedding.
     Enter ROSALIND, CELIA, *and* OLIVER.
 Ros. To you I give myself, for I am yours.—
To you I give myself, for I am yours.
 Duke. If there be truth in sight, you are my daughter!
 Orlan. If there be truth in sight, you are my Rosalind!
 Ros. I'll have no father, if you be not he.—
I'll have no husband, if you be not he.
 Duke. O my dear niece! welcome thou art to me!
Even daughter, welcome in no less degree!
First, in this forest, let us do those ends
That here were well begun, and well begot:
And after, every of this happy number
That have endured shrewd days and nights with us,
Shall share the good of our returnèd fortune,
According to the measure of their states.
Meantime, forget this new-fall'n dignity,
And fall into our rustic revelry.
 Jaques. Sir, by your patience: If I heard you rightly,
The Duke hath put on a religious life,
And thrown into neglect the pompous court?
 Jaques de B. He hath.
 Jaques. To him will I: out of these convertites
There is much matter to be heard and learned.—
So, to your pleasures;
I am for other than for dancing measures.
 Duke. Stay, Jaques, stay.
 Jaques. To see no pastime, I: what you would have,
I'll stay to know at your abandoned cave.   [*Exit Jaques.*
 Duke. Proceed, proceed; we will begin these rites,
As we do trust they'll end, in true delights.   SHAKESPEARE.

SELECTIONS FROM "PYGMALION AND GALATEA."

(*By permission of the Author.*)
Scene: *Pygmalion's Studio.*

I.

PYGMALION (a Sculptor), CYNISCA (his Wife), and GALATEA (a Marble Statue).

Cyn. It all but breathes! Now mark thou this, Pygmalion, while I'm away from thee: there stands my only representative, and I charge you, sir, be faithful unto her, as unto me. If thoughts of love should haply crowd on thee, there stands my other self; tell them to her—she'll listen well, *she* hath no temper, sir, and hath no tongue. Thou hast thy license, make good use of it: already I'm half jealous—p'sha! the thing is but a statue after all. Pygmalion, farewell!

Pyg. Farewell, Cynisca! [*Exit Cynisca.*] "The thing is but a statue after all!" Cynisca little thought that in these words she touched the key-note of my discontent. True, I have powers denied to other men. Give me a block of senseless marble; well, it shall contain a man, a woman, child—a dozen men and women, if I will. So far the gods and I run neck and neck. Nay, so far, I can beat them at their trade. I am no bungler; all the men I make are straight-limbed fellows, all my women goddesses, in outward form. But there's my tether: I can go so far, and go no further; at that point I stop. To curse the bonds that hold me sternly back, to curse the arrogance of those proud gods who say, thou shalt be greatest among men, and yet infinitesimally small.

Gal. Pygmalion!
Pyg. Who called?
Gal. Pygmalion!!
Pyg. Ye gods! I have my prayer.

Gal. Pygmalion !!!

Pyg. It speaks! It lives!! My Galatea breathes!!!

Gal. Where am I? Give me thy hand—both hands. How soft and warm. Whence came I?

Pyg. From yonder pedestal.

Gal. And where am I now?

Pyg. Born into the world, by miracle!

Gal. But how came I to be?

Pyg. Well, let me see—I modelled you in clay; my artisans then roughed you out in marble; I brought my artistic skill to bear on you, and made you what you are, in all but life. The gods they finished what I had begun, and gave the only gift I could not give—life.

Gal. Then, this is life?

Pyg. It is.

Gal. And not long since I was a cold, dull stone.

Pyg. And now thou art a woman, perfect in thy loveliness.

Gal. Am I a woman?

Pyg. There's no doubt of that.

Gal. Art thou a woman?

Pyg. No, I am a man.

Gal. What is a man?

Pyg. A being strongly framed to wait on woman,—to work and toil for her that she may rest; to fight and die for her that she may live.

Gal. And, for these, men work, and toil, and fight, and die?

Pyg. Man works for those he loves.

Gal. Then, by thy work, I know thou lovest me.

Pyg. Indeed, I love thee.

Gal. With what kind of love?

Pyg. I love thee, as a sculptor loves his work.

Gal. My love is different in kind to thine: I am no sculptor, and I've done no work,—yet I do love thee! Say, what love is mine?

SELECTIONS FROM "PYGMALION AND GALATEA."

Pyg. Tell me its symptoms, then I'll answer thee.

Gal. Its symptoms! Let me call them as they come: a sense that I am made by thee, for thee—that I have life, that I may live for thee—that I am thine—that thou and I are one. Say, what kind of love is that?

Pyg. A kind of love that I shall run some risk in dealing with.

Gal. And why, Pygmalion?

Pyg. Such love as thine a man may not receive, except from one who is, or is to be his wife.

Gal. Then *I* will be thy wife.

Pyg. That may not be; I have a wife.

Gal. And yet thou lovest me?

Pyg. Who could look on that fair face and stifle love?

Gal. Then I am beautiful?

Pyg. Indeed thou art.

Gal. I wish that I could look upon my face. But that's impossible.

Pyg. Not so. This mirror will reflect thy face.

Gal. How beautiful! Believe me, love, I could look in this mirror all day long. O happy maid! to be so passing fair; and happier still, Pygmalion, who can gaze at will upon so beautiful a face.

Pyg. Hush, Galatea! In thine innocence thou sayest things which others would reprove.

Gal. Then is it wrong to think that one is exquisitely beautiful?

Pyg. Well, it's a sentiment which every woman shares with thee; they think it, but they keep it to themselves.

Gal. Is thy wife within?

Pyg. No, she's not within.

Gal. But she'll come back?

Pyg. Oh yes, she will come back.

Gal. How pleased she'll be when she returns, to know that there was some one here to fill her place.

Pyg. Yes, she'll be *extremely* pleased.

Gal. There is something in thy voice which says that thou art jesting. Is it possible to say one thing and mean another?

Pyg. It's sometimes done.

Gal. How very wonderful! Teach me the art.

Pyg. The art will come in time. (*Aside:* Let me be brave, and put an end to this.) My wife will not be pleased. I may not love thee. I must send thee hence.

Gal. Was it for this that Heaven gave me life? Thou tellest me of one who claims thy love—that thou hast love for her alone. Alas! I know not of these things; I only know that Heaven, who sent me here, has given me one all-absorbing duty to discharge—to love thee, and to make thee love again.

Pyg. Galatea! it may not be. My sister shall provide thee with a home; her house is close at hand. [*Exeunt.*

II.

CHRYSOS (an Art Patron), DAPHNE (his Wife), PYGMALION, GALATEA, and CYNISCA.

Chry. Where is the statue that I saw last time?

Pyg. Oh, it's unfinished—a clumsy thing; I'm ashamed of it.

Chry. I know it isn't good. There's want of tone, air and motion, light and shade.

Daph. Bethink yourself, my dear; that's said of painting—this is sculpture.

Chry. Eh? it's the same thing, the principle's the same. Now for the cost; let's see. What will it weigh?—a ton or thereabouts? Suppose we say a thousand drachmas!

Pyg. No, no, my lord, the work wants tone; and then, remember, sir, the light and shade.

Chry. Oh, it's horrible! But never mind, although the thing is poor, 'twill do to hold a candle in my hall.

Pyg. Excuse me, sir; poor though that statue be, I value it beyond all price.

Chry. Young man, are you aware I gave but fifteen hundred for an Apollo twice as big as that?

Pyg. Pardon me, sir; a sculptor does not test the beauty of a figure by its bulk.

Daph. Young man, I'll not stay to hear my husband bullied. —My dear, I'll wait for you outside. [*Exit Daphne*

Chry. I tell ye, sir, I will not be denied.

Pyg. And I tell you, sir, the statue's not for sale.

[*Exit Pygmalion.*

Chry. Look here, young man. Why, the fellow's gone! If a patron of the arts is thus to be dictated to by art, what comes of that art patron's patronage? O upstart vanity of human kind! O pride of worms! O ponderosity of atoms! O substantiality of nothingness! He must be taught a lesson. Where's the statue? Why, it's gone! [*Enter Galatea.*] Bless us! what's this?

Gal. Are you unwell?

Chry. No, I'm not unwell. I only fancied—pooh, pooh! ridiculous! And yet—it's very like. I should know your face. Haven't I seen you in—

Gal. In marble? Very probably.

Chry. Oh, now I understand—Pygmalion's model.

Gal. Tell me, what are you?

Chry. What am I?

Gal. Yes; I mean, are you a man?

Chry. Well, I'm told so.

Gal. Then believe them not, they've been deceiving you.

Chry. Oh, indeed!

Gal. Yes. A man is tall, and straight, and strong, with big brave eyes, and tender voice. I've seen one.

Chry. Have you?

Gal. Yes. You are not a man.

Chry. D'ye take me for a woman?

Gal. A woman? No! a woman's soft, and weak, and exquisitely beautiful: I'm a woman. You are not like me: you are so round, and red, your eyes so small, your face so seared with lines; and then you are so little, and so fat.

Chry. This is a most peculiar girl.

Gal. How awkwardly you sit. Pygmalion does not sit like that; he always puts his arms around my waist.

Chry. Does he?

Gal. Yes; but you do not. Perhaps you don't know how?

Chry. Oh yes; I do know how.

Gal. Well! do it then.

Chry. It's a strange whim, but I'll humour her.

[*Enter Daphne.*

Daph. Can I believe my eyes! Who's this woman?

Chry. Calm yourself, my dear. You know the statue Galatea—it has come to life; behold it here!

Daph. Bah! D'ye think me mad? [*Enter Pygmalion.*] Young man, who is this woman?

Pyg. She is my statue, Galatea, come to life.

Chry. [*Aside to Pygmalion*] That's very good! go on, keep it up. [*Enter Cynisca.*

Cyn. I beg your pardon; I thought my husband was alone.

Daph. No doubt; I also thought *my* husband was alone.

Cyn. What's this? Impossible! and yet the statue's gone! Pygmalion!—canst thou not speak?

Gal. O madam! in every word, in every thought, he has obeyed thy wish. Thou bad'st him speak to me as unto thee, and he and I have sat as lovingly as if thou hadst been here.

Cyn. Pygmalion! Art thou dumb?

Gal. Bear with him, madam; he's not like this when he and I are sitting here alone: he has two voices, and two faces, madam.

Cyn. Thy wife against thine eyes. These are the stakes. Thou hast played thy game; and thou hast lost.

Pyg. Hear me, Cynisca! In an evil hour I prayed for power to give that statue life. My impious prayer aroused the outraged gods; they are my judges. Leave me in their hands; I have been false to them, but not to thee.—Spare me, Cynisca!

Cyn. Oh, pitiful adventurer! he dares to lose, but does not dare to pay. Hear me, ye gods! Ere I remember how I loved that man,—if he in thought or word hath been untrue—be just, and let him pay the penalty! [*Pygmalion is struck blind.*

Gal. O madam, pity him!

Cyn. I know no pity, woman! The act that thawed thee into flesh has hardened me into the stone from which thou cam'st. We have changed places: from this time forth be thou the wife, and I the senseless stone. W. S. GILBERT.

SACRED READINGS.

O GOD OF BETHEL.

O God of Bethel! by whose hand
    Thy people still are fed;
Who through this weary pilgrimage
    Hast all our fathers led:
Our vows, our pray'rs, we now present
    Before thy throne of grace:
God of our fathers! be the God
    Of their succeeding race.

Through each perplexing path of life
    Our wand'ring footsteps guide;
Give us each day our daily bread,
    And raiment fit provide.
O spread thy cov'ring wings around,
    Till all our wand'rings cease,
And at our Father's lov'd abode
    Our souls arrive in peace.

Such blessings from thy gracious hand
    Our humble pray'rs implore;
And thou shalt be our chosen God,
    And portion evermore.

PSALM C.

All people that on earth do dwell,
Sing to the Lord with cheerful voice.
Him serve with mirth, his praise forth tell,
Come ye before him, and rejoice.
Know that the Lord is God indeed;
Without our aid he did us make:
We are his flock, he doth us feed,
And for his sheep he doth us take.

O enter then his gates with praise!
Approach with joy his courts unto!
Praise, laud, and bless his name always,
For it is seemly so to do.
For why? the Lord our God is good,
His mercy is for ever sure;
His truth at all times firmly stood,
And shall from age to age endure.

PSALM XXIII.

The Lord is my shepherd; I shall not want. He maketh me to lie down in green pastures: he leadeth me beside the still waters. He restoreth my soul: he leadeth me in the paths of righteousness, for his name's sake. Yea, though I walk through the valley of the shadow of death, I will fear no evil: for thou art with me; thy rod and thy staff they comfort me. Thou preparest a table before me in the presence of mine enemies: thou anointest my head with oil; my cup runneth over. Surely goodness and mercy shall follow me all the days of my life: and I will dwell in the house of the Lord for ever.

ECCLESIASTES XII. 1-7.

Remember now thy Creator in the days of thy youth, while the evil days come not, nor the years draw nigh, when thou shalt say, I have no pleasure in them; while the sun, or the light, or the moon, or the stars, be not darkened, nor the clouds return after the rain: in the day when the keepers of the house shall tremble, and the strong men shall bow themselves, and the grinders cease because they are few, and those that look out of the windows be darkened, and the doors shall be shut in the streets, when the sound of the grinding is low, and he shall rise up at the voice of the bird, and all the daughters of music shall be brought low; also when they shall be afraid of that which is high, and fears shall be in the way, and the almond tree shall flourish, and the grasshopper shall be a burden, and desire shall fail: because man goeth to his long home, and the mourners go about the streets: or ever the silver cord be loosed, or the golden bowl be broken, or the pitcher be broken at the fountain, or the wheel broken at the cistern. Then shall the dust return to the earth as it was: and the spirit shall return unto God who gave it.

PART OF ISAIAH XL.

Comfort ye, comfort ye my people, saith your God. Speak ye comfortably to Jerusalem, and cry unto her, that her warfare is accomplished, that her iniquity is pardoned: for she hath received of the Lord's hand double for all her sins. The voice of him that crieth in the wilderness,

Prepare ye the way of the Lord, make straight in the desert a highway for our God.

Every valley shall be exalted, and every mountain and hill shall be made low: and the crooked shall be made straight, and the rough places plain: and the glory of the Lord shall be revealed, and all flesh shall see it together: for the mouth of the Lord hath spoken it. The voice said, Cry! And he said, What shall I cry? All flesh is grass, and all the goodliness thereof is as the flower of the field: the grass withereth, the flower fadeth, because the Spirit of the Lord bloweth upon it: surely the people is grass. The grass withereth, the flower fadeth: but the word of our God shall stand for ever. O Zion, that bringest good tidings, get thee up into the high mountain; O Jerusalem, that bringest good tidings, lift up thy voice with strength; lift it up, be not afraid; say unto the cities of Judah, Behold your God!

Behold, the Lord God will come with strong hand, and his arm shall rule for him: behold, his reward is with him, and his work before him.

He shall feed his flock like a shepherd: he shall gather the lambs with his arm, and carry them in his bosom, and shall gently lead those that are with young. Who hath measured the waters in the hollow of his hand, and meted out heaven with the span, and comprehended the dust of the earth in a measure, and weighed the mountains in scales, and the hills in a balance? All nations before him are as nothing; and they are counted to him less than nothing, and vanity. To whom then will ye liken me, or shall I be equal? saith the Holy One. Hast thou not known? hast thou not heard, that the everlasting God, the Lord, the Creator of the ends of the earth, fainteth not, neither is weary? there is no searching of his understanding. He giveth power to the faint; and to them that have no might he increaseth strength. Even the youths shall faint and be weary, and the young men shall utterly fall: but they that wait upon the Lord shall renew their strength; they shall mount up with wings as eagles; they shall run, and not be weary; and they shall walk, and not faint.

LUKE XV. 11-32.

And he said, A certain man had two sons: and the younger of them said to his father, Father, give me the portion of goods that falleth to me. And he divided unto them his living. And not many days after, the younger son gathered all together, and took his journey into a far country; and there wasted his substance with riotous living. And when he had spent all, there arose a mighty famine in that land; and he began to be in want. And he went and joined himself to a citizen of that country; and he sent him into his fields to feed swine. And he would fain have filled his belly with the husks that the swine did eat: and no man gave unto him. And when he came to himself, he said, How many hired servants of my father's have bread enough, and to spare, and I perish with hunger! I will arise, and go to my father, and will say unto him, Father, I have sinned against heaven, and before thee, and am no more worthy to be called thy son: make me as one of thy hired servants. And he arose, and came to his father. But when he was yet a great way off, his father saw him, and had compassion, and ran, and fell on his neck, and kissed him. And the son said unto him, Father, I have sinned against heaven, and in thy sight, and am no more worthy to be called thy son. But the father said to his servants, Bring forth the best robe, and put it on him; and put a ring on his hand, and shoes on his feet: and bring hither the fatted calf, and kill it;

and let us eat and be merry : for this my son was dead, and is alive again; he was lost, and is found. And they began to be merry. Now his elder son was in the field : and as he came and drew nigh to the house, he heard music and dancing. And he called one of the servants, and asked what these things meant. And he said unto him, Thy brother is come; and thy father hath killed the fatted calf, because he hath received him safe and sound. And he was angry, and would not go in : therefore came his father out, and entreated him. And he answering said to his father, Lo, these many years do I serve thee, neither transgressed I at any time thy commandment : and yet thou never gavest me a kid, that I might make merry with my friends : but as soon as this thy son was come, which hath devoured thy living with harlots, thou hast killed for him the fatted calf. And he said unto him, Son, thou art ever with me, and all that I have is thine. It was meet that we should make merry, and be glad; for this thy brother was dead, and is alive again; and was lost, and is found.

1 CORINTHIANS XIII.

Though I speak with the tongues of men and of angels, and have not charity, I am become as sounding brass, or a tinkling cymbal. And though I have the gift of prophecy, and understand all mysteries, and all knowledge; and though I have all faith, so that I could remove mountains, and have not charity, I am nothing. And though I bestow all my goods to feed the poor, and though I give my body to be burned, and have not charity, it profiteth me nothing. Charity suffereth long, and is kind; charity envieth not; charity vaunteth not itself, is not puffed up, doth not behave itself unseemly, seeketh not her own, is not easily provoked, thinketh no evil; rejoiceth not in iniquity, but rejoiceth in the truth; beareth all things, believeth all things, hopeth all things, endureth all things. Charity never faileth : but whether there be prophecies, they shall fail; whether there be tongues, they shall cease; whether there be knowledge, it shall vanish away. For we know in part, and we prophesy in part. But when that which is perfect is come, then that which is in part shall be done away. When I was a child, I spake as a child, I understood as a child, I thought as a child: but when I became a man, I put away childish things. For now we see through a glass, darkly; but then face to face : now I know in part; but then shall I know, even as also I am known. And now abideth faith, hope, charity, these three; but the greatest of these is charity

LEAD, KINDLY LIGHT!

Lead, kindly Light! amid the encircling gloom,
 Lead thou me on;
The night is dark, and I am far from home,
 Lead thou me on;

Keep thou my feet; I do not ask to see
The distant scene; one step, enough for me.

I was not ever thus, nor prayed that thou
  Shouldst lead me on;
I loved to choose and see my path; but now
  Lead thou me on;
I loved the garish day, and, spite of fears,
Pride ruled my will—remember not past years.

So long thy power has blest me, sure it still
  Will lead me on
O'er moor and fen, o'er crag and torrent, till
  The night is gone;
And with the morn, those angel-faces smile,
Which I have loved long since, and lost awhile.
J. H. NEWMAN.

THE COMFORTER.

Our blest Redeemer, ere he breathed
  His tender, last farewell,
A Guide, a Comforter, bequeathed
  With us to dwell.

He came sweet influence to impart,
  A gracious, willing guest,

While he can find one humble heart
    Wherein to rest.

And his that gentle voice we hear,
    Soft as the breath of even,
That checks each thought, that calms each fear,
    And speaks of Heaven.

And every virtue we possess,
    And every conquest won,
And every thought of holiness,
    Are his alone.

Spirit of purity and grace,
    Our weakness, pitying, see;
O make our hearts thy dwelling-place,
    And worthier thee.

O praise the Father; praise the Son;
    Blest Spirit, praise to thee;
All praise to God, the Three in One,
    The One in Three.

H. AUBER.

ADDITIONAL STUDIES IN ELOCUTION.

POETRY.

THE MOUSE.

I'M only a poor little mouse, ma'am!
I live in a wall of your house, ma'am!
With a fragment of cheese, and a very few peas,
I was having a little carouse, ma'am!

No mischief at all I intended, ma'am!
I hope you will act as my friend, ma'am!
If my life you should take, many hearts it would break,
And the trouble would be without end, ma'am!

My wife lives in there in the crack, ma'am!
She's waiting for me to come back, ma'am,
She hoped I might find a bit of a rind,
For the children their dinner do lack, ma'am!

'Tis hard living there in the wall, ma'am!
For plaster and mortar will pall, ma'am,
On the minds of the young, and when specially
Hungry, upon their poor father they'll fall, ma'am!

I never was given to strife, ma'am!
(Don't look at that terrible knife, ma'am!)

The noise overhead that disturbs you in bed,
'Tis the rats, I will venture my life, ma'am!

In your eyes I see mercy, I'm sure, ma'am!
Oh, there's no need to open the door, ma'am!
I'll slip through the crack, and I'll never come back,
Oh, I'll never come back any more, ma'am.

THE DEAD DOLL.

You needn't be trying to comfort me; I tell you my dolly is dead!
There's no use in saying she isn't, with a crack like that in her head.
It's just like you said it wouldn't hurt much to have my tooth out that day;
And then, when the man 'most pulled my head off, you hadn't a word to say.

You surely must think I'm a baby, when you say you can mend it with glue!
As if I didn't know better than that! Why, just suppose it was you.
You might make her look all mended; but what do I care for looks?
Why, glue's for chairs and tables, and toys, and the backs of books!

My dolly, my own little daughter! Oh, but it's the awfullest crack!
It makes me sick to think of the sound when her poor little head went whack
Against that horrible brass thing that holds up the little shelf.
Now, Nursey, what makes you remind me? I know that I did it myself!

I think you must be crazy—you'll get her another head!
What good would forty heads do her? I tell you my dolly is dead!

And to think I hadn't quite finished her elegant new spring hat!
And I took a sweet ribbon of hers last night to tie on that horrid cat!

When my mamma gave me that ribbon—I was playing in the yard—
She said to me most expressly, "Here's a ribbon for Hildegarde."
And I went and put it on Tabby, and Hildegarde saw me do it;
But I said to myself, "Oh, never mind, I don't believe she knew it."

But I know that she knew it now, and I just believe, I do,
That her poor little heart was broken, and so her head broke too.
Oh, my baby, my little baby! I wish my head had been hit!
For I've hit it over and over, and it hasn't cracked a bit.

But since the darling is dead, she'll want to be buried, of course:
We will take my little waggon, Nurse, and you shall be the horse;
And I'll walk behind and cry, and we'll put her in this, you see—
This dear little box, and we'll bury her then, under the maple tree.

And papa will make me a tombstone, like the one he made for my bird;
And he'll put what I tell him on it—yes, every single word!
I shall say—"Here lies Hildegarde, a beautiful doll, who is dead;
She died of a broken heart, and a dreadful crack in her head."

American Magazine.

SOMEBODY'S MOTHER.

The woman was old, and ragged, and gray,
And bent with the chill of the winter's day;
The street was wet with a recent snow,
And the woman's feet were aged and slow.

She stood at the crossing and waited long,
Alone, uncared for, amid the throng
Of human beings who passed her by,
Nor heeded the glance of her anxious eye.

Down the street, with laughter and shout,
Glad in the freedom of "school let out."
Came the boys, like a flock of sheep,
Hailing the snow piled white and deep.

Past the woman so old and gray
Hastened the children on their way,
Nor offered a helping hand to her,
So meek, so timid, afraid to stir,

Lest the carriage wheels or the horses' feet
Should crowd her down in the slippery street.
At last came one of the merry troop—
The gayest laddie of all the group;

He paused beside her, and whispered low,
"I'll help you across, if you wish to go."
Her aged hand on his strong young arm
She placed, and so, without hurt or harm,

He guided the trembling feet along,
Proud that his own were firm and strong.
Then back again to his friends he went,
His young heart happy and well content.

"She's somebody's mother, boys, you know,
For all she's aged, and poor, and slow;
And I hope some fellow will lend a hand
To help *my* mother, you understand,
If ever she's poor, and old, and gray,
When her own dear boy is far away."

And " somebody's mother " bowed low her head
In her home that night, and the prayer she said
Was, " God, be kind to the noble boy,
Who is somebody's son, and pride, and joy!"

GUILTY, OR NOT GUILTY?

She stood at the bar of justice, a creature wan and wild,
In form too small for a woman, in feature too old for a child;
For a look so worn and pathetic was stamped on her poor young face,
It seemed long years of suffering must have left that silent trace.
" Your name," said the judge, as he eyed her, with kindly look, yet keen,
" Is—" " Mary Maguire, if you please, sir." " And your age?" "I am turned fifteen."
" Well, Mary,"—and then from a paper he slowly and gravely read,—
" You are charged here—I am sorry to say it—with stealing three loaves of bread.
You look not like an old offender, and I hope that you can show
The charge to be false. Now, tell me, are you guilty of this, or no?"
A passionate burst of weeping was at first her sole reply;
But she dried her tears in a moment, and looked in the judge's eye.
" I will tell you just how it was, sir:—My father and mother are dead,
And my little brothers and sisters were hungry, and asked me for bread.
At first I earned it for them, by working hard all day,
But somehow the times were hard, sir, and the work all fell away.

I could get no more employment; the weather was bitter cold;
The young ones cried and shivered (little Johnnie's but four years old);—
So what was I to do, sir? I am guilty, but do not condemn;
I *took*—oh! was it *stealing?*—the bread to give to them."
Every man in the court-room—gray-beard and thoughtless youth—
Knew, as he looked upon her, that the prisoner spoke the truth.
Out from their pockets came 'kerchiefs, out from their eyes sprung tears,
And out from old, faded wallets treasures hoarded for years.
The judge's face was a study, the strangest you ever saw,
As he cleared his throat and murmured *something* about the *law;*
For one so learned in such matters, so wise in dealing with men,
He seemed, on a simple question, sorely puzzled just then.
But no one blamed him, or wondered when at last these words they heard:
"The sentence of this young prisoner is for the present deferred."
And no one blamed him or wondered when he went to her and smiled,
And tenderly led from the court-room, himself, the "guilty" child.
　　　　　　　　　　　　　　　　　　　　ANON.

"NAY; I'LL STAY WITH THE LAD."

 Six hundred souls one summer's day
  Worked in the deep, dark Hutton seams;
 Men were hewing the coal away,
  Boys were guiding the loaded teams.

"NAY; I'LL STAY WITH THE LAD."

Horror of darkness was everywhere—
  It was coal above, and coal below;
Only the miner's guarded lamp
  Made in the gloom a passing glow.

Down in the deep, black Hutton seams
  There came a flowery, balmy breath;[*]
Men dropped their tools, and left their teams—
  They knew the balmy air meant death—
And fled before the earthquake shock,
  The cruel fire-damp's fatal course,
That tore apart the roof and walls,
  And buried by fifties man and horse.

"The shaft! the shaft!" they wildly cried;
  And as they ran they passed a cave
Where stood a father by his son—
  The child had found a living grave,
And lay among the shattered coal,
  His little life had almost sped.
"Fly, fly! for there may yet be time!"
  The father calmly, firmly said:
    "Nay; I'll stay with the lad."

He had no hurt—he yet might reach
  The blessed sun and light again;
But at his feet his child lay bound,
  And every hope of help was vain.
He let deliverance pass him by,
  He stooped and kissed the little face—
"I will not leave thee by thysel';
  Ah, lad, this is thy father's place."

---

[*] The fire-damp is frequently heralded by a balmy-scented air, warm, and having an odour of flowers.

So Self before sweet Love lay slain.
  In the deep mine again was told
The story of a father's love,
  Older than mortal man is old;
For though they urged him o'er and o'er,
  To every prayer he only had
The answer he had found at first,
  "Nay; I'll stay with the lad!"

And when some weary days had passed,
  And men durst venture near the place,
They lay where Death had found them both,
  But hand in hand, and face to face.
And men were better for that sight,
  And told the tale with tearful breath;
There was not one but inly felt
  The man had touched a noble death,
And left this thought for all to keep—
  If earthly fathers can so love,
Ah, surely we may safely lean
  Upon the Fatherhood above!

Lillie E. Barr.

NOTTMAN.

(By kind permission of the Author.)

That was Nottman waving at me,
But the steam fell down, so you could not see;
He is out to-day with the fast express,
And running a mile in the minute, I guess.

Danger? None in the least, for the way
Is good, though the curves are sharp, as you say;
But, bless you! when trains are a little behind,
They thunder around them—a match for the wind.

Nottman himself is a keen one to drive,
But cool and steady, and ever alive
To whatever danger is looming in front,
When a train has run hard, to gain time for a shunt.

But he once got a fear, though, that shook him with pain,
Like sleepers beneath the weight of a train.
I remember the story well, for you see
His stoker, Jack Martin, told it to me.

Nottman had sent down the wife for a change
To the old folks living at Riverly Grange—
A quiet, sleepy sort of a town,
Save when the engines went up and down;

For close behind it the railway ran
In a mile of a straight, if a single span;
Three bridges were over the straight, and between
Two, the distant signal was seen.

She had with her her boy—a nice little chit
Full of romp and mischief, and childish wit;
And every time that we thundered by,
Both were out on the watch, for Nottman and I.

"Well, one day," said Jack, "on our journey down,
Coming round on the straight, at the back of the town,
I saw right ahead—in front of our track—
In the haze—on the rail—something dim-like and black.

"I looked over at Nottman, but, ere I could speak,
He shut off the steam, and with one wild shriek
A whistle took to the air, with a bound,
But—the object ahead—never stirred at the sound.

"In a moment he flung himself down on his knee,
   Leant over the side of the engine to see,—
Took one look—then sprang up, crying, breathless and pale:
   'Brake, Jack! it's some one asleep on the rail!'

"The rear-brakes were whistled on in a trice,
   While I screwed on the tender-brake, firm as a vice;
But still we tore on, with this terrible thought
   Sending fear to our hearts—'Can we stop her, or not?'

"I took one look again, then sung out to my mate—
   'We can never draw up; we've seen it too late!'
When, sudden and swift, like the change in a dream,
   Nottman drew back the lever, and flung on the steam.

"The great wheels staggered, and span with the strain,
   While the spray from the steam fell around us like rain;
But we slackened our speed, till we saw with a wild
   Throb at the heart—right before us—a child!

"It was lying asleep, on the rail—with no fear
   Of the terrible death, that was looming so near;—
The sweat on us both broke as cold as the dew
   Of death—as we questioned, 'What can we do?'

"It was done—swift as acts that take place in a dream—
   Nottman rushed to the front, and knelt down on the beam;
Put one foot in the couplings, the other he kept
   Right in front of the wheel, for the child that still slept.

"'Saved!' I burst forth, my heart leaping with pride,
   For one touch of his foot sent the child to the side;
But Nottman looked up, his lips white as with foam,
   'My God! Jack,' he cried, 'it's my own little Tom.'

"He shrunk—would have slipped, but one grasp of my hand
Held him firm, till the engine was brought to a stand,
Then I heard from behind a shriek take to the air,
And I knew that the voice of a *mother* was there.

"The boy was all right, and got off with a scratch;
He had crept through the fence in his frolic, to watch
For his father; but wearied with mischief and play,
Had fallen asleep on the rail where he lay.

"For days after that, on our journey down,
Ere we came to the straight, at the back of the town,
As if the signal were up, with its gleam
Of red, Nottman always shut off the steam."

ALEX. ANDERSON.

JACK CHIDDY.

(By kind permission of the Author.)

Brave Jack Chiddy! O well, you may sneer,
For the name isn't one that sounds nice to the ear;
But a name is a sound—nothing more—deeds are best,
And Jack had the soul of a man in his breast.

Jack Chiddy—there you're smiling again
At the name, which, I own, is both common and plain—
Jack Chiddy, I say, wrought along with his mates,
Year in and year out, on a section of plates.

Simple enough was the work, with no change
But to see that both lines were in gauge and range;
Fasten a key there, and tighten a bolt,
All to save fast trains from giving a jolt.

Strange, when one thinks, where a hero may rise,
Say, at times, in a moment, before our eyes,

Or right from our side, ere we know it, and do
The task of a giant—and pass from our view.

But the story, you say; well—I'm coming to that,
Though I wander a little—now, where was I at?
Let me see—can you catch, shining round and clear,
The mouth of Breslington tunnel, from here?

You see it? Well, there on the bank, at the top,
When stacking some blocks, all at once down the slope
A huge slab of stone from the rest shore its way,
And fell right on the down-line of metals, and lay—

One sharp cry of terror burst forth from us all,
As we saw the huge mass topple over and fall;
And we stood as if bound to the spot dumb of speech,
Reading horror and doubt in the faces of each.

Then one of our mates snatched a glance at his watch,
Gave a start and a look that made each of us catch
At our breath—then a cry that thrilled our hearts through,
"My God! the 'Flying Dutchman' is overdue!"

Hark! Right over the hill we could hear
A dull sound coming faint on the ear,
Then a short sharp whistle that told with its blast
That the "Dutchman" was into the tunnel at last.

And there, on the rail, lay that huge block of stone,
With the "Dutchman" behind coming thundering on;
In a minute, or less, she would come with a dash,
And a hundred lives would be lost in the crash.

"Now for your life, Jack!" For Chiddy had flown
Down the bank, and three leaps brought him right to the stone;

Not for his own life, for wife and child's sake, thought he,
But the hundreds that now were at stake.

'Twas the work of a moment : with terrible strength
And a heave of the shoulder, the slab moved at length—
Slipped clear of the rail, when, half muffled in smoke,
From the mouth of the tunnel, the " Dutchman " broke.

There was one short whistle, a roar and a crash
Of wheels ringing clear on the rail, and a cloud
Of coiling smoke, and a glitter and gleam of iron and steel,
And then down fell the steam.

Not a breath could we draw, but stood blank with dismay
As the train tore along, making up for delay,
Till at last, from us all, burst a shout and a cheer,
When we knew that the " Dutchman " was past and clear.

" And Chiddy ? "   Ah, well—you will pardon these tears,
For Jack was my mate on the rails, many years—
When we found him, one look was enough to reveal
That his life's-blood was red on the engine-wheel.

" Brave Jack Chiddy ! "   *Now*, you don't sneer
At the name, which, I own, is but harsh to the ear ;
But a name is a sound—nothing more—deeds are best,
And Jack had the heart of a man in his breast.

ALEX. ANDERSON.

THE FIREMAN'S WEDDING.

(By kind permission of the Author.)

" What are we looking at, guv'nor ?—
  Well, you see these carriages there ?
It's a wedding—that's what it is, sir ;
  And aren't they a beautiful pair ?

THE FIREMAN'S WEDDING.

"They don't want no marrow-bone music,
 There's the fireman's band come to play;
It's a fireman that's going to get married,
 And you don't see such sights every day.

"They're in the church now, and we're waiting
 To give them a cheer as they come;
And the grumbler that wouldn't join in it
 Deserves all his life to go dumb.

"They won't be out for a minute,
 So if you've time and will stay,
I'll tell you right from the beginning
 About this 'ere wedding to-day.

"One night I was fast getting drowsy,
 And thinking of going to bed,
When I heard such a clattering and shouting:
 'That sounds like an engine!' I said.

"So I jumped up and opened the window:
 'It's a fire, sure enough, wife,' says I;
For the people were running and shouting,
 And the red glare quite lit up the sky.

"I kicked off my old carpet slippers,
 And on with my boots in a jiff;
I stuck up my pipe in a corner
 Without waiting to have the last whiff.

"The wife, she just grumbled a wee bit,
 But I didn't take notice of that;
For I on with my coat in a minute,
 And sprang down the stairs like a cat.

THE FIREMAN'S WEDDING.

" I followed the crowd, and it brought me
 In front of the house in a blaze;
At first I could see nothing clearly,
 For the smoke made it all of a haze.

" The firemen were shouting their loudest,
 And unwinding great lengths of hose;
The p'licemen were pushing the people,
 And treading on every one's toes.

" I got pushed with some more in a corner,
 Where I couldn't move, try as I might;
But little I cared for the squeezing
 So long as I had a good sight.

" Ah, sir, it was grand, but 'twas awful!
 The flames leaped up higher and higher;
The wind seemed to get underneath them,
 Till they roared like a great blacksmith's fire!

" I was just looking round at the people,
 With their faces lit up by the glare,
When I heard some one cry, hoarse with terror,
 ' Oh, look, look—there's a woman up there!'

" I shall never forget the excitement,
 My heart beat as loud as a clock;
I looked at the crowd—they were standing
 As if turned into stone by the shock.

" And there was the face at the window,
 With its blank look of haggard despair;
Her hands were clasped tight on her bosom,
 And her white lips were moving in prayer.

"The staircase was burnt to a cinder,
　　There wasn't a fire-escape near;
But a ladder was brought from a builder's,
　　And the crowd gave a half-frightened cheer.

"The ladder was put to the window,
　　While the flames were still raging below;
I looked, with my heart in my mouth, then,
　　To see who would offer to go!

"When up sprang a sturdy young fireman,
　　As a sailor would climb up a mast;
We saw him go in at the window,
　　And we cheered as though danger were past.

"We saw nothing more for a moment,
　　But the sparks flying round us like rain;
And then, as we breathlessly waited,
　　He came to the window again.

"And on his broad shoulder was lying
　　The face of that poor fainting thing,
And we gave him a cheer as we never
　　Yet gave to a prince or a king.

"He got on the top of the ladder—
　　I can see him there now, noble lad!
And the flames underneath seemed to know it,
　　For they leaped at that ladder like mad.

"But just as he got to the middle,
　　I could see it begin to give way,
For the flames had got hold of it now, sir!
　　I could see the thing tremble and sway.

"He came but a step or two lower,
    Then sprang with a cry to the ground;
And then, we could hardly believe it,
    He stood with the girl safe and sound!

"And now they're in church getting married—
    I bet you she'll make a good wife;
And who has the most right to have her?
    Why, the brave fellow who saved her young life.

"A beauty? I believe you, sir.—
    Stand back, lads! stand back! here they are!
We'll give 'em the cheer that we promised;
    Now, lads, with a hip, hip, hurrah!"

W. E. EATON.

KARL THE MARTYR.

It was the closing of a summer's day,
And trellised branches from encircling trees
Threw silver shadows o'er the golden space,
Where groups of merry-hearted sons of toil
Were met to celebrate a village feast,
Casting away, in frolic sport, the cares
That ever press and crowd and leave their mark
Upon the brows of all whose bread is earned
By daily labour. 'Twas, perchance, the feast
Of fav'rite saint, or anniversary
Of one of bounteous Nature's season gifts
To grateful husbandry—no matter what
The cause of their uniting. Joy beamed forth
On every face, and the sweet echoes rang
With sounds of honest mirth, too rarely heard
In the vast workshop man has made his world,
Where months of toil must pay one day of song.

Somewhat apart from the assembled throng
There sat a swarthy giant, with a face
So nobly grand, that though (unlike the rest)
He wore nor festal garb nor laughing mien,
Yet was he study for the painter's art.
He joined not in their sports, but rather seemed
To please his eye with sight of others' joy.
There was a cast of sorrow on his brow,
As though it had been early there. He sat
In listless attitude, yet not devoid
Of gentlest grace, as down his stalwart form
He bent, to catch the playful whisperings
And note the movements of a bright-haired child
Who danced before him in the evening sun,
Holding a tiny brother by the hand.
He was the village smith (the rolled-up sleeves
And the well-charred leathern apron showed his craft);
Karl was his name—a man beloved by all.

He was not of the district. He had come
Amongst them ere his forehead bore one trace
Of age or suffering. A wife and child
He had brought with him; but the wife was dead.
Not so the child, who danced before him now,
And held a tiny brother by the hand—
Their mother's last and priceless legacy!
So Karl was happy still that these two lived,
And laughed and danced before him in the sun.

The frolics pause: now Casper's laughing head
Rests wearily against his father's knee
In trusting lovingness; while Trudchen runs
To snatch a hasty kiss (the little man,
It may be, wonders if the tiny hand
With which he strives to reach his father's neck

Will ever grow so big and brown as that
He sees imbedded in his sister's curls);
When quick as lightning's flash up starts the smith,
Huddles the frightened children in his arms,
Thrusts them far back, extends his giant frame,
And covers them as with Goliath's shield.

Now, hark! a rushing, yelping, panting sound,
So terrible that all stood chilled with fear;
And in the midst of that late joyous throng
Leaped an infuriate hound, with flaming eyes,
Half-open mouth, and fiercely bristling hair,
Proving that madness drove the brute to death.
One spring from Karl, and the wild thing was seized,
Fast prisoned in the stalwart Vulcan's grip.
A sharp, shrill cry of agony from Karl
Was mingled with the hound's low fevered growl;
And all, with horror, saw the creature's teeth
Fixed in the blacksmith's shoulder. None had power
To rescue him; for scarcely could you count
A moment's space ere both had disappeared—
The man and dog. The smith had leaped a fence,
And gained the forest with a frantic rush,
Bearing the hideous mischief in his arms.

A long receding cry came on the ear,
Showing how swift their flight, and fainter grew
The sound. Ere well a man had time to think
What might be done for help, the sound was hushed—
Lost in the very distance; women crouched
And huddled up their children in their arms,
Men flew to seek their weapons—'twas a change
So swift and fearful none could realize
Its actual horrors for a time; but now,
The panic past, to rescue and pursuit!

Crash through the brake into the forest-track ;
But pitchy darkness, caused by closing night
And foliage dense, impedes the avengers' way,
When, lo ! they trip o'er something in their path—
It was the bleeding body of the hound,
Warm, but quite dead. No other trace of Karl
Was near at hand ; they called his name in vain,
They sought him in the forest all night through—
Living or dead he was not to be found.

At break of day they left the fruitless search.
Next morning, as an anxious village group
Stood meditating plans what best to do,
Came little Trudchen, who, in simple tones,
Said, "Father's at the forge ; I heard him there
Working long hours ago, but he is angry.
I raised the latch ; he bade me to be-gone.
What have I done to make him chide me so ?"
And then her bright blue eyes ran o'er with tears.
"The child's been dreaming through this troubled night,"
Said a kind dame, and drew the child towards her ;
But the sad answers of the girl were such
As led them all to seek her father's forge.
It lay beyond the village some short span ;
They forced the door, and there beheld the smith.
His sinewy frame was drawn to its full height,
And round his loins a double chain of iron,
Wrought with true workman skill, was riveted
Fast to an anvil of enormous weight.
He stood as pale and statue-like as death.
Now let his own words close the hapless tale.

"I killed the hound, you know, but not until
His maddening venom through my veins had passed ;
I know full well the death in store for me,

And would not answer when you called my name,
But crouched among the brushwood while I thought
Over some plan. I know my giant strength,
And dare not trust it after reason's loss;
Why, I might turn and rend whom most I love.
I've made all fast now. 'Tis a hideous death.
I thought to plunge me into the deep, still pool
That skirts the forest, to avoid it; but
I thought that for the suicide's poor shift
I would not throw away my chance of heaven,
And meeting one who made earth heaven to me.
So I came home and forged these chains about me—
Full well I know no human hand can rend them—
And now am safe from harming those I love.
Keep off, good friends! Should God prolong my life,
Throw me such food as nature may require;
Look to my babes: *this* you are bound to do;
For by my deadly grasp on that poor hound
How many of you have I saved from death
Such as *I* now await? But hence, away!
The poison works! These chains must try their strength:
My brain's on fire! With me 'twill soon be night."

Too true his words: the brave, great-hearted Karl—
A raving maniac—battled with his chains
For three fierce days. The fourth day saw him free;
For Death's strong hand had loosed the martyr's bonds.

THE BRIDGE OF SIGHS.

One more unfortunate, weary of breath, rashly importunate, gone to her death! Take her up tenderly—lift her with care: fashioned so slenderly, young, and so fair! Look at her garments, clinging like cerements; whilst the wave constantly drips from her clothing. Take her up instantly, loving, not loathing. Touch her not scornfully, think of her mournfully, gently and humanly; not of the stains of her:—all that remains of her now is pure womanly. Make no deep scrutiny into her mutiny, rash and undutiful: past all dishonour. Death has left on her only the beautiful. Still,—for all slips of hers, one of Eve's family,—wipe those poor lips of hers, oozing so clammily. Loop up her tresses escaped from the comb—her fair auburn tresses!—whilst wonderment guesses, Where was her home? who was her father? who was her mother? had she a sister? had she a brother? or was there a dearer one still, and a nearer one yet than all other? Alas for the rarity of Christian charity under the sun! Oh, it was pitiful! near a whole city-full, home she had none. Sisterly, brotherly, fatherly, motherly feelings had changed: love, by harsh evidence, thrown from its eminence: even God's providence seeming estranged!

Where the lamps quiver so far in the river, with many a light from window and casement, from garret to basement, she stood with amazement, houseless by night. The bleak wind of March made her tremble and shiver; but not the dark arch, or the black-flowing river: mad from life's history, glad to death's mystery; swift to be hurled anywhere, anywhere, out of the world! In she plunged boldly, no matter how coldly the rough river ran:—over the brink of it, picture it, think of it, dissolute Man! lave in it, drink of it, then, if you can!

Take her up tenderly, lift her with care: fashioned so slenderly, young, and so fair! Ere her limbs frigidly stiffen too rigidly, decently, kindly, smooth and compose them; and her eyes—close them, staring so blindly! Dreadfully staring through muddy impurity; as when with the daring last look of despairing, fixed on futurity. Perishing gloomily, spurned by contumely, cold inhumanity, burning insanity, into her rest. Cross her hands humbly, as if praying dumbly, over her breast; owning her weakness, her evil behaviour—and leaving, with meekness, her sins to her Saviour.   HOOD.

THE EXECUTION OF MONTROSE.

Come hither, Evan Cameron, come, stand beside my knee;
I hear the river roaring down towards the wintry sea.
There's shouting on the mountain-side, there's war within the blast.
Old faces look upon me, old forms go trooping past.
I hear the pibroch wailing amidst the din of fight,
And my dim spirit wakes again upon the verge of night.

'Twas I that led the Highland host through wild Lochaber's snows,
What time the plaided clans came down to battle with Montrose.
I've told thee how the Southrons fell beneath the broad claymore,
And how we smote the Campbell clan by Inverlochy's shore;
I've told thee how we swept Dundee, and tamed the Lindsays' pride;
But never have I told thee yet how the great marquis died.

A traitor sold him to his foes—oh, deed of deathless shame!
I charge thee, boy, if e'er thou meet with one of Assynt's name—
Be it upon the mountain's side, or yet within the glen,
Stand he in martial gear alone, or backed by armèd men—
Face him as thou wouldst face the man who wronged thy sire's renown;
Remember of what blood thou art, and strike the caitiff down!

They brought him to the Watergate, hard bound with hempen span,
As though they held a lion there, and not a 'fenceless man.
They set him high upon a cart—the hangman rode below—
They drew his hands behind his back, and bared his noble brow.
Then, as a hound is slipped from leash, they cheered,—the common throng,
And blew the note with yell and shout, and bade him pass along.

It would have made a brave man's heart grow sad and sick that day,
To watch the keen malignant eyes bent down on that array.
But when he came, though pale and wan, he looked so great and high,
So noble was his manly front, so calm his steadfast eye,
The rabble rout forbore to shout, and each man held his breath,
For well they knew the hero's soul was face to face with death.
    But onwards—always onwards, in silence and in gloom,
The dreary pageant laboured, till it reached the house of doom.
Then, as the Græme looked upwards, he saw the ugly smile
Of him who sold his king for gold—the master-fiend, Argyll!
And a Saxon soldier cried aloud, "Back, coward, from thy place!
For seven long years thou hast not dared to look him in the face."
    Had I been there, with sword in hand, and fifty Camerons by,
That day through high Dunedin's streets had pealed the slogan-cry;
Not all their troops of trampling horse, nor might of mailèd men,
Not all the rebels in the South had borne us backwards then!
Once more his foot on Highland heath had trod as free as air,
Or I, and all who bore my name, been laid around him there!
    It might not be. They placed him next within the solemn hall,
Where once the Scottish kings were throned amidst their nobles all.
With savage glee came Warristoun to read the murderous doom;
And then uprose the great Montrose in the middle of the room.
"Now, by my faith as belted knight, and by the name I bear,
And by the bright St. Andrew's cross that waves above us there—

THE EXECUTION OF MONTROSE.

I have not sought in battle-field a wreath of such renown,
Nor dared I hope on my dying day to win the martyr's crown
There is a chamber far away, where sleep the good and brave,
But a better place ye have named for me than by my father's grave;
For truth and right, 'gainst treason's might, this hand hath always striven,
And ye raise it up for a witness still, in the eye of earth and heaven.
Then nail my head on yonder tower—give every town a limb—
And God, who made, shall gather them: I go from you to him!"

  Ah, boy, that ghastly gibbet! how dismal 'tis to see
The great tall spectral skeleton, the ladder, and the tree!
Hark! hark! it is the clash of arms—the bells begin to toll—
"He is coming! he is coming! God's mercy on his soul!"
There was colour in his visage, though the cheeks of all were wan,
And they marvelled as they saw him pass, that great and goodly man.
He mounted up the scaffold, and he turned him to the crowd;
But they dared not trust the people, so he might not speak aloud.
But he looked upon the heavens, and they were clear and blue,
And in the liquid ether the eye of God shone through;
Yet a black and murky battlement lay resting on the hill,
As though the thunder slept within—all else was calm and still.
  A beam of light fell o'er him, like a glory round the shriven,
And he climbed the lofty ladder as it were the path to heaven.
Then came a flash from out the cloud, and a stunning thunder-roll!
And no man dared to look aloft, for fear was on every soul.
There was *another* heavy sound, a hush, and then a groan;
And darkness swept across the sky—the work of death was done!
AYTOUN.

THE FIELD OF WATERLOO.

Stop!—for thy tread is on an empire's dust!
An earthquake's spoil is sepulchred below!
Is the spot marked with no colossal bust?
Nor column trophied for triumphal show?
None; but the moral's truth tells simpler so.
As the ground was before, thus let it be;—
How that red rain hath made the harvest grow!
And is this all the world hath gained by thee,
Thou first and last of fields! king-making victory?

There was a sound of revelry by night,
And Belgium's capital had gathered then
Her beauty and her chivalry, and bright
The lamps shone o'er fair women and brave men:
A thousand hearts beat happily; and when
Music arose with its voluptuous swell,
Soft eyes looked love to eyes which spake again,
And all went merry as a marriage bell;—
But hush! hark! a deep sound strikes like a rising knell.

Did ye not hear it?—No; 'twas but the wind,
Or the car rattling o'er the stony street:
On with the dance! let joy be unconfined;
No sleep till morn, when youth and pleasure meet,
To chase the glowing hours with flying feet:—
But hark! that heavy sound breaks in once more,
As if the clouds its echo would repeat;
And nearer, clearer, deadlier than before!—
Arm! arm! it is—it is—the cannon's opening roar!

Within a windowed niche of that high hall
Sat Brunswick's fated chieftain: he did hear
That sound the first amidst the festival,

And caught its tone with Death's prophetic ear;
And when they smiled, because he deemed it near,
His heart more truly knew that peal too well
Which stretched his father on a bloody bier,
And roused the vengeance blood alone could quell:
He rushed into the field, and, foremost fighting, fell!

Ah! then and there was hurrying to and fro,
And gathering tears, and tremblings of distress,
And cheeks all pale, which but an hour ago
Blushed at the praise of their own loveliness;
And there were sudden partings, such as press
The life from out young hearts; and choking sighs
Which ne'er might be repeated;—who could guess
If ever more should meet those mutual eyes,
Since upon night so sweet such awful morn could rise?

And there was mounting in hot haste: the steed,
The mustering squadron, and the clattering car,
Went pouring forward with impetuous speed,
And swiftly forming in the ranks of war;
And the deep thunder, peal on peal afar;
And near, the beat of the alarming drum
Roused up the soldier ere the morning star;
While thronged the citizens with terror dumb,
Or whispering, with white lips—"The foe! they come, they come!"

And wild and high the "Camerons' gathering" rose!
The war-note of Lochiel, which Albyn's hills
Have heard—and heard too have her Saxon foes.
How in the noon of night that pibroch thrills,
Savage and shrill! but with the breath which fills
Their mountain-pipe, so fill the mountaineers
With the fierce native daring which instils

The stirring memory of a thousand years;
And Evan's, Donald's fame, rings in each clansman's ears!

And Ardennes waves above them her green leaves,
Dewy with Nature's tear-drops, as they pass,
Grieving, if aught inanimate e'er grieves,
Over the unreturning brave—alas!
Ere evening to be trodden like the grass,
Which now beneath them, but above shall grow
In its next verdure, when this fiery mass
Of living valour, rolling on the foe,
And burning with high hope, shall moulder cold and low.

Last noon beheld them full of lusty life;
Last eve, in Beauty's circle proudly gay;
The midnight brought the signal-sound of strife;
The morn, the marshalling of arms; the day,
Battle's magnificently stern array!
The thunder-clouds close o'er it, which, when rent,
The earth is covered thick with other clay,
Which her own clay shall cover,—heaped and pent,
Rider and horse, friend, foe, in one red burial blent!
BYRON.

HORATIUS.

The Fathers of the City, they sat all night and day,
For every hour some horsemen came with tidings of dismay.
They held a council standing before the River-Gate;
Short time was there, ye well may guess, for musing or debate.

Out spake the Consul roundly: "The bridge must straight go down;
For since Janiculum is lost, naught else can save the town."
Just then a scout came flying, all wild with haste and fear—
"To arms! to arms! Sir Consul; Lars Porsena is here!"

On the low hills to westward the Consul fixed his eye,
And saw the swarthy storm of dust rise fast along the sky.
"Their van will be upon us before the bridge goes down;
And if they once may win the bridge, what hope to save the town?"

Then out spake brave Horatius, the Captain of the Gate:
"To every man upon this earth death cometh soon or late;
And how can man die better than facing fearful odds,
For the ashes of his fathers, and the temples of his gods?

"Hew down the bridge, Sir Consul, with all the speed ye may;
I, with *two* more to help me, will hold the foe in play.
In yon strait path a *thousand* may well be stopped by *three;*—
Now, who will stand on either hand, and keep the bridge with me?"

Then out spake Spurius Lartius—a Ramnian proud was he:
"Lo, I will stand at thy *right* hand, and keep the bridge with thee."
And out spake strong Herminius—of Titian blood was he:
"I will abide on thy *left* side, and keep the bridge with thee."

"Horatius," quoth the Consul, "as thou say'st, so let it be."
And straight against that great array forth went the dauntless Three.

The Three stood calm and silent, and looked upon the foes,
And a great shout of laughter from all the vanguard rose:
And forth three chiefs came spurring before that deep array;
  To earth they sprang, their swords they drew,
  And lifted high their shields, and flew
   To win the narrow way.

Stout Lartius hurled down Aunus into the stream beneath:
Herminius struck at Seius, and clove him to the teeth;

At Picus brave Horatius darted one fiery thrust,
And the proud Umbrian's gilded arms clashed in the bloody
　　dust.

But hark! the cry is "Astur;" and lo! the ranks divide,
And the great Lord of Luna comes with his stately stride.
He smiled on those bold Romans a smile serene and high;
He eyed the flinching Tuscans, and scorn was in his eye.

Then, whirling up his broadsword with both hands to the height,
He rushed against Horatius, and smote with all his might.
With shield and blade Horatius right deftly turned the blow.
　　The blow, though turned, came yet too nigh;
　　It missed his helm, but gashed his thigh.

He reeled, and on Herminius he leaned one breathing-space;
Then, like a wild-cat mad with wounds, sprang right at
　　Astur's face.
Through teeth, and skull, and helmet, so fierce a thrust he sped,
The good sword stood a handbreadth out behind the
　　Tuscan's head!
And the great Lord of Luna fell at that deadly stroke,
As falls on Mount Alvernus the thunder-smitten oak.

But meanwhile axe and lever have manfully been plied;
And now the bridge hangs tottering above the boiling tide.
"Come back, come back, Horatius!" loud cried the Fathers all;
'Back, Lartius! back, Herminius! back, ere the ruin fall!"

Back darted Spurius Lartius; Herminius darted back;
And, as they passed, beneath their feet they felt the timbers
　　crack:
But when they turned their faces, and on the farther shore
Saw brave Horatius stand alone, they would have crossed
　　once more.

But with a crash like thunder fell every loosened beam,
And, like a dam, the mighty wreck lay right athwart the stream ;
And a long shout of triumph rose from the walls of Rome,
As to the highest turret-tops was splashed the yellow foam.

Alone stood brave Horatius,—but constant still in mind,—
Thrice thirty thousand foes before, and the broad flood behind.
"Down with him!" cried false Sextus, with a smile on his pale face.
"Now yield thee," cried Lars Porsena, "now yield thee to our grace."

Round turned he, as not deigning those craven ranks to see ;
Naught spake he to Lars Porsena, to Sextus naught spake he ;
But he saw on Palatinus the white porch of his home,
And he spake to the noble river that rolls by the towers of Rome.

"O Tiber! father Tiber! to whom the Romans pray,
A Roman's life, a Roman's arms, take thou in charge this day!"
So he spake, and speaking, sheathed the good sword by his side,
And with his harness on his back, plunged headlong in the tide.

No sound of joy or sorrow was heard from either bank ;
   But friends and foes, in dumb surprise,
   With parted lips and straining eyes,
     Stood gazing where he sank :
And when above the surges they saw his crest appear,
   All Rome sent forth a rapturous cry,
   And even the ranks of Tuscany
     Could scarce forbear to cheer.
But fiercely ran the current, swollen high by months of rain :
And fast his blood was flowing ; and he was sore in pain.

Never, I ween, did swimmer, in such an evil case,
Struggle through such a raging flood, safe to the landing-place ;
But his limbs were borne up bravely, by the brave heart within,
And our good father Tiber bare bravely up his chin.

And now he feels the bottom ; now on dry earth he stands ;
Now round him throng the Fathers, to press his gory hands ;
And now with shouts and clapping, and noise of weeping loud,
He enters through the River-Gate, borne by the joyous crowd.

When the goodman mends his armour, and trims his helmet's plume ;
When the goodwife's shuttle merrily goes flashing through the loom ;—
With weeping and with laughter still is the story told,
How well Horatius kept the bridge in the brave days of old.

LORD MACAULAY.

VIRGINIA.

Over the Alban mountains the light of morning broke ;
From all the roofs of the Seven Hills curled the thin wreaths of smoke :
The city gates were opened ; the Forum, all alive
With buyers and with sellers, was humming like a hive :
Blithely on brass and timber the craftsman's stroke was ringing,
And blithely o'er her panniers the market-girl was singing ;
And blithely young Virginia came smiling from her home—
Ah ! woe for young Virginia, the sweetest maid in Rome.
With her small tablets in her hand, and her satchel on her arm,
Forth she went bounding to the school, nor dreamed of shame or harm.
She crossed the Forum, shining with the stalls in alleys gay,
And just had reached the very spot whereon I stand this day,

When up the varlet Marcus came; not such as when, erewhile,
He crouched behind his patron's heels, with the true client smile:
He came with lowering forehead, swollen features, and clenched fist,
And strode across Virginia's path, and caught her by the wrist.
Hard strove the frighted maiden, and screamed with look aghast,
And at her scream from right and left the folk came running fast;
And the strong smith Muræna gave Marcus such a blow,
The caitiff reeled three paces back, and let the maiden go:
Yet glared he fiercely round him, and growled, in harsh, fell tone,—
" She's mine, and I will have her; I seek but for mine own.
She is my slave, born in my house, and stolen away and sold,
The year of the sore sickness, ere she was twelve years old.
I wait on Appius Claudius; I waited on his sire:
Let him who works the client wrong, beware the patron's ire!"
—But ere the varlet Marcus again might seize the maid,
Who clung tight to Muræna's skirt and sobbed and shrieked for aid,
Forth through the throng of gazers the young Icilius pressed,
And stamped his foot and rent his gown and smote upon his breast,
And beckoned to the people, and, in bold voice and clear,
Poured thick and fast the burning words which tyrants quake to hear:—

"Now by your children's cradles, now by your fathers' graves,
Be men to-day, Quirites, or be for ever slaves!
Oh for that ancient spirit which curbed the Senate's will!
Oh for the tents which in old time whitened the Sacred Hill!
In those brave days our fathers stood firmly side by side;
They faced the Marcian fury, they tamed the Fabian pride;

They drove the fiercest Quintius an outcast forth from Rome;
They sent the haughtiest Claudius with shivered fasces home.
But what their care bequeathed us, our madness flung away;
All the ripe fruit of threescore years is blighted in a day.
Exult, ye proud patricians! the hard-fought fight is o'er:
We strove for honour—'twas in vain; for freedom—'tis no more.
Our very hearts, that were so high, sink down beneath your will;
Riches and lands and power and state, ye have them—keep them still!
Heap heavier still the fetters, bar closer still the grate;
Patient as sheep we yield us up unto your cruel hate:—
But, by the shades beneath us, and by the gods above,
Add not unto your cruel hate your yet more cruel love!
Have ye not graceful ladies, whose spotless lineage springs
From consuls, and high pontiffs, and ancient Alban kings?—
Ladies, who deign not on our paths to set their tender feet;
Who from their cars look down with scorn upon the wondering street;
Who in Corinthian mirrors their own proud smiles behold,
And breathe of Capuan odours, and shine with Spanish gold?
Then leave the poor plebeian his single tie to life—
The sweet, sweet love of daughter, of sister, and of wife;
Spare us the inexpiable wrong, the unutterable shame,
That turns the coward's heart to steel, the sluggard's blood to flame;
Lest, when our latest hope is fled, ye taste of our despair,
And learn, by proof, in some wild hour, how much the wretched dare!"

* * * * *

Straightway Virginius led the maid a little space aside,
To where the reeking shambles stood, piled up with horn and hide.
Hard by, a flesher on a block had laid his whittle down;
Virginius caught the whittle up, and hid it in his gown.

And then his eyes grew very dim, and his throat began to swell,
And in a hoarse, changed voice he spake: "Farewell, sweet child, farewell!
Oh, how I loved my darling! Though stern I sometimes be,
To thee, thou know'st, I was not so; who could be so to thee?
And how my darling lovèd me! how glad she was to hear
My footstep on the threshold, when I came back last year!
And how she danced with pleasure to see my civic crown,
And took my sword and hung it up, and brought me forth my gown!
Now all those things are over—yes, all thy pretty ways,
Thy needlework, thy prattle, thy snatches of old lays;
And none will grieve when I go forth, or smile when I return,
Or watch beside the old man's bed, or weep upon his urn.
The house that was the happiest within the Roman walls,
The house that envied not the wealth of Capua's marble halls,
Now, for the brightness of thy smile, must have eternal gloom,
And for the music of thy voice, the silence of the tomb.
The time is come! See how he points his eager hand this way!
See how his eyes gloat on thy grief, like a kite's upon the prey!
With all his wit he little deems that, spurned, betrayed, bereft,
Thy father hath, in his despair, one fearful refuge left.
He little deems that in this hand I clutch what still can save
Thy gentle youth from taunts and blows, the portion of the slave;
Yea, and from nameless evil, that passeth taunt and blow—
Foul outrage, which thou knowest not, which thou shalt never know!
Then clasp me round the neck once more, and give me one more kiss;
And now, mine own dear little girl, there is no way—but this!"
—With that he lifted high the steel, and smote her in the side,
And in her blood she sank to earth, and with one sob she died!

When Appius Claudius saw that deed, he shuddered and sank
    down,
And hid his face some little space with the corner of his gown,
Till, with white lips and blood-shot eyes, Virginius tottered
    nigh,
And stood before the judgment-seat and held the knife on high:
" O dwellers in the nether gloom, avengers of the slain,
By this dear blood I cry to you, do right between us twain ;
And even as Appius Claudius hath dealt by me and mine,
Deal you by Appius Claudius, and all the Claudian line!"
Then up sprang Appius Claudius: "Stop him, alive or dead!
Ten thousand pounds of copper to the man who brings his
    head!"
He looked upon his clients, but none would work his will ;
He looked upon his lictors, but they trembled and stood still.
And as Virginius through the press his way in silence cleft,
Ever the mighty multitude fell back to right and left:
And he hath passed in safety unto his woful home,
And there ta'en horse to tell the camp what deeds are done in
    Rome. LORD MACAULAY.

THE RAVEN.

Once upon a midnight dreary, while I pondered, weak and
    weary,
Over many a quaint and curious volume of forgotten lore—
While I nodded, nearly napping, suddenly there came a
    tapping,
As of some one gently rapping, rapping at my chamber door.
" 'Tis some visitor," I muttered, "tapping at my chamber door—
    Only this, and nothing more."

Ah! distinctly I remember, it was in the bleak December,
And each separate dying ember wrought its ghost upon the
    floor :

Eagerly I wished the morrow; vainly I had sought to borrow
From my books surcease of sorrow, sorrow for the lost
   Lenore—
For the rare and radiant maiden whom the angels name
   Lenore—
      Nameless here for evermore.

And the silken, sad, uncertain rustling of each purple curtain
Thrilled me—filled me with fantastic terrors never felt before;
So that now, to still the beating of my heart, I stood repeating,
" 'Tis some visitor entreating entrance at my chamber door—
Some late visitor entreating entrance at my chamber door:
      This it is, and nothing more."

Presently my soul grew stronger; hesitating then no longer,
" Sir," said I, " or madam, truly your forgiveness I implore;
But the fact is, I was napping, and so gently you came rapping,
And so faintly you came tapping, tapping at my chamber door,
That I scarce was sure I heard you." Here I opened wide
   the door—
      Darkness there, and nothing more.

Deep into that darkness peering, long I stood there, wondering, fearing,
Doubting, dreaming dreams no mortal ever dared to dream
   before;
But the silence was unbroken, and the stillness gave no token,
And the only word there spoken was the whispered word,
   " Lenore!"
This *I* whispered, and an echo murmured back the word,
   " Lenore!"
      Merely this, and nothing more.

Back into my chamber turning, all my soul within me burning,
Soon again I heard a tapping, something louder than before.

"Surely," said I, "surely that is something at my window
    lattice;
Let me see then what thereat is, and this mystery explore—
Let my heart be still a moment, and this mystery explore.
        'Tis the wind, and nothing more."

Open here I flung the shutter, when, with many a flirt and
    flutter,
In there stepped a stately raven, of the saintly days of yore;
Not the least obeisance made he, not a minute stopped or
    stayed he;
But with mien of lord or lady, perched above my chamber
    door—
Perched above a bust of Pallas, just above my chamber door—
        Perched, and sat, and nothing more.

Then this ebony bird beguiling my sad fancy into smiling,
By the grave and stern decorum of the countenance it wore—
"Though thy crest be shorn and shaven, thou," I said, "art
    sure no craven;
Ghastly, grim, and ancient raven, wandering from the nightly
    shore,
Tell me what thy lordly name is on the night's Plutonian
    shore."
        Quoth the raven, "Nevermore."

Much I marvelled this ungainly fowl to hear discourse so
    plainly,
Though its answer little meaning, little relevancy bore;
For we cannot help agreeing that no living human being
Ever yet was blessed with seeing bird above his chamber door
        With such name as "Nevermore."

But the raven, sitting lonely on that placid bust, spoke only
That one word, as if his soul in that one word he did outpour;

Nothing further then he uttered, not a feather then he fluttered,
Till I scarcely more than muttered—" Other friends have flown before;
On the morrow *he* will leave me, as my hopes have flown before."
    Then the bird said, " Nevermore."

Startled by the stillness broken by reply so aptly spoken,
" Doubtless," said I, " what it utters is its only stock and store,
Caught from some unhappy master, whom unmerciful disaster
Followed fast and followed faster, till his songs one burden bore—
Till the dirges of his hope that melancholy burden bore
    Of 'Never—nevermore.'"

But the raven still beguiling all my sad soul into smiling,
Straight I wheeled a cushioned seat in front of bird, and bust, and door;
Then upon the velvet sinking, I betook myself to linking
Fancy unto fancy, thinking what this ominous bird of yore—
What this grim, ungainly, ghastly, gaunt, and ominous bird of yore
    Meant in croaking " Nevermore."

This I sat engaged in guessing, but no syllable expressing
To the fowl whose fiery eyes now burned into my bosom's core;
This and more I sat divining, with my head at ease reclining
On the cushion's velvet lining, that the lamp-light gloated o'er,
But whose velvet violet lining, with the lamp-light gloating o'er,
    She shall press, ah, nevermore!

Then methought the air grew denser, perfumed from an unseen censer
Swung by seraphim, whose footfalls tinkled on the tufted floor.
" Wretch," I cried, " thy God hath lent thee, by these angels he hath sent thee,

Respite—respite and nepenthe from thy memories of Lenore;
Quaff, oh quaff this kind nepenthe, and forget this lost
  Lenore!"
    Quoth the raven, "Nevermore."

"Prophet," said I, "thing of evil—prophet still, if bird or
  devil!
Whether tempter sent, or whether tempest tossed thee here
  ashore—
Desolate, yet all undaunted, on this desert land enchanted,
On this home by horror haunted—tell me truly, I implore,
Is there—*is* there balm in Gilead? tell me—tell me—I
  implore!"
    Quoth the raven, "Nevermore."

"Prophet," said I, "thing of evil—prophet still, if bird or devil!
By that heaven that bends above us, by that God we both
  adore,
Tell this soul, with sorrow laden, if within the distant Aiden
It shall clasp a sainted maiden whom the angels name Lenore—
Clasp a rare and radiant maiden whom the angels name
  Lenore?"
    Quoth the raven, "Nevermore."

"Be that word our sign of parting, bird or fiend!" I shrieked
  upstarting—
"Get thee back into the tempest and the night's Plutonian shore!
Leave no black plume as a token of that lie thy soul hath
  spoken!
Leave my loneliness unbroken! quit the bust above my door!
Take thy beak from out my heart, and take thy form from
  off my door!"
    Quoth the raven, "Nevermore."

And the raven, never flitting, still is sitting, still is sitting
On the pallid bust of Pallas just above my chamber door;

And his eyes have all the seeming of a demon's that is dreaming,
And the lamp-light o'er him streaming throws his shadow on the floor;
And my soul from out that shadow, that lies floating on the floor,
Shall be lifted—nevermore!   E. A. POE.

PROSE.

JUD. BROWNIN' ON RUBENSTEIN'S PLAYING.

"Jud., they say you heard Rubenstein play, when you were in New York."

"I did, last fall."

"Well, tell us about it."

"What! me? I might's well tell you about the creation of the world."

"Come, now; no mock modesty. Go ahead."

"Wal, sir, he had the blamedest, biggest, cattycorneredest pianner you ever laid eyes on—somethin' like a distracted billiard-table on three legs. The lid was h'isted. If it hadn't been, he'd a tore the entire insides clean out, and scattered 'em to the four winds of heaven."

"Played well, did he?"

"You bet, he did. When he first sat down, he 'peared to keer mighty little 'bout playin', and wisht he hadn't come. He tweedle-eedled a little on the treble, and twoodle-oodled some on the bass—jest foolin' and boxin' the thing's jaws for bein' in his way. And I says to a man sittin' next to me, says I: 'What sort o' fool playin' is that?' And he says, 'Heish!' But presently his hands commenced chasin' one 'nother up and down the keys, like a passel o' rats scamperin' through a garret very swift.

"'Now,' I says to my neighbour, 'he's a-showin' off. He thinks he's a-doin' of it, but he ain't got no idee, no plan of nothin'. If he'd play me a tune of some kind or other, I'd—'

"But my neighbour says, 'Heish!' very impatient.

"I got up to go home, bein' tired of that foolishness, when I heerd a little bird wakin' up away off in the woods, and callin' sleepy-like to his mate, and I looked up, and I see that Rubin was beginning to take some interest in his business, and I sat down again. It was the peep o' day. The light came faint from the east, the breeze blowed gentle and fresh, some more birds waked up in the orchard, then some more in the trees near the house, and all began singin' together. People began to stir, and the gal opened the shutters. Jest then the first beam o' the sun fell upon the blossoms; a leetle more and it techt the roses on the bushes; the next thing it was broad day: the sun fairly blazed, the birds sang like they'd split their little throats; all the leaves were movin', and flashin' diamonds of dew, and the whole wide world was bright and happy as a king. Seemed to me like there was a good breakfast in every house in the land, and not a sick child or woman anywhere. It was a fine mornin'.

"And I says to my neighbour: 'That's music, that is.'

"But he glared at me like he'd like to cut my throat.

"Then the sun went down—it got dark; the wind moaned and wept, like a lost child for its dead mother. There wasn't a thing in the world left to live for; and yet I didn't want that music to stop one bit. It was happier to be miserable, than to be happy without being miserable. I couldn't understand it. I hung down my head, and pulled out my handkerchief, and blowed my nose, loud, to keep from cryin'. My eyes are weak any way. I didn't want anybody to be a-gazin' at me a-sniv'lin', and it's nobody's business what I do with my nose. It's mine.

"Then, all of a sudden, old Rubin changed his tune. He ripped and rar'd, he tipped and tar'd. 'Peared to me that all the gas in the house was turned on at once, things got so bright. It was a circus, and a brass band, and a big ball, all a-goin' on at the same time. He lit into them keys like a thousand of bricks; he set every livin' j'int in me a-goin'; and not bein' able to stand it no longer, I jumped spang on to my seat, and jest hollered:

"'Go it, my Rube!'

"Every man, woman, and child in the house riz on me, and shouted: 'Put him out! put him out! put him out!!'

"'Put your great-grandmother's grizzly-gray-greenish cat into the middle of next month!' I says. 'Tech me if you dar! I've paid my money, and I'm bound to hear old Rube out—or die!'

"He had changed his tune again. He played soft, and low, and solemn. I heard the old church-bells over the hills. The candles in heaven were lit, one by one; I saw the stars rise. The great organ of eternity began to play, from the world's end to the world's end; and the angels went to prayers...... Then the music changed to water, full of feelin' that couldn't be thought, and began to drip, drop—drip, drop—drip, drop—clear and sweet, like tears of joy fallin' into a lake of glory. It was as sweet as a sweet-heart, sweetened with white sugar, mixed with powdered silver, and seed diamonds. It was too sweet.

"Then he run his fingers through his hair, he shoved up his sleeve, he dug up his stool, he leaned over, and, sir, he jest went for that old pianner. He slapped her face, he boxed her jaws, he pulled her nose, he pinched her ears, and he scratched her cheeks till she fairly yelled. He knocked her down, and he stamped on her shameful. She bellowed like a bull, she bleated like a calf, she howled like a hound, she squealed like a pig, she shrieked like a rat, and *then* he wouldn't let her up. He crossed over first gentleman, he chassade right and left, back to your places, he all hands around, ladies to the right, promenade all, in and out, here and there, back and forth, up and down, turned and tacked and tangled into forty-'leven thousand double bow-knots.

"By jings! it was a mixtery. And *then* he wouldn't let the old pianner go. He fetched up his right wing, he fetched up his left wing, he fetched up his centre, he fetched up his reserves. He fired by file, by platoons, by companies, by regiments, and by brigades. He opened his cannon—siege-guns down thar, Napoleons here, twelve-pounders yonder—big guns, little guns, middle-sized guns, round shot, shells, shrapnels, grape, canister, mortar, mines and magazines, every livin' battery and bomb a-goin' at the same time. The house trembled, the lights danced, the walls shook, the floor come up, the ceilin' come down, the sky split, the ground rocked—heaven and earth, creation, sweet-potatoes, ninepences, tenpenny nails, roodle-oodle-oodle-oodle—ruddle-uddle-uddle-uddle—raddle-addle-addle-addle—riddle-iddle-iddle-iddle—reedle-eedle-eedle-eedle—p-r-r-r-lang! Bang! lang! per-ling! p-r-r-r-r-r!! Bang!!!

"With that bang, sir, he lifted himself bodily into the air, and he comes down with his knees, his ten fingers, his ten toes, his elbows, and his nose, strikin' every single solitary key on that pianner at the same time. The thing busted—and went off into seventeen hunderd and fifty-seven thousand five hunderd and forty-two, hemi-demi-semi-quavers, and I knowed no more." M. ADAMS.

THE BABIES.

Speech of Mark Twain at the banquet given in honour of Gen. Grant, by the Army of the Tennessee, at the Palmer House, Chicago, Nov. 14, 1879.

TOAST:

"*The Babies—As they comfort us in our sorrows, let us not forget them in our festivities.*"

I like that. We haven't all had the good fortune to be ladies; we haven't all been generals, or poets, or statesmen; but when the toast works down to the babies, we stand on common ground, for we have all been babies. It is a shame that, for a thousand years the world's banquets have utterly ignored the baby — as if *he* didn't amount to anything! If you gentlemen will stop and think a minute, — if you will go back fifty or a hundred years, to your early married life, and recontemplate your first baby, you will remember that he amounted to a good deal, and even something over. You soldiers all know that when that little fellow arrived at family head-quarters you had to hand in your resignation. He took entire command. You became his lackey, his mere body-servant, and you had to stand around, too. He was not a commander who made allowances for time, distance, weather, or anything else. You had to execute his order whether it was possible or not. And there was only one form of marching in his manual of tactics, and that was the double-quick. He treated you with every sort of insolence and disrespect, and the bravest of you didn't dare to say a word. You could face the death-storm of Donelson and Vicksburg, and give back blow for blow; but when he clawed your whiskers, and pulled your hair, and twisted your nose, you had to take it. When the thunders of war were sounding in your ears, you set your faces toward the batteries, and advanced with steady tread; but when he turned on the terrors of his war-whoop, you advanced in the other direction — and mighty glad of the chance, too. When he called for soothing syrup, did you venture to throw out any side remarks about certain services unbecoming an officer and a gentleman? No; you got up and got it. If he ordered his bottle, and it wasn't warm, did you talk back? Not you; you went to work and warmed it. You even descended so far in your menial office as to take a suck at that warm, insipid stuff yourself, to see if it was right, — three parts water to one of milk, a touch of sugar to modify the colic, and a drop of peppermint to kill those immortal hickups. I can taste that stuff yet. And how many things you learned as you went along; sentimental young folks still took stock in that beautiful old saying that when the baby smiles in his sleep, it is because the angels are whispering to him. Very pretty, but "too thin,"—simply wind on the stomach, my friends! If the baby proposed to take a walk at his usual hour, 2.30 in the morning, didn't you rise up promptly and remark—with a mental addition which wouldn't improve a Sunday-school book much—that that was the very thing you were about to propose yourself! Oh, you were under good discipline! And as you went fluttering up and down the room in your "undress uniform," you not only prattled undignified baby-talk, but even tuned up your martial voices and tried to sing "Rockaby baby in a tree-top," for instance. What a spectacle for an Army of the Tennessee! And what an affliction for the neighbours, too! for it isn't everybody within a mile around that likes military music at three in the morning. And when you had been keeping this sort of thing up two or three hours, and your little velvet-head intimated that nothing suited him like exercise and noise,—"Go on!"—what did you do? You simply *went* on, till you disappeared in the last ditch.

The idea that a baby doesn't amount to anything! Why, *one* baby is just a house and a front-yard full by itself. One baby can furnish more business than you and your whole interior department can attend to. He is enterprising, irrepressible, brimful of lawless activities. Do what you please, you can't make him stay on the reservation. Sufficient unto the day is one baby; as long as you are in your mind, don't you ever pray for twins.

Yes, it was high time for a toast-master to recognize the importance of the babies. Think what is in store for the present crop. Fifty years hence we shall all be dead, I trust, and then this flag, if it still survive—and let us hope it may—will be floating over a republic numbering 200,000,000 souls, according to the settled laws of our increase; our present schooner of state will have grown into a political leviathan— a *Great Eastern*—and the cradled babies of to-day will be on deck. Let them be well trained, for we are going to leave a big contract on their hands. Among the three or four million cradles now rocking in the land are some which this nation would preserve for ages as sacred things, if we could know which ones they are. In one of these cradles the unconscious Farragut of the future is at this moment *teething*—think of it! —and putting in a world of dead-earnest, unarticulated, but perfectly justifiable profanity over it, too; in another the future great historian is lying—and doubtless he will continue to lie until his earthly mission is ended; in another the future president is busying himself with no profounder problem of state than what the mischief has become of his hair so early: and in a mighty array of other cradles there are now some 60,000 future office-seekers getting ready to furnish him occasion to grapple with that same old problem a second time; and in still one more cradle, somewhere under the flag, the future illustrious commander-in-chief of the American armies is so little burdened with his approaching grandeurs and responsibilities as to be giving his whole strategic mind, at this moment, to trying to find out some way to get his own big toe into his mouth,—an achievement which (meaning no disrespect) the illustrious guest of this evening turned *his* whole attention to some fifty-six years ago. And if the child is but the prophecy of the man, there are mighty few will doubt that he succeeded. MARK TWAIN.

THE RAPIDS.

[ADAPTED.]

I remember once riding from Buffalo to the Niagara Falls; and I said to a gentleman, "What river is that, sir?"

"That is the Niagara river," he said.

"Well, it is a beautiful stream, bright, and fair, and glassy. How far off are the rapids?"

"Only a mile or two."

THE RAPIDS.

"Is it possible, that only a mile from here, we shall find the water in the turbulence which it must show when near the falls?"

"You will find it so, sir."

And so I found it; and that first sight of the Niagara I shall never forget.

Now, young men, launch your bark on that Niagara river. It is bright, smooth, beautiful, and glassy. The ripple at the bow, the silvery wake you leave behind, add to your enjoyment. Down the stream you glide, oars, sail, and helm in proper trim, and you set out on your pleasure excursion.

Suddenly some one cries out from the bank, "Young men, ahoy!"

"What is it?"

"The rapids are below you."

"Oh, we've heard of the rapids, but we're not such fools as to get there! If we go too fast, we'll up with the helm, and steer for the shore; we'll set the mast in the socket, hoist the sail, and speed to land. Then on, boys, on! don't be alarmed; there's no danger."

"Young men, ahoy!!"

"Well, what is it?"

"The rapids are below you."

"Ha! ha! ha!! Another old fool told us that. Bother the rapids! We'll laugh and quaff; all things delight us. What care *we* for the future? No man ever saw it! Sufficient for the day is the evil thereof. We'll enjoy life while we may; we'll catch pleasure as it flies. This—this is enjoyment—"

"Young men, ahoy!!!"

"Well, well, what is it now?"

"Beware! beware!! The rapids are below you!! Look how fast you pass that point!! See the water foaming all around you there!!"

"Ah!!! so it is!!!—Up with the helm!! Now turn!! Pull hard—quick! quick! Pull for your lives—pull! till the blood starts from the nostrils, and the veins stand like whipcord upon the brow. Set the mast—pull! pull!! hoist the sail—pull!! pull!!!"

Ah!!—it is too late!! too late!! Shrieking! howling! cursing! blaspheming!—OVER YOU GO.   J. B. GOUGH.

EUROPEAN GUIDES.

(*By kind permission of* Messrs. CHATTO AND WINDUS.)

European guides know about enough English, to tangle everything up so, that a man can make neither head nor tail of it. The guides in Génoa are delighted to secure an American party, because Americans so much wonder, and deal so much in sentiment and emotion before any relic of Columbus. Our guide there, jumped about us, as if he had swallowed—a springmattress—he was full of animation, full of impatience. He said, "Coom vis me, zhenteelmans; I show you ze letter-writing by Christopher Colombo—write eet heemself! write vis his own hand! coom!!" After much impressive fumbling of keys, and opening of locks, the stained and aged document was spread before us. Our guide's eyes sparkled, he danced about us, and tapped the parchment with his fingers. "Vat I tell you, zhenteelmans!! ees eet not so? Hand-writeeng, Christopher Colombo—write eet heemself!! Write vis hees own hand."

The doctor, one of our party, usually asks the questions, because he can keep his countenance better, and look more like—an inspired idiot—than any man living; it comes natural to him. He put up his eye-glass, and said, without any show of interest, "Ah! what did you say was the name of the gentleman who wrote this?"

"Christopher Colombo!!! Ze gret Christopher Colombo!!!"

"Christopher Columbus! the great Christopher Columbus! ah,—did he write himself?"

"He write eet heemself!! Christopher Colombo, hees own hand-writeeng, write by heemself!!!"

"Well, Ferguson, I've seen boys in New York, only fourteen years old, could write a better hand than that."

"But zis ees ze gret Christopher Colombo!!!"

"I don't care who it is—it's the worst writing I ever saw. If you've got any specimens of penmanship of real merit, trot 'em out; if you haven't, drive on."

He drove on. Our guide was considerably shaken up. He made one more venture; he said, "Ah, zhenteelmans, you coom vis me. I show you, Bee-u-ti-ful!! Grand! Magneeficent!! Bust—Christopher Colombo!!!"

"I say, Ferguson, what did you say was the name of this gentleman?"

"Christopher Colombo!! ze gret Christopher Colombo!!!"

"Christopher Colombo, the great Christopher Colombo; well, what did he do?"

"Discöver America!! discóver America!!!"

"No, Ferguson, no; that statement will hardly wash. We are just from America ourselves. We heard nothing about it. Christopher Columbus!! Pleasant name; is he—ah—dead?"

"Dead? been dead tree hundred year!!!"

"What did he die of?"

"I do not know. I cannot tell."

"Small-pox, think?"

"I do not know, zhenteelmans; I cannot tell *vat* he die of."

"Measles, likely."

"Maybe, maybe. I sink he die of—some sings."

"Very likely. Parents living?"

"Imposseeble!!"

"Which is the bust, and which is the pedestal?"

"*Zis* de bust!!! *Zis* de pedestal!!!"

"Ah, I see. Happy combination, very happy combination. Is this the first time this gentleman was ever on a bust?"— That joke was lost on the foreigner. European guides cannot master the subtleties of the American joke. Our guide walked his legs off, nearly, in hunting up extraordinary things, but it was a failure. He had reserved what he considered to be his greatest wonder, till the last—a Royal Egyptian Mummy—the best preserved in the world, perhaps. He said,—

"See, zhenteelmans, see!!! 'Mummy!! Mummy!!'"

"Ah, Ferguson, what did you say was the gentleman's name?"

"Name!!! he got no name—Mummy!!! 'Gyp-ti-an Mummy!!!"

"Yes, yes. Born here?"

"No!! no!! 'Gyptian Mummy!!!"

"Just so. Frenchman, I presume."

"No, no!! *not* French-man!! *not* Ro-man!! born in E-gyp-ta!! born in E-gyp-ta!!!"

"Born in Egypta. Never heard of Egypta before. Foreign locality, likely. Mummy, mummy—how calm he looks—how self-possessed! Is he—dead?"

"*Santa Maria!!* been dead tree tousan' year!!"

"Now look here, Ferguson! What d'ye mean by such conduct as this? Trying to impose your vile second-hand carcasses on us. If you've got a nice *fresh* corpse—fetch him out—or, by George!! I'll brain you." MARK TWAIN.

EXAMINATION OF MR. WINKLE AND SAM WELLER.

[ADAPTED FROM "THE PICKWICK PAPERS."]

Judge. What is the first case on the file, Brother Buzfuz?
Buzfuz. Bardell *versus* Pickwick, my Lud.
Judge. Who is your first witness?
Buz. Samuel Weller, my Lud.
Judge. Call Samuel Weller.

Sam Weller, upon hearing his name, stepped briskly into the witness-box, put his hat on the floor, his arms on the rail, and took a bird's-eye view of the assembled court.

Judge. What's your name, Sir?

Sam. Sam Weller, my Lord.

Judge. Do you spell it with a V or a W?

Sam. That depends upon the taste and fancy of the speller, my Lord. I never had occasion to spell it more than once or twice in my life, but I spells it with a V.

Here a voice in the gallery exclaimed aloud: "Quite right, too, Samivel; quite right.—Put it down a we, my Lord, put it down a we."

Judge. Do you know who that is who has dared to address the court?

Sam. I rayther suspect it is my father, my Lord.

Judge. Do you see him here now?

Sam. "No, I don't, my Lord," replied Sam, staring right up into the lantern in the roof of the court.

Judge. If you could have pointed him out, I would have committed him instantly.

Sam bowed his acknowledgments, and turned with unimpaired cheerfulness of countenance towards Sergeant Buzfuz.

Buz. Now, Mr. Weller.

Sam. Now, sir.

Buz. I believe you are in the service of Mr. Pickwick? Speak up, if you please, Mr. Weller.

Sam. I mean to speak up, sir. I am in the service of that 'ere gen'l'man, and a wery good service it is.

Buz. Little to do, and plenty to get, I suppose?

Sam. Oh, quite enough to get, sir, as the soldier said ven they ordered him three hundred and fifty lashes.

Judge. You must not tell us what the soldier, or any other man, said, sir; it's not evidence.

Sam. Wery good, my Lord.

Buz. Do you recollect anything particular happening on the morning when you were first engaged by the defendant? Eh, Mr. Weller?

Sam. Yes, I do, sir.

Buz. Have the goodness to tell the jury what it was.

Sam. I had a reg'lar new fit out o' clothes that mornin', gen'l'men of the jury, and that was a wery partickler and uncommon circumstance vith me in those days.

Judge. You had better be careful, sir.

Sam. So Mr. Pickwick said at the time, my Lord, and I was wery careful o' that 'ere suit o' clothes; wery careful, indeed, my Lord.

The Judge looked sternly at Sam for full two minutes; but Sam's features were so perfectly calm and serene that the Judge said nothing, and motioned Sergeant Buzfuz to proceed.

Buz. Do you mean to tell me, Mr. Weller—do you mean to tell me, that you saw nothing of the fainting on the part of the plaintiff in the arms of the defendant?

Sam. Certainly not. I was in the passage till they called me up, and then the old lady wasn't there.

Buz. Now, attend, Mr. Weller. You were in the passage till they called you up, and yet saw nothing of what was going forward! Have you a pair of eyes, Mr. Weller?

Sam. Yes, I have a pair o' eyes, and that's just it. If they was a pair o' patent double million magnifyin' gas microscopes of hextra power, p'raps I might be able to see through a flight o' stairs, and a deal door; but bein' only eyes, you see, my wision's limited.

Buz. It's perfectly useless, my Lud, attempting to get at any evidence, through the impenetrable stupidity of this witness. —Stand down, sir.

Sam. Would any other gen'l'man like to ask me anythin'?

Buz. Go down, sir ! ! !

Sam went down accordingly.

Judge. Who is your next witness, Brother Buzfuz?

Buz. Nathaniel Winkle, my Lud.

Judge. Call Nathaniel Winkle.

Mr. Winkle entered the witness-box, and bowed to the judge.

Judge. Don't look at me, sir; look at the jury.

Mr. Winkle obeyed the mandate.

Judge. What's your name, sir?

Winkle. W-Winkle.

Judge. What's your Christian name, sir?

Winkle. Na-thaniel, sir.

Judge. Daniel; any other name?

Winkle. Na-thaniel, sir.

Judge. Nathaniel Daniel, or Daniel Nathaniel?

Winkle. No, my Lord, only Na-thaniel—not Daniel at all.

Judge. Why did you tell me it was Daniel, then?

Winkle. I d-didn't, my Lord.

Judge. You did, sir; how could I have got Daniel in my notes, unless you had told me so?

Buz. Now, Mr. Winkle, attend to me, if you please. I believe you are a particular friend of Mr. Pickwick, are you not?

Winkle. I—I have known Mr. Pickwick, now—as well as I can recollect at this moment, nearly—

Buz. Pray, Mr. Winkle, do not evade the question. Are you, or are you not, a particular friend of Mr. Pickwick?

Winkle. I—I was just about to say, that—

Buz. Will you, or will you not, answer my question?

Judge. If you don't answer the question, sir, you'll be committed.

Buz. Come, sir, yes or no, if you please.

Winkle. Y-Yes—I am.

Buz. Yes, you are!! And why couldn't you say so at once, sir? Perhaps you know Mrs. Bardell, too—eh, Mr. Winkle?

Winkle. I—I don't know her—I—I've seen her.

Buz. Oh, you don't know her, but you've seen her. What do you mean by that, Mr. Winkle?

Winkle. I—mean that I am not intimate with her, but that

I have seen her, when I went to call upon my friend, Mr. P-Pickwick, in G-Goswell Street.

Judge. Will you stop that stammering, Mr. Winkle!!!

Winkle. My Lord, it's a natural impediment in my sp-speech —which I c-can by no p-possibility g-get over.

Buz. Oh, get down, Mr. Winkle. CHARLES DICKENS.

"SAM WELLER'S VALENTINE."

[*Adapted from " The Pickwick Papers."*]

SAM WELLER and MR. WELLER, Senior.

Old Weller. Vell, Sammy!!

Sam. Vell, my Prooshan Blue; what's the last bulletin about mother-in-law?

Old W. Mrs. Veller passed a wery good night, but is uncommon perwerse, and unpleasant this mornin'. Signed upon oath, S. Veller, Esquire, Senior. That's the last vun as was issued, Sammy.

Sam. No better yet?

Old W. All the symptoms aggerawated. But what's that you're a-doin' of? pursuit of knowledge under difficulties— eh, Sammy?

Sam. I've done now, father; I've been a-writin'.

Old W. So I see. Not to any young 'ooman, I hope, Sammy?

Sam. Why, it's no use a-sayin' it ain't. It's a walentine.

Old W. A what!!

Sam. A walentine.

Old W. Samivel! Samivel! I didn't think you'd ha' done it!! Arter the warnin' you've had o' your father's wicious propensities; arter all I've said to you upon this here wery subject; arter activally seein' and bein' in the company of your own mother-in-law, vich I should ha' thought was a moral

lesson as no man could never ha' forgotten to his dyin' day!!
I didn't think you'd ha' done it, Sammy!! I didn't think
you'd ha' done it!!

Sam. Wot's the matter now?

Old W. Nev'r mind, Sammy. It'll be a wery agonizin' trial
to me at my time o' life; but I'm pretty tough, as the wery old
turkey remarked, wen the farmer said he was afeard he'd be
obliged to kill him, for the London market.

Sam. Wot'll be a trial?

Old W. To see you married, Sammy. To see you a deluded
wictim, and you thinkin,' in your innocence, that it's all wery
capital. It's a dreadful trial to a father's feelin's, that 'ere
Sammy.

Sam. Nonsense!! I ain't a-goin' to get married; don't fret
yourself about that. I know you're a judge o' these things.
Order in your pipe, and I'll read you the letter—there!!

Old W. All right, Sammy, fire away!!!

Sam. [*Reading*] "Lovely creetur—"

Old W. Stop. 'Tain't in poetry, is it?

Sam. No, no.

Old W. Wery glad to hear it, Sammy. Poetry's unnat'ral.
No man ever talked poetry 'cept a beadle on boxin' day—or
Warren's blackin'—or Rowland's oil—or some o' them low
fellows. Never you let yourself down to talk poetry, my
boy. Begin agin, Sammy.

Sam. "Lovely creetur, I feel myself a—I feel myself a—"

Old W. You feel yourself a wot, Sammy?

Sam. There's a blot here. Oh—it's "shamed." "I feel
myself ashamed."

Old W. Wery good, Sammy; go on.

Sam. "Feel myself ashamed and completely cir—" I forget
wot this here word is.

Old W. Why don't you look at it then?

Sam. So I am a-lookin' at it, but there's another blot.
Here's a "c," and a "i," and a "d."

Old W. Circumwented, p'raps.

Sam. No, it ain't that—"circumscribed;" that's it.

Old W. That ain't as good a word as circumwented, Sammy.

Sam. Think not?

Old W. Nothin' like it.

Sam. But don't you think it means more?

Old W. Vell, p'raps it is a more tenderer word. Go on, Sammy.

Sam. "Feel myself ashamed and completely circumscribed in a dressin' of you, for you *are* a nice gal and nothin' but it."

Old W. That's a wery pretty sentiment, Sammy.

Sam. Yes; I think it is rayther good.

Old W. Wot I like in that 'ere style o' writin', is, that there ain't no callin' names in it—no Wenuses, nor nothin' o' that kind. Wot's the good o' callin' a young 'ooman a Wenus or a angel, Sammy? You might jist as well call her a griffin, or a unicorn, or a king's arms at once, vich is wery well known to be a col-lection o' fabulous animals. Drive on, Sammy.

Sam. "Afore I see you I thought all women was alike."

Old W. So they are.

Sam. "But now I find what a reg'lar soft-headed, inkred'lous turnip I must ha' been; for there ain't nobody like you, though *I* like you better than nothin' at all."

Old W. I'm afeard that werges on the poetical, Sammy.

Sam. No, it don't. "Except of me Mary my dear as your walentine and think over what I've said.—My dear Mary I will now conclude." That's all.

Old W. That's rayther a sudden pull up, ain't it, Sammy?

Sam. Not a bit on it. She'll vish there was more, and that's the great art o' letter-writin'.

Old W. Vell, there's somethin' in that; an' I wish your mother-in-law 'ud only conduct her conwersation on the same genteel principle. CHARLES DICKENS.

FROM "HAMLET."

Enter ROSENCRANTZ, GUILDENSTERN, and HAMLET.

Guil. Good my lord, vouchsafe me a word with you.
Ham. Sir, a whole history.
Guil. The king, sir,—
Ham. Ay, sir, what of him?
Guil. Is in his retirement marvellously distempered.
Ham. With drink, sir?
Guil. No, my lord, rather with choler.
Ham. Your wisdom should show itself more richer to signify this to his doctor; for, for me to put him to his purgation, would perhaps plunge him into more choler.
Guil. Good my lord, put your discourse into some frame, and start not so wildly from my affair.
Ham. I am tame, sir: pronounce.
Guil. The queen, your mother, in most great affliction of spirit, hath sent me to you.
Ham. You are welcome.
Guil. Nay, good my lord, this courtesy is not of the right breed. If it shall please you to make me a wholesome answer, I will do your mother's commandment; if not, your pardon and my return shall be the end of my business.
Ham. Sir, I cannot.
Guil. What, my lord?
Ham. Make you a wholesome answer; my wit's diseased: but, sir, such answer as I can make, you shall command; or, rather, as you say, my mother; therefore no more, but to the matter: My mother, you say,—
Ros. Then, thus she says: Your behaviour hath struck her into amazement and admiration.
Ham. O wonderful son, that can so astonish a mother!
Ros. She desires to speak with you in her closet, ere you go to bed.

Ham. We shall obey, were she ten times our mother. Have you any further trade with us?

Ros. My lord, you once did love me.

Ham. And do still, by these pickers and stealers.

Ros. Good my lord, what is your cause of distemper? you do, surely, but bar the door upon your own liberty, if you deny your griefs to your friend.

Ham. Sir, I lack advancement.

Ros. How can that be, when you have the voice of the king himself for your succession in Denmark?

Ham. Ay, sir, but, *While the grass grows*—the proverb is something musty. Why do you go about to recover the wind of me, as if you would drive me into a toil?

Guil. O my lord, if my duty be too bold, my love is too unmannerly.

Ham. I do not well understand that. Will you play upon this pipe?

Guil. My lord, I cannot.

Ham. I pray you.

Guil. Believe me, I cannot.

Ham. I do beseech you.

Guil. I know no touch of it, my lord.

Ham. 'Tis as easy as lying: govern these ventages with your fingers and thumb, give it breath with your mouth, and it will discourse most eloquent music. Look you, these are the stops.

Guil. But these cannot I command to any utterance of harmony; I have not the skill.

Ham. Why, look you now, how unworthy a thing you make of me! You would play upon me; you would seem to know my stops; you would pluck out the heart of my mystery; you would sound me from my lowest note to the top of my compass: and there is much music, excellent voice in this little organ; yet cannot you make it speak. Why! do you think I am easier to be played on than a pipe? Call me what instrument you will, though you can fret me, you cannot play upon me.

Enter POLONIUS.

Pol. My lord, the queen would speak with you, and presently.

Ham. Do you see yonder cloud that's almost in shape of a camel?

Pol. By the mass, and 'tis like a camel, indeed.

Ham. Methinks it is like a weasel.

Pol. It is backed like a weasel.

Ham. Or like a whale?

Pol. Very like a whale.

Ham. Then I will come to my mother by-and-by.—They fool me to the top of my bent.—I will come by-and-by.

Pol. I will say so.

Ham. By-and-by is easily said. [*Exit Polonius.*]—Leave me, friends. [*Exeunt Rosencrantz and Guildenstern.*
'Tis now the very witching time of night,
When churchyards yawn, and hell itself breathes out
Contagion to this world. Now could I drink hot blood,
And do such bitter business as the day
Would quake to look on. Soft! now to my mother.—
O heart, lose not thy nature; let not ever
The soul of Nero enter this firm bosom:
Let me be cruel, not unnatural:
I will speak daggers to her, but use none. [*Exit.*

Enter HAMLET and QUEEN.

Hamlet. Now, mother, what's the matter?

Queen. Hamlet, thou hast thy father much offended.

Hamlet. Mother, you have my father much offended.

Queen. Come, come, you answer with an idle tongue.

Hamlet. Go, go, you question with a wicked tongue.

Queen. Why, how now, Hamlet?

Hamlet. What's the matter now?

Queen. Have you forgot me?

Hamlet. No, by the rood, not so: you are the queen, your

husband's brother's wife; and—would it were not so!—you are my mother.

Queen. Nay, then, I'll set those to you that can speak.

Hamlet. Come, come, and sit you down; you shall not budge; you go not till I set you up a glass where you may see the inmost part of you.

Queen. What wilt thou do? thou wilt not murder me?

Hamlet. Leave wringing of your hands: peace! sit you down, and let me wring your heart; for so I shall, if it be made of penetrable stuff, if wicked custom have not brazed it so that it is proof and bulwark against sense.

Queen. What have I done, that thou darest wag thy tongue in noise so rude against me?

Hamlet. Such an act, that blurs the grace and blush of modesty; calls virtue, hypocrite; takes off the rose from the fair forehead of an innocent love, and sets a blister there; makes marriage-vows as false as dicers' oaths: oh, such a deed as from the body of contraction plucks the very soul, and sweet religion makes a rhapsody of words! Ah me! that act!

Queen. Ah me, what act, that roars so loud, and thunders in the index?

Hamlet. Look here, upon this picture, and on this, the counterfeit presentment of two brothers. See, what a grace was seated on this brow; Hyperion's curls; the front of Jove himself; an eye like Mars, to threaten and command; a station like the herald Mercury, new-lighted on a heaven-kissing hill; a combination and a form indeed, where every god did seem to set his seal, to give the world assurance of a man: this *was* your husband.—Look you now, what follows: here *is* your husband; like a mildewed ear, blasting his wholesome brother.

Queen. Oh, speak to me no more; these words, like daggers, enter into mine ears; no more, sweet Hamlet!

Hamlet. A murderer and a villain; a slave that is not twentieth part the tithe of your precedent lord: a vice of kings; a cutpurse of the empire and the rule, that from a shelf the precious diadem stole, and put it in his pocket!

Queen. No more.

Hamlet. A king of shreds and patches,—[*Enter Ghost.*] Save me, and hover o'er me with your wings, you heavenly guards!— What would your gracious figure?

Queen. Alas, he's mad!

Hamlet. Do you not come your tardy son to chide, that, lapsed in time and passion, lets go by the important acting of your dread command? Oh, say!

Ghost. Do not forget: this visitation is but to whet thy almost blunted purpose.—But, look! amazement on thy mother sits: oh, step between her and her fighting soul; speak to her, Hamlet.

Hamlet. How is it with you, lady?

Queen. Alas, how is't with *you*, that you do bend your eye on vacancy, and with the incorporeal air do hold discourse? O gentle son! upon the heat and flame of thy distemper, sprinkle cool patience. Whereon do you look?

Hamlet. On him, on him! Look you, how pale he glares! His form and cause conjoined, preaching to stones, would make them capable.—Do not look upon me; lest, with this piteous action, you convert my stern effects: then what I have to do will want true colour; tears, perchance, for blood.

Queen. To whom do you speak this?

Hamlet. Do you see nothing there?

Queen. Nothing at all; yet all that is I see.

Hamlet. Nor did you nothing hear?

Queen. No, nothing but ourselves.

Hamlet. Why, look you there! look, how it steals away! My father, in his habit as he lived! Look, where he goes, even now, out at the portal! [*Exit Ghost.*

Queen. This is the very coinage of your brain: this bodiless creation, ecstasy is very cunning in.

Hamlet. Ecstasy! My pulse, as yours, doth temperately

keep time, and makes as healthful music: it is not madness that I have uttered: bring me to the test, and I the matter will re-word; which madness would gambol from. Mother, for love of grace, lay not that flattering unction to your soul, that not your trespass, but my madness, speaks: it will but skin and film the ulcerous place, whiles rank corruption, mining all within, infects unseen. Confess yourself to heaven; repent what's past; avoid what is to come.

Queen. O Hamlet, thou hast cleft my heart in twain.

Hamlet. Oh, throw away the worser part of it, and live the purer with the other half. Good night! And when you are desirous to be blessed, I'll blessing beg of you. So, again, good night. I must be cruel, only to be kind: thus bad begins, and worse remains behind.　　　　　　　　　SHAKESPEARE.

FROM "MACBETH."

Macb. Is this a dagger which I see before me,
The handle toward my hand? Come, let me clutch thee.—
I have thee not, and yet I see thee still.
Art thou not, fatal vision, sensible
To feeling as to sight? or art thou but
A dagger of the mind, a false creation,
Proceeding from the heat-oppressèd brain?
I see thee yet, in form as palpable
As this which now I draw.
Thou marshall'st me the way that I was going;
And such an instrument I was to use.
Mine eyes are made the fools o' the other senses,
Or else worth all the rest; I see thee still,
And on thy blade and dudgeon gouts of blood,
Which was not so before.—There's no such thing:
It is the bloody business which informs
Thus to mine eyes.—Now o'er the one half-world

Nature seems dead, and wicked dreams abuse
The curtained sleep; witchcraft celebrates
Pale Hecate's offerings, and withered Murder,
Alarumed by his sentinel, the wolf,
Whose howl's his watch, thus with his stealthy pace,
With Tarquin's ravishing strides, towards his design
Moves like a ghost.—Thou sure and firm-set earth,
Hear not my steps, which way they walk, for fear
Thy very stones prate of my whereabout,
And take the present horror from the time,
Which now suits with it.—Whiles I threat, he lives:
Words to the heat of deeds too cold breath gives.
[*A bell rings.*
I go, and it is done; the bell invites me.
Hear it not, Duncan; for it is a knell
That summons thee to heaven or to hell. [*Exit.*

Enter LADY MACBETH.

Lady M. That which hath made them drunk hath made me bold;
What hath quenched them hath given me fire.—Hark!—Peace!
It was the owl that shrieked, the fatal bellman,
Which gives the stern'st good-night.—He is about it:
The doors are open; and the surfeited grooms
Do mock their charge with snores: I have drugged their possets—
Macb. [*Within*] Who's there?
Lady M. Alack, I am afraid they have awaked,
And 'tis not done. The attempt and not the deed
Confounds us.—Hark!—I laid their daggers ready;
He could not miss 'em. Had he not resembled
My father as he slept, I had done't.

Enter MACBETH.

Macb. I have done the deed. Didst thou not hear a noise?

Lady M. I heard the owl scream and the crickets cry. Did not you speak ?
Macb. When ?
Lady M. Now.
Macb. As I descended ?
Lady M. Ay.
Macb. Methought I heard a voice cry, "Sleep no more !
Macbeth does murder sleep,"—the innocent sleep,
Sleep that knits up the ravelled sleave of care,
The death of each day's life, sore labour's bath,
Balm of hurt minds, great nature's second course,
Chief nourisher in life's feast,—
Lady M. What do you mean ?
Macb. Still it cried "Sleep no more ! " to all the house :
" Glamis hath murdered sleep, and therefore Cawdor
Shall sleep no more ; Macbeth shall sleep no more."
Lady M. Who was it that thus cried ? Why, worthy thane,
You do unbend your noble strength, to think
So brainsickly of things. Go get some water,
And wash this filthy witness from your hand.
Why did you bring these daggers from the place ?
They must lie *there :* go carry them ; and smear
The sleepy grooms with blood.
Macb. I'll go no more :
I am afraid to think what I have done ;
Look on't again I dare not.
Lady M. Infirm of purpose !
Give me the daggers : the sleeping and the dead
Are but as pictures : 'tis the eye of childhood
That fears a painted devil. If he do bleed,
I'll gild the faces of the grooms withal ;
For it must seem their guilt. [*Exit. Knocking within.*
Macb. Whence is that knocking ?
How is't with me, when every noise appals me ?

What hands are here? ha! they pluck out mine eyes.
Will all great Neptune's ocean wash this blood
Clean from my hand? No, this my hand will rather
The multitudinous seas incarnadine,
Making the green one red.

Re-enter LADY MACBETH.

Lady M. My hands are of *your* colour; but I shame
To wear a heart so white.—[*Knocking within.*] I hear a knocking
At the south entry: retire we to our chamber:
A little water clears us of this deed:
How easy is it, then! [*Knocking within.*
Hark! more knocking.
Be not lost
So poorly in your thoughts.
    Macb. To know my deed, 'twere best not know myself.
[*Knocking within.*
Wake Duncan with thy knocking! I would thou couldst!
[*Exeunt.*
SHAKESPEARE.

FROM "JULIUS CÆSAR."

BRUTUS AND CASSIUS.

Cas. That you have wronged me doth appear in this: you have condemned and noted Lucius Pella, for taking bribes here of the Sardians; wherein my letters (praying on his side, because I knew the man) were slighted of.

Bru. You wronged yourself, to write in such a case.

Cas. In such a time as this, it is not meet that every nice offence should bear its comment.

Bru. Yet let me tell you, Cassius, you yourself are much condemned to have an itching palm; to sell and mart your offices for gold, to undeservers.

Cas. I an itching palm! You know that you are Brutus that speak this; or, by the gods, this speech were else your last!

Bru. The name of Cassius honours this corruption, and chastisement doth therefore hide its head.

Cas. Chastisement!

Bru. Remember March, the ides of March, remember! Did not great Julius bleed for justice' sake? What villain touched his body, that did stab, and not for justice? What! shall one of us, that struck the foremost man of all this world, but for supporting robbers,—shall we now contaminate our fingers with base bribes, and sell the mighty space of our large honours, for so much trash as may be graspèd thus? I had rather be a dog, and bay the moon, than such a Roman.

Cas. Brutus, bay not me;—I'll not endure it: you forget yourself, to hedge me in. I am a soldier, I, older in practice, abler than yourself to make conditions.

Bru. Go to; you are not, Cassius.

Cas. I am!

Bru. I say you are not.

Cas. Urge me no more, I shall forget myself; have mind upon your health, tempt me no further.

Bru. Away, slight man!

Cas. Is't possible?

Bru. Hear me, for I will speak. Must I give way and room to your rash choler? Shall I be frighted when a madman stares?

Cas. O gods, ye gods! must I endure all this?

Bru. All this! ay, more. Fret, till your proud heart break; go, show your slaves how choleric you are, and make your bondmen tremble. Must I budge? must I observe you? must I stand and crouch under your testy humour? By the gods, you shall digest the venom of your spleen, though it do split you; for, from this day forth, I'll use you for my mirth, yea, for my laughter, when you are waspish.

Cas. Is it come to this?

Bru. You say you are a better soldier: let it appear so; make your vaunting true, and it shall please me well. For mine own part, I shall be glad to learn of noble men.

Cas. You wrong me every way; you wrong me, Brutus: I said, an elder soldier, not a better: did I say "better"?

Bru. If you did, I care not.

Cas. When Cæsar lived, he durst not thus have moved me!

Bru. Peace, peace! you durst not so have tempted him.

Cas. I durst not!

Bru. No.

Cas. What, durst not tempt him!

Bru. For your life you durst not.

Cas. Do not presume too much upon my love; I may do that I shall be sorry for.

Bru. You have done that you should be sorry for. There is no terror, Cassius, in your threats; for I am armed so strong in honesty, that they pass by me as the idle wind, which I respect not. I did send to you for certain sums of gold, which you denied me; for I can raise no money by vile means. I had rather coin my heart, and drop my blood for drachmas, than to wring, from the hard hands of peasants, their vile trash, by any indirection. I did send to you for gold to pay my legions, which you denied me: was that done like Cassius? Should I have answered Caius Cassius so? When Marcus Brutus grows so covetous, to lock such rascal counters from his friends, be ready, gods, with all your thunderbolts; dash him to pieces!

Cas. I denied you not.

Bru. You did.

Cas. I did not: he was but a fool that brought my answer back.—Brutus hath rived my heart: a friend should bear his friend's infirmities, but Brutus makes mine greater than they are.

Bru. I do not, till you practise them on me.

Cas. You love me not.

Bru. I do not like your faults.

Cas. A friendly eye could never see such faults.

Bru. A flatterer's would not, though they do appear as huge as high Olympus!

Cas. Come, Antony, and young Octavius, come! revenge yourselves alone on Cassius, for Cassius is a-weary of the world; hated by one he loves; braved by his brother; checked like a bondman; all his faults observed, set in a note-book, learned, and conned by rote, to cast into my teeth. Oh, I could weep my spirit from mine eyes!—There is my dagger, and here my naked breast; within, a heart dearer than Plutus's mine, richer than gold: if that thou be'st a Roman, take it forth; I, that denied thee gold, will give my heart: strike, as thou didst at Cæsar; for, I know, when thou didst hate him worst, thou lovedst him better than ever thou lovedst Cassius.

Bru. Sheathe your dagger: be angry when you will, it shall have scope; do what you will, dishonour shall be humour. O Cassius, you are yokèd with a lamb, that carries anger as the flint bears fire: which, much enforcèd, shows a hasty spark, and straight is cold again.

Cas. Hath Cassius lived to be but mirth and laughter to his Brutus, when grief, and blood | ill-tempered, vexeth him?

Bru. When I spoke that, I was ill-tempered too.

Cas. Do you confess so much? Give me your hand.

Bru. And my heart too.

Cas. O Brutus! Have you not love enough to bear with me, when that rash humour which my mother gave me, makes me forgetful?

Bru. Yes, Cassius; and, from henceforth, when you are over-earnest with your Brutus, he'll think your mother chides, and leave you so. SHAKESPEARE.

FROM "THE MERCHANT OF VENICE."

SHYLOCK ON REVENGE.

Shylock. How now, Tubal! what news from Genoa? hast thou found my daughter?

Tubal. I often came where I did hear of her, but cannot find her.

Shy. Why, there, there, there, there! a diamond gone, cost me two thousand ducats in Frankfort! The curse never fell on our nation till now; I never felt it till now:—two thousand ducats in that; and other precious, precious jewels.—I would my daughter were dead at my foot, and the jewels in her ear! would she were hearsed at my foot, and the ducats in her coffin! No news of them?—Why, thou loss upon loss! the thief gone with so much, and so much to find the thief; and no satisfaction, no revenge! nor no ill luck stirring, but what lights on my shoulders; no sighs, but of my breathing; no tears, but of my shedding.

Tub. Yes, other men have ill luck too: Antonio, as I heard in Genoa—

Shy. What, what, what? ill luck, ill luck?

Tub. Hath an argosy cast away, coming from Tripolis.

Shy. I thank God, I thank God! Is't true, is't true?

Tub. I spoke with some of the sailors that escaped the wreck.

Shy. I thank thee, good Tubal:—good news, good news! ha, ha!—where? in Genoa?

Tub. Your daughter spent in Genoa, as I heard, in one night fourscore ducats.

Shy. Thou stickest a dagger in me:—I shall never see my gold again. Fourscore ducats at a sitting! fourscore ducats!

Tub. There came divers of Antonio's creditors in my company to Venice, that swear he cannot choose but break.

Shy. I am very glad of it: I'll plague him, I'll torture him: I am glad of it.

FROM "THE MERCHANT OF VENICE."

Tub. One of them showed me a ring he had of your daughter, for a monkey.

Shy. Out upon her! Thou torturest me, Tubal. It was my turquoise; I had it of Leah, when I was a bachelor: I would not have given it for a wilderness of monkeys!!!

Tub. But Antonio is certainly undone.

Shy. Nay, that's true, that's very true! I will have the heart of him, if he forfeit!! Go, go, Tubal; meet me at our synagogue. Go, good Tubal; at our synagogue, Tubal.

[*Exit Tubal.*

Enter SALARINO.

Sal. How now, Shylock! what news among the merchants?

Shy. You knew, none so well, none so well as you, of my daughter's flight.

Sal. That's certain: I knew the tailor that made the wings she flew withal. But say, do you hear whether Antonio have had any loss at sea or no?

Shy. There I have another bad match: a bankrupt, a prodigal, who dare scarce show his head on the Rialto; a beggar, that was used to come so smug upon the mart; let him look to his bond! he was wont to call me usurer; let him look to his bond!! he was wont to lend money for a Christian courtesy; let him look to his bond!!!

Sal. Why, if he forfeit, thou wilt not take his flesh? What's that good for?

Shy. To bait fish withal. If it will feed nothing else, it will feed my revenge!! He hath disgraced me, and hindered me half-a-million; laughed at my losses, mocked at my gains, scorned my nation, thwarted my bargains, cooled my friends, heated mine enemies; and what's his reason? I am a Jew. Hath not a Jew eyes? hath not a Jew hands, organs, dimensions, senses, affections, passions? fed with the same food, hurt with the same weapons, subject to the same diseases, healed by the same means, warmed and cooled by the same winter and summer, as a Christian is? If you prick us, do we not bleed? if you tickle us, do we not laugh? if you poison us, do we not die? and if you wrong us, shall we not revenge? If we are like you in the rest, we will resemble you in that. If a Jew wrong a Christian, what is his humility? Revenge!! If a Christian wrong a Jew, what should his sufferance be by Christian example? Why, revenge!!! The villany you teach me, I will execute; and it shall go hard but I will better the instruction.

SHAKESPEARE.

THE TWO GRAVE-DIGGERS IN "HAMLET."

1st G. D. Is she to be buried in Christian burial, that wilfully seeks her own salvation?

2nd G. D. I tell thee she is; therefore make her grave straight. The crowner hath sat on her, and finds it Christian burial.

1st G. D. How can that be, unless she drowned herself in her own defence?

2nd G. D. Why, 'tis found so.

1st G. D. It must be *se offendendo;* * it cannot be else, for here lies the point: if I drown myself wittingly, it argues an act; and an act hath three branches—it is, to act, to do, and to perform; *argal,*† she drowned herself wittingly.

2nd G. D. Nay, but hear you, goodman delver.

1st G. D. Give *me* leave. Here lies the water; good. Here stands the man; good. If the man go to this water, and drown himself, it is, will he, nill he, he goes—mark you that; but if the water come to him, and drown him, he drowns not himself: *argal,* he that is not guilty of his own death, shortens not his own life.—Come, my spade.—There is no ancient gentlemen, but gardeners, ditchers, and grave-makers: they hold up Adam's profession.

2nd G. D. Was he a gentleman?

* By offending herself.
† The grave-digger's corruption of *ergo,* therefore.

1st G. D. He was the first that ever bore arms.

2nd G. D. Why, he had none.

1st G. D. What! art a heathen? How dost thou understand the Scripture? The Scripture says, "Adam digged." Could he dig without arms? I'll put another question to thee: What is he that builds stronger than either the mason, the shipwright, or the carpenter?

2nd G. D. The gallows-maker; for that frame outlives a thousand tenants.

1st G. D. I like thy wit well, in good faith: the gallows does well; but how does it well? it does well to those that do ill: *argal*, the gallows may do well to thee. To't again; come.

2nd G. D. What is he that builds stronger than a mason, a shipwright, or a carpenter?

1st G. D. Ay, tell me that, and unyoke.

2nd G. D. Marry, now I can tell—mass, I cannot tell.

Enter HAMLET *and* HORATIO.

1st G. D. Cudgel thy brains no more about it, for your dull ass will not mend his pace with beating; and when you are asked this question next, say "a grave-maker,"—for the houses that he makes last till doomsday. Go, get thee to Yaughan, and fetch me a stoup of liquor.   [*Exit 2nd Grave-digger.*

1st G. D. [*digs and sings*]—

> "In youth, when I did love, did love,
>   Methought it was very sweet,
> Oh, a pit of clay for to be made
>   For such a guest is meet."

Hamlet. I will speak to this fellow.—Whose grave's this, sir?

1st G. D. Mine, sir.

Hamlet. I think it be thine indeed; for thou liest in't.

1st G. D. You lie out on't, sir, and therefore it is not yours; for my part, I do not lie in't, and yet it is mine.

Hamlet. Thou dost lie in't, to be in't, and say it is thine. 'Tis for the dead, not for the quick; therefore thou liest.

1st G. D. 'Tis a quick lie, sir; 'twill away again, from me to you.
Hamlet. What man dost thou dig it for?
1st G. D. For no man, sir.
Hamlet. What woman, then?
1st G. D. For none, neither.
Hamlet. Who is to be buried in't?
1st G. D. One that *was* a woman, sir; but, rest her soul, she's dead.
Hamlet. How long hast thou been a grave-maker?
1st G. D. Of all the days i' the year, I came to't that very day our last king Hamlet overcame Fortinbras.
Hamlet. How long is that since?
1st G. D. Cannot you tell that? every fool can tell that. It was the very day that young Hamlet was born; he that is mad, and sent into England.
Hamlet. Ay, marry.—Why was he sent into England?
1st G. D. Why, because he was mad : he shall recover his wits there; or, if he do not, 'tis no great matter there.
Hamlet. Why?
1st G. D. 'Twill not be seen in him there. There the men are as mad as he.
Hamlet. How came he mad?
1st G. D. Very strangely, they say.
Hamlet. How strangely?
1st G. D. 'Faith, e'en with losing his wits.
Hamlet. Upon what ground?
1st G. D. Why, here in Denmark. I have been sexton here, man and boy, thirty years.
Hamlet. How long will a man lie i' the earth ere he rot?
1st G. D. I' faith, he will last you some eight year or nine year : a tanner will last you nine year.
Hamlet. Why he, more than another?
1st G. D. Why, sir, his hide is so tanned with his trade, that he will keep out water a great while. Here's a skull now; this skull hath lain i' the earth three-and-twenty years.

Hamlet. Whose was it?

1st G. D. A queer mad fellow's it was. Whose do you think it was?

Hamlet. Nay, I know not.

1st G. D. A pestilence on him for a mad rogue! a' poured a flagon o' Rhenish on my head once. This same skull, sir, was Yorick's skull, the king's jester.

Hamlet. This?

1st G. D. E'en that.

Hamlet. Let me see.—[*Takes the skull.*] Alas, poor Yorick!— I knew him, Horatio: a fellow of infinite jest, of most excellent fancy; he hath borne me on his back a thousand times; and now, how abhorrèd in my imagination it is! my gorge rises at it. Here hung those lips that I have kissed, I know not how oft. Where be your gibes now? your gambols? your songs? your flashes of merriment, that were wont to set the table on a roar? Not one now, to mock your own grinning? quite chapfallen? Now get you to my lady's chamber, and tell her, let her paint an inch thick, to this favour she must come.

SHAKESPEARE.

FROM "THE RIVALS."

SIR LUCIUS O'TRIGGER AND BOB ACRES.

I.—*The Challenge.*

Sir Lucius. Mr. Acres, I am delighted to embrace you.

Acres. My dear Sir Lucius, I kiss your hands.

Sir L. Pray, my friend, what has brought you so suddenly to Bath?

Acres. 'Faith I have followed Cupid's Jack-a-lantern, and find myself in a quagmire at last. In short, I have been very ill-used, Sir Lucius. I don't choose to mention names, but look on me as a very ill-used gentleman.

Sir L. Pray, what is the case? I ask no names.

Acres. Mark me, Sir Lucius. I fall as deep as need be in love with a young lady—her friends take my part—I follow her to Bath—send word of my arrival—and receive for answer, that the lady is to be otherwise disposed of. This, Sir Lucius, I call being ill-used.

Sir L. Very ill, upon my conscience! Pray, can you divine the cause of it?

Acres. Why, there's the matter! She has another lover, one Beverley, who, I am told, is now in Bath.—Odds slanders and lies! he must be at the bottom of it.

Sir L. A rival in the case, is there? and you think he has supplanted you unfairly?

Acres. Unfairly! to be sure he has. He never could have done it fairly.

Sir L. Then sure you know what is to be done?

Acres. Done—not I.

Sir L. We wear no swords here—but you understand me.

Acres. What! fight him?

Sir L. Ay, to be sure; what can I mean else?

Acres. But he has given me no provocation.

Sir L. Now I think he has given you the greatest provocation in the world. Can a man commit a more heinous offence against another, than to fall in love with the same woman? It is the most unpardonable breach of friendship.

Acres. Breach of friendship! Ay, ay; but I have no acquaintance with this man. I never saw him in my life.

Sir L. That's no argument at all; he has the less right, then, to take such a liberty.

Acres. That's true: I grow full of anger, Sir Lucius—I fire apace! Odds hilts and blades! I find a man may have a deal of valour in him, and not know it. But couldn't I contrive to have a little right on my side?

Sir L. What signifies *right* when your *honour* is concerned? Do you think Achilles, or my little Alexander the Great, ever inquired where the right lay? No, they drew their broadswords, and left the lazy sons of peace to settle the justice of it.

Acres. Your words are a grenadier's march to my heart: I believe courage must be catching! I certainly do feel a kind of valour arising, as it were—a kind of courage, as I may say. Odds flints, pans, and triggers! I'll challenge him directly.

Sir L. Ah, my little friend, if we had Blunderbuss Hall here, I could show you a range of ancestry, in the O'Trigger line, that would furnish the New Room, every one of whom had killed his man. For though the mansion-house and dirty acres have slipped through my fingers, our honour and the family pictures are as fresh as ever.

Acres. O Sir Lucius, I have had ancestors too — every man of them colonel, or captain in the militia! Odds balls and barrels! say no more—I'm braced for it. The thunder of your words has soured the milk of human kindness in my breast! Zounds! as the man in the play says, "I could do such deeds "—

Sir L. Come, come, there must be no passion at all in the case; these things should always be done civilly.

Acres. I must be in a passion, Sir Lucius—I must be in a rage! Dear Sir Lucius, let me be in a rage if you love me. Come, here's pen and paper. Indite, I say, indite. How shall I begin? Odds bullets and blades! I'll write a good bold hand, however.

Sir L. Pray, compose yourself. Begin now. "Sir "—

Acres. That's too civil by half.

Sir L. "To prevent the confusion which might arise "—

Acres. "To prevent the confusion which might arise "— Well?

Sir L. "From our both addressing the same lady "—

Acres. Ay, Sir Lucius; that's the reason — "same lady." Well?

Sir L. "I shall expect the honour of your company "—

Acres. Zounds, I'm not asking him to dinner!

Sir L. Pray, be easy.

Acres. Well, then, "honour of your company"—

Sir L. "To settle our pretensions"—

Acres. "To settle our pretensions"—Well?

Sir L. Let me see—ay, "in King's Mead-fields."

Acres. "In King's Mead-fields." So, that's down: my own crest; a hand and dagger shall be the seal.

Sir L. You see now, this little explanation will put a stop at once to all confusion or misunderstanding that might arise between you.

Acres. Ay, we fight to prevent any misunderstanding.

Sir L. I'll leave you to fix your own time. Take my advice, and you'll decide it this evening, if you can; then, let the worst come of it, 'twill be off your mind in the morning.

Acres. Very true.

Sir L. Remember now, when you meet your antagonist, do everything in a mild and agreeable manner. Let your courage be as keen, but at the same time as polished as your sword. Good-morning, Mr. Acres.

Acres. Good-morning, Sir Lucius. [*Exit Sir Lucius.*] If the worst comes to the worst, it certainly *shall* be off my mind in the morning.

II.—*The Duel.*

Acres. By my valour! then, Sir Lucius, forty yards is a good distance. Odds levels and aims! I say it is a good distance.

Sir L. It is for muskets, or small field-pieces. Upon my conscience, Mr. Acres, you must leave these things to me. Stay, now—I'll show you. [*Measures six paces.*] There, now, that is a very pretty distance—a pretty gentleman's distance.

Acres. We might as well fight in a sentry-box! I tell you, Sir Lucius, the farther he is off, the cooler I shall take my aim.

Sir L. I suppose you would aim at him best of all if he was out of sight?

Acres. No, Sir Lucius; but I should think forty, or eight-and-thirty yards—

Sir L. Pho, pho! nonsense! three or four feet between the mouths of your pistols is as good as a mile.

Acres. Odds bullets, no! By my valour, there is no merit in killing him so near. Do, my dear Sir Lucius, let me bring him down at a long shot: a long shot, Sir Lucius, if you love me!

Sir L. Well, the gentleman's friend and I must settle that. But tell me now, Mr. Acres, in case of an accident, is there any little will or commission I could execute for you?

Acres. I am much obliged to you, Sir Lucius, but I don't understand—

Sir L. Why, you may think there's no being shot at without a little risk; and if an unlucky bullet should carry a quietus with it—I say, it will be no time then to be bothering you about family matters.

Acres. A quietus!

Sir L. For instance, now, if that should be the case, would you choose to be pickled, and sent home? or would it be the same to you to lie here in the Abbey? I'm told there is very snug lying in the Abbey.

Acres. Pickled! Snug lying in the Abbey! Odds tremors! Sir Lucius, don't talk so!

Sir L. I suppose, Mr. Acres, you never were engaged in an affair of this kind before?

Acres. No, Sir Lucius, never before, [*aside*] and never will again, if I get out of this.

Sir L. Ah, that's a pity! there's nothing like being used to a thing. Pray, now, how would you receive the gentleman's shot?

Acres. Odds files! I've practised that. There, Sir Lucius, there—a side-front, hey? Odd! I'll make myself small enough; I'll stand edgeways.

Sir L. Now, you're quite out; for if you stand so when I take my aim—

FROM "THE RIVALS."

Acres. Zounds, Sir Lucius! are you sure it is not cocked?

Sir L. Never fear

Acres. But—you don't know—it may go off of its own head!

Sir L. Pho! be easy. Well, now if I hit you in the body, my bullet has a double chance; for if it misses a vital part on your right side, 'twill be very hard if it don't succeed on the left.

Acres. A vital part!

Sir L. But, there—fix yourself so; let him see the broadside of your full front. Oh, bother! do you call that the broadside of your front? There! now a ball or two may pass clean through your body, and never do you any harm at all.

Acres. Clean through me! a ball or two clean through me!

Sir L. Ay, may they; and it is much the genteelest attitude into the bargain.

Acres. Look ye! Sir Lucius, I'd just as lief be shot in an awkward posture as a genteel one; so, by my valour, I will stand edgeways.

Sir L. Sure they don't mean to disappoint us.

Acres. [*Aside*] I hope they do.

Sir L. I think I see them coming.

Acres. Hey? what—coming!

Sir L. Ay; who are those yonder, getting over the stile?

Acres. There are two of them, indeed! well, let them come—hey, Sir Lucius?—we—we—we—we—won't run.

Sir L. Run.

Acres. No, I say—we *won't* run, by my valour!

Sir L. What's the matter with you?

Acres. Nothing—nothing—my dear friend—my dear Sir Lucius; but I—I—I don't feel quite so bold, somehow, as I did.

Sir L. Oh, fie! consider your honour.

Acres. Ay, true, my honour; do, Sir Lucius, edge in a word or two, every now and then, about my honour.

Sir L. Well, here they're coming.

Acres. Sir Lucius, if I wa'n't with you, I should almost think I was afraid. If my valour should leave me! valour will come and go.

Sir L. Then pray keep it fast, while you have it.

Acres. Sir Lucius, I doubt it is going—yes, my valour is certainly going! it is sneaking off! I feel it oozing out, as it were, at the palms of my hands!

Sir L. Your honour—your honour. Here they are.

Acres. Then I'm off. [*Exit Acres.*

Sir L. Well! upon my conscience, his valour has certainly oozed away with a vengeance. SHERIDAN.

FROM "ROB ROY."

Scene: A Cell in the Tolbooth of Glasgow.

BAILIE NICOL JARVIE, ROB ROY, MR. OWEN, FRANCIS OSBALDISTONE.

Bailie. [*Looking back*] I'll ca' when I want ye, Stanchells. Dougal shall mak' a' fast, or I'll mak' him fast, the scoundrel! A bonnie thing, and beseemin', that I should be kept at the door half-an-hour, knockin' as hard to get into jail as onybody else would be to get out o't. How's this? Strangers in the Tolbooth after lock-up hours! Keep the door lockit, you Dougal cratur'; I'll sune talk to these gentlemen, but I maun first hae a crack wi' an auld acquaintance.—Mr. Owen, Mr. Owen, how's a' wi' ye, man?

Owen. Pretty well in body, Mr. Jarvie, I thank you, but sore afflicted in spirit.

Bailie. Ay, ay, we're a' subject to downfa's, Mr. Owen, as my worthy faither, the Deacon—rest and bless him!—used to say. "Nick," said he (ye maun ken his name was Nicol, as weel as mine, so the folks in their daffin used to ca' us Young Nick and Auld Nick)—"Young Nick," said he, "never put oot your arm farther than you can draw it easily back again."

Owen. You need not have called these things to my memory in such a situation, Mr. Nicol Jarvie.

Bailie. What! do you think I cam' oot at sic a time o' nicht to tell a fa'in' man of his backslidin's? No, no, that's no Bailie Jarvie's way, nor his worthy faither's, the Deacon—rest and bless him!—afore him. I sune discovered what lodgings your *freends* had provided you, Mr. Owen. But gi'e us your list, man, and let us see how things stand between us, while I rest my shanks. [*Rob Roy sits on table and whistles.*] That's a vera queer chiel'; he seems unco near his ain fireside. Sit still, sir; I'll talk to you by-and-by.

Owen. There, sir, you'll find the balance in the wrong column —for us—but you'll please to consider—

Bailie. There's nae time to consider, Mr. Owen—it's plain you owe me siller; but I canna see how you'll clear it aff by snorin' here in the Tolbooth. Noo, sir, if you'll promise no to flee the country, you shall be at liberty in the mornin'.

Owen. O sir! O Mr. Jarvie!

Bailie. I'm a carefu' man as ony in the Sautmarket, and I'm a prudent man, as my worthy faither the Deacon was before me; but rather than that double-faced dog, MacVittie, shall keep an honest, civil gentleman by the heels, I'se be your bail mysel'. There, there, you've said enough. But, in the name o' misrule, how got ye companions?—Eh! my conscience! it's impossible! and yet—I'm clean bambaized! *You!* ye robber— ye cateran—ye cheat-the-gallows rogue!

Owen. Bless me! it's my poor friend, Mr. Campbell—a very honest man, Mr. Jarv—

Bailie. Honest! my conscience! *you* in the Glasgow Tolbooth! What d'ye think's the value o' your head?

Rob. Umph! why, fairly weighed, and Dutch weight, one Provost, four Bailies, a Town-clerk, and sax Deacons.

Bailie. Sax Deacons! Was there ever sic a born deevil? But tell owre your sins, sir, for if I but say the word—

Rob. True, Bailie, but ye will **never say that word.**

Bailie. And why suld I not, sir? why suld I not?

Rob. For three sufficient reasons, Bailie Jarvie: first, for auld langsyne.

Bailie. Ay, Rab!

Rob. Second, for the goodwife ayont the fire, that made some mixture of our bluids—

Bailie. Weel, Rab?

Rob. And lastly, Bailie—

Bailie. Ay, Rab?

Rob. Because, if I saw a sign o' your betraying me, I would plaster that wa' with your brains, ere the hand of man could rescue you.

Owen. Oh dear!

Bailie. My conscience! Weel, weel, Rab, it would be quite as unpleasant for me to hae my head knocked aboot, as it would be discreditable to string up a kinsman in a hempen cravat; but if it hadna been yoursel', Rab, I'd hae grippit the best man in the Highlands.

Rob. Ye wad hae tried, Bailie.

Bailie. Ay, "I wad hae tried, Bailie." But wha's this? [*To Francis.*] Anither honest man, I reckon.

Owen. This, good Sir, is Mr. Francis Osbaldistone.

Bailie. Oh, I've heard o' this spark—run away from his faither, in pure dislike to the labour an honest man should live by. Weel, sir, what do you say to your handiwork?

Francis. My dislike to the commercial profession, Mr. Jarvie, is a feeling of which I am the best, and sole judge.

Owen. Oh dear!

Rob. It's manfully spoken, and I honour the callant for his contempt of weavers and spinners, and sic-like mechanical persons.—Mr. Osbaldistone, you must visit me in the glens; and cousin, if you daur venture to show him the way—

Bailie. Catch me!

Rob. And eat a leg o' red-deer venison wi' me—

Bailie. No, thank ye, Rab.

Rob. I'll pay you the two hundred pounds I owe you; and you can leave Mr. Owen the while, to do the best he can in Glasgow.

Bailie. Say nae mair, Rab, say nae mair. I'll gang wi' you; but you maun guarantee me safe hame again to the Sautmarket.

Rob. There's my thumb, I'll ne'er beguile you. But I must be budging, Cousin, for the air of the Glasgow Tolbooth is not ower salutary to a Highlander's constitution.

Bailie. Noo, to think that I should be aidin' and abettin' an escape frae justice. It'll be a disgrace to me and mine, and the memory o' my worthy faither the Deacon—rest and bless him!—for ever.

Rob. Hout, tout, man! when the dirt's dry it will rub out again. Your faither could look ower a friend's faults, and why not your faither's son?

Bailie. So he could, Robin, so he could; he was a gude man, the Deacon. Ye mind him, Rab, dinna ye?

Rob. Troth, do I: he was a weaver, and wrought my first pair o' hose.

Bailie. Tak' care his son doesna weave your last cravat. Ye've a lang craig for a gibbet, Rab. But whaur's that Dougal cratur'?

Rob. If he is the lad I think him, he has not waited your thanks for his share of this night's work.

Bailie. What! gane, and left me locked up in a jail for a nicht? I'll hang the Hieland blackguard as high as Haman.

Rob. When ye catch him, Bailie, when ye catch him. But see, he ken'd an open door wad serve me at a pinch. Come, Bailie, speak the password.

Bailie. Stanchells, let this stranger out; he—he's—

Rob. He's a what?

Bailie. He's a friend o' mine. My conscience! an' a bonny friend he is.

Rob. Fare-ye-weel! Be early wi' me at Aberfoyle.

> "Come fill up my cup, come fill up my can,
> Come saddle my horses, and call up my men,
> Come open your gates, and let me gae free,
> I daurna stay langer in bonny Dundee."
>
> [*Exit Rob Roy.*

Bailie. So that Dougal cratur' was an agent o' Rab's! I shouldna wonder if he has ane in ilka jail in Scotland. [*Whistling without.*] Do you hear them out there whistlin', without ony regard for Sunday or Saturday? I fancy they think themsells on the tap o' Ben Lomond already. Weel, I hae dune things this blessed nicht that my worthy faither the Deacon—rest and bless him!—wadna hae believed. But there's balm in Gilead; there's balm in Gilead! Mr. Owen, I hope to see you at breakfast in the mornin'. Eh? why, the man's fast.

Francis. And the sooner we depart, and follow his example, sir, the better, for it must be near midnight.

Bailie. Midnicht! My conscience! Sir Walter Scott.

THE CONSEQUENCES OF SIN.

(By kind permission of the Author.)

The consequences of sin are *inevitable;* the punishment of sin is *impartial.* There is a form of self-deception common to all of us, by which we admit this general law, but try to shirk its personal, individual application.

It is the old, old story of Eden over again, in the case of every one of us; the serpent, creeping up to us, all glitter and fascination, all dulcet flattery and sinuous glide, whispering, "See the fruit, how fair it is, how much to be desired; be as a god, knowing good and evil; thou shalt not surely die;" and so the boy and the youth, healthy, and bright, and gay, and even, in his folly, the grown man believes, that it shall not be so with *him;* that *he* is the darling of Providence, *he* the favourite of Heaven, *he* the one who may sin, and shall not suffer. If *others* handle pitch, *they* shall be defiled; if *others* take fire into their bosom, *they* shall be burned; but God will indulge *him;* out of special favour to *him*, "this adamantine chain of moral gravitation, more lasting and binding than that by which the stars are held in their spheres, will be snapped; (that) sin for him will change its nature," and at his approach, the Gehenna of punishment be transformed into a garden of delight.

Is it so? Has there been any human being yet, since time began, however noble, however gifted, who has sinned with impunity?

No! God is no respecter of persons. Fire burns, and water drowns, whether the sufferer be a worthless villain, or a fair and gentle child; and so the *moral* law works, whether the sinner be a "David or a Judas, whether he be publican or priest."......

In the *physical* world, there is no forgiveness of sins. "Sin and punishment walk this world with their heads tied together;" and the rivet that links their iron link is a rivet of adamant.

Yes, the punishment of sin *is* inevitable and impartial; there is a frightful resemblance between the penalty and the transgression; an awful germ of identity in the seed and in the fruit. We recognize the sown wind, in the harvest whirlwind. It needs no gathered lightning, no divine intervention, no miraculous message, to avenge in us God's violated laws. They avenge *themselves*. Sin coming after men, with leaden footsteps, and gathering form, and towering over them, smites them at last, with the iron hand of its *own* revenge......

As there are some men whose sins are open, going before to judgment, so there are some men whose sins follow after. There are men, everywhere—who, ever as they walk through life, hear footsteps behind them—on whom the stars seem to look down as spies—men, whose faces blanch if they be suddenly accosted—who tremble, if a steady gaze be fixed upon them—who never again, in this world, shall sleep the sleep of the innocent—for whom the "furies have taken their seats upon the midnight pillow."

Have none of you felt the working of this law? Have you known, but for one hour, what it is to be utterly, miserably, intolerably ashamed of yourself? It is the glare of illumination, which the conscience flings over the soul, after a deed of darkness. It is the revulsion | of feeling | on which we did not calculate, when we have done with the *sin*, but the *sin* has not *done* with *us*. It is the Dead Sea apple, shrivelling into hideousness, the moment it has been tasted. It is the horror of the murderer, when his passion of revenge is spent, and the cold-gray-dawn reveals the face of his murdered victim!......

But *let* conscience, for a time, be dead; *let* life, for years, be prosperous; *let* there be no intervention, no sickness, no detection, no shame even; no fear, no outward and visible punishment of any kind. Does sin escape, *then?* Is the sinner happy, *then?* Nay! this is God's worst, severest punishment; "Ephraim is joined to idols, *let him alone!*"

Let *sin* be the deadliest executioner, the most merciless avenger of sin. Let the acute pang, become the chronic malady; let the thought, become the wish, and the wish, the act, and the act, the habit. Let the solitary, become the frequent, the frequent the incessant. Let *crime* awake him! Let greed become theft and swindling; let ambition become conspiracy; let hatred become murder. Ah! when God sends forth a *besetting sin*, a *guilty habit*, to be his executioner, the case is most awful, most hopeless then; God only, by Christ's redemption, can save from the body of that death.

ARCHDEACON FARRAR.

GOD IS LOVE.

Where shall we go for manifestations of the tenderness, the sympathy, the benignity of God? The Philosopher of this world leads us to Nature, its benevolent final causes, and kind contrivances to increase the sum of animal happiness; and there he stops—with *half* his demonstration! But the Apostle leads us to the Gift, bestowed by the Father, for the recovery of man's intellectual and moral nature, and to the Cross, endured by the Son, on this high behalf. Go to the heavens, which canopy man with grandeur, cheer his steps with successive light, and mark his festivals by their chronology; go to the atmosphere, which invigorates his spirits, and is to him the breath of life; go to the smiling fields, decked with verdure for his eye, and covered with fruits for his sustenance; go to every scene which spreads beauty before his gaze, which is made harmoniously vocal to his ear, which fills and delights the imagination, by its glow or by its greatness: we travel with you, we admire with you, we feel and enjoy with you, we adore with you,—but we stay not with you. We hasten onwards, in search of a demonstration *more* convincing, that "God is love:" we rest not till we press into the strange, the mournful, the joyful scenes of Calvary; and amidst the throng of invisible and astonished angels, weeping disciples, and the mocking multitude, under the arch of the darkened heaven, and with earth trembling beneath our feet, we gaze upon the meek, the resigned, but fainting Sufferer; and exclaim, "Herein is love!"—herein, and *nowhere else*, is it so affectingly, so unequivocally, demonstrated,—"not that *we* loved God, but that *God* loved us, and sent his Son to be the propitiation for our sins."   RICHARD WATSON.

"LOVE ONE ANOTHER."

Would you make men trustworthy? *Trust* them. Would you make men true? *Believe* them.

This was the real force of that sublime battle-cry, which no Englishman hears without emotion. When the sailors of the British fleet, knew that they were *expected* to do their duty, they *did* their duty. They went to serve a country which *expected* from them great things, and they *did* great things. Those pregnant words raised an enthusiasm for the man who had *trusted* them, which a double line of hostile ships, could not appal, nor decks drenched in blood, extinguish.

On this principle, Christ wins the hearts of his redeemed. He trusted the doubting Thomas; and the doubter arose with a faith worthy of "his Lord and his God." He would not suffer | even the lie of Peter, to shake his conviction that Peter might love him yet; and Peter answered nobly, to that sublime forgiveness. His last prayer, was in extenuation and hope, for the race who had rejected him.

Come what may, hold fast to love. Learn the new commandment of the Son of God; not to love merely, but to love *as he loved.* Though men should rend your heart, let them not embitter or harden it; we win by tenderness; we conquer by forgiveness. Go forth in this spirit to your life duties; go forth, soldiers of the Cross, and win victories for God, by the conquering power of a love like his.

F. W. ROBERTSON.

THE FIELD IS THE WORLD.

(By permission of the Author.)

A great imaginative writer has tried to picture the scene which we should behold, if, rising higher than the stork or the eagle, as they lean upon the wind, we could gaze down upon the variegated mosaic of the earth's surface. The blue Mediterranean lying beneath us, with Syria, Greece, Spain, and Italy sleeping in the sun. Northwards, mountain-rock, purple-moor, and bleak islands of stormy seas. Northwards still, a wall of ice sets death-like its white teeth against us out of the polar twilight. Southwards, from the glow and glories of the broad tropic belt of the world, down to where the volcanoes of the Antarctic darken the awful desolation with their grim canopies of smoke. Here, a tropic forest rushes in one day into crimson fragrance; there, the northern lights incarnadine the white solitudes of everlasting snow. Here, the warm air is brightened with living gems of fire-fly and humming-bird; there, leviathan tempests with mighty wallowings the ice-encumbered seas: yet, with whole systems and galaxies from which to choose,— worlds bursting with chaotic forces like our sun; worlds dead and done with like our moon; worlds but yet mid-way in their life-history like our earth,—we might well imagine that in mere outward aspect there would be but little amid a firmament which glows with living sapphires to guide to this small planet an angel's flight. But how different is the interest of the earth when we think of it as the abode of man—man whom God made in his own image, after his likeness; man, whose nature was worn by the Son of man, who was the Son of God; man, for whom Christ died.

What a strange spectacle to an angel's gaze would be this world of man! The boundless complexity and rushing hurry of our modern life, with its science and inventions; the glittering wave of civilization, with its black fringe of misery and vice. Northward, men struggling against the hostile forces of nature for bare life; the sledge of the Laplander, whirled by reindeer; the Esquimaux, tossed on the stormy foam in his boat of skin. Southwards, the glad peasants stripping their purple vintage. In Asia, the Arab, scouring the desert on his swift steed; the long train of camels on their way to Mecca; the Hindoo, worshipping by his ancient rivers; the Chinese, toiling in his fields of rice. In Africa, the negroes, tortured by the slave-trade; in America, the sons of the Old World developing their inexhaustible energies in the New. It is on these—on these strange heirs of immortality—that an angel would gaze, according to his knowledge, with aching or exulting heart, while he sighed forth, "How poor, how rich, how abject, how august, how complicate, how wonderful is man! helpless, immortal! insect infinite! a worm! a god!"

For he would see that the nations of the world have felt after God, and, for the most part, have not found him. The gospel of Christ was the remedy for that vast failure. It has proved its mission by its unique supremacy. Humanity has groped in blindness after God; in Christ alone has it learned the love of his Fatherhood, and that was why the risen Saviour said to his apostles, "Go ye into all the world, and make disciples of all nations."

To whom did he give that high command? To a handful of poor, unlearned, helpless, persecuted Galilean peasants. There was not a Pharisee, there was not a ruler among them; all kings, all priests, all philosophers were against them; all that called itself orthodoxy, all that called itself government, all that called itself intellect was against them. Rome and Jerusalem, Antioch and Athens spurned their teaching. Wealth and rank disowned them; thirty legions held them in execration and contempt. And yet the irresistible might of their weakness shook the world; and before three centuries had passed, their hated Cross had displaced the victorious eagles, and the monogram of Christ took the place of the world-renowned motto * on the banners of imperial Rome.

ARCHDEACON FARRAR.

* S. P. Q. R.
Senatus Populus que Romanus.
(*The Senate and the Roman People.*)

ADDITIONAL STUDIES.

SECOND SERIES.

THE MAISTER AND THE BAIRNS.

The Maister sat in a wee cot-hoose
    Tae the Jordan's waters near,
An' the fisher folk crushed an' crooded roond
    The Maister's words tae hear.

An' even the bairns frae the near-haund streets
    Were mixin' in wi' the thrang,
Laddies an' lassies wi' wee bare feet
    Jinkin' the crood amang.

An' ane o' the Twal at the Maister's side
    Rose up an' cried aloud,
"Come, come, bairns, this is nae place for you,
    Rin awa' hame oot the crood."

But the Maister said, as they turned awa',
    "Let the wee bairns come tae Me!"
An' He gathered them roond Him where He sat,
    An' lifted ane up on His knee.

Ay, He gathered them roond Him where He sat,
    An' straiked their curly hair,
An' He said tae the wonderin' fisher folk
    That crooded aroond Him there:

"Send na the weans awa' frae Me;
   But rather this lesson learn—
That nane 'll won in at heaven's yett
   That isna as pure as a bairn!"

An' He that wisna oor kith an' kin,
   But a Prince o' the Far Awa',
Gathered the wee anes in His airms,
   An' blessed them ane an' a'.

W. Thomson.

THE COTTER'S SATURDAY NIGHT.

November chill blaws loud wi' angry sugh;
   The short'ning winter day is near a close;
The miry beasts retreating frae the pleugh;
   The black'ning trains o' craws to their repose;
The toil-worn cotter frae his labour goes,
   (This night his weekly moil is at an end,)
Collects his spades, his mattocks, and his hoes,
   Hoping the morn in ease and rest to spend,
And, weary, o'er the moor his course does homeward bend.

At length his lonely cot appears in view,
   Beneath the shelter of an aged tree;
Th' expectant wee things, toddlin', stacher through
   To meet their dad, wi' flichterin' noise and glee.
His wee bit ingle blinkin' bonnily,
   His clean hearthstane, his thrifty wifie's smile,
The lisping infant prattling on his knee,
   Does a' his weary carking cares beguile,
And makes him quite forget his labour and his toil.

Belyve the elder bairns come drapping in—
   At service out, among the farmers roun';

THE COTTER'S SATURDAY NIGHT.

Some ca' the pleugh, some herd, some tentie rin
  A canny errand to a neibor town:
Their eldest hope, their Jenny, woman grown,
  In youthfu' bloom, love sparkling in her ee,
Comes hame, perhaps to show a braw new gown
  Or deposit her sair-won penny-fee,
To help her parents dear, if they in hardship be.

Wi' joy unfeigned, brothers and sisters meet,
  And each for other's weelfare kindly spiers.
The social hours, swift-winged, unnoticed, fleet:
  Each tells the uncos that he sees or hears.
The parents, partial, eye their hopeful years;
  Anticipation forward points the view.
The mother, wi' her needle and her shears,
  Gars auld claes look amaist as weel's the new;
The father mixes a' wi' admonition due.

But, hark! a rap comes gently to the door;
  Jenny, wha kens the meaning o' the same,
Tells how a neibor lad cam o'er the moor,
  To do some errands, and convoy her hame.
The wily mother sees the conscious flame
  Sparkle in Jenny's ee, and flush her cheek,
Wi' heart-struck anxious care, inquires his name,
  While Jenny hafflins is afraid to speak;
Weel pleased the mother hears it's nae wild, worthless
    rake.

Wi' kindly welcome, Jenny brings him ben;
  A strappin' youth, he taks the mother's eye.
Blithe Jenny sees the visit's no ill ta'en;
  The father cracks of horses, pleughs, and kye.
The youngster's artless heart o'erflows wi' joy,
  But blate and lathefu', scarce can weel behave;

The mother, wi' a woman's wiles, can spy
    What makes the youth sae bashfu' and sae grave;
Weel pleased to think her bairn's respected like the lave.

O happy love!—where love like this is found!—
    O heart-felt raptures! bliss beyond compare!
I've pacëd much this weary, mortal round,
    And sage experience bids me this declare,—
"If Heaven a draught of heavenly pleasure spare,
    One cordial in this melancholy vale,
'Tis when a youthful, loving, modest pair,
    In other's arms, breathe out the tender tale,
Beneath the milk-white thorn that scents the evening gale!"

But now the supper crowns their simple board,
    The halesome parritch, chief of Scotia's food;
The soupe their only hawkie does afford,
    That 'yont the hallan snugly chows her cood.
The dame brings forth, in complimental mood,
    To grace the lad, her weel-hained kebbuck fell;
And aft he's prest, and aft he ca's it guid:
    The frugal wifie, garrulous, will tell,
How 'twas a towmond auld, sin' lint was i' the bell.

The cheerfu' supper done, wi' serious face,
    They round the ingle form a circle wide;
The sire turns o'er, wi' patriarchal grace,
    The big ha' Bible, ance his father's pride;
His bonnet rev'rently is laid aside.
    His lyart haffets wearin' thin and bare;
Those strains that once did sweet in Zion glide,
    He wales a portion with judicious care;
And "Let us worship God!" he says, with solemn air.

They chant their artless notes in simple guise;
    They tune their hearts, by far the noblest aim;

THE COTTER'S SATURDAY NIGHT.

Perhaps " Dundee's " wild-warbling measures rise,
   Or plaintive " Martyrs," worthy of the name ;
Or noble " Elgin " beets the heaven-ward flame—
   The sweetest far of Scotia's holy lays.
Compared with these, Italian trills are tame ;
   The tickled ear no heartfelt raptures raise ;
Nae unison hae they with our Creator's praise.

Perhaps the Christian volume is the theme,—
   How guiltless blood for guilty man was shed ;
How He, who bore in heaven the second name,
   Had not on earth whereon to lay His head ;
How His first followers and servants sped
   The precepts sage they wrote to many a land ;
How he who lone in Patmos banishëd
   Saw in the sun a mighty angel stand,
And heard great Bab'lon's doom pronounced by Heaven's command.

Then kneeling down, to heaven's eternal King
   The saint, the father, and the husband prays :
Hope "springs exulting on triumphant wing,"
   That thus they all shall meet in future days ;
There ever bask in uncreated rays,
   No more to sigh or shed the bitter tear,
Together hymning their Creator's praise,
   In such society, yet still more dear ;
While circling time moves round in an eternal sphere.

Compared with this, how poor religion's pride,
   In all the pomp of method and of art,
When men display to congregations wide
   Devotion's every grace, except the heart !
The Power, incensed, the pageant will desert,
   The pompous strain, the sacerdotal stole ;

But, haply, in some cottage far apart,
  May hear, well-pleased, the language of the soul,
And in His book of life the inmates poor enrol.

Then homeward all take off their several way;
  The youngling cottagers retire to rest;
The parent-pair their secret homage pay,
  And proffer up to Heaven the warm request
That He who stills the raven's clamorous nest,
  And decks the lily fair in flow'ry pride,
Would, in the way His wisdom sees the best,
  For them and for their little ones provide;
But chiefly in their hearts with grace divine preside.

From scenes like these old Scotia's grandeur springs,
  That makes her loved at home, revered abroad.
Princes and lords are but the breath of kings,
  "An honest man's the noblest work of God:"
And certes, in fair virtue's heavenly road,
  The cottage leaves the palace far behind.
What is a lordling's pomp?—a cumbrous load,
  Disguising oft the wretch of human kind,
Studied in arts of hell, in wickedness refined!

O Scotia! my dear, my native soil,
  For whom my warmest wish to Heaven is sent!
Long may thy hardy sons of rustic toil
  Be blest with health, and peace, and sweet content!
And, oh! may Heaven their simple lives prevent
  From luxury's contagion, weak and vile!
Then, howe'er crowns and coronets be rent,
  A virtuous populace may rise the while,
And stand a wall of fire around their much-loved isle.

ROBERT BURNS.

SCOTS WHA HAE.

Scots wha hae wi' Wallace bled,
Scots wham Bruce has aften led,
Welcome to your gory bed,
    Or to victory!

Now's the day, and now's the hour!
See the front of battle lŏwer!
See approach proud Edward's power—
    Chains and slavery!

Wha will be a traitor knave?
Wha can fill a coward's grave?
Wha sae base as be a slave?
    Let him turn and flee!

Wha for Scotland's king and law
Freedom's sword will strongly draw,
Freeman stand or freeman fa'?
    Let him follow me!

By oppression's woes and pains!
By your sons in servile chains!
We will drain our dearest veins,
    But they shall be free!

Lay the proud usurpers low!
Tyrants fall in every foe!
Liberty's in every blow!
    Let us do, or die!
                ROBERT BURNS.

THE DOWIE DENS O' YARROW.

Late at e'en, drinking the wine, and ere they paid the lawing,
They set a combat them between, to fight it in the daw'ing.
" You took our sister for your wife, and thought her not your marrow :
You stole her frae her father's back, when she was the Rose o' Yarrow."—
" I took your sister for my wife, and I made her my marrow ;
I gat her frae her father's hand, and she's still the Rose o' Yarrow."—

" What though you be our sister's lord, we'll cross our swords to-morrow."—
" And though my wife your sister be, I'll meet wi' you on Yarrow."
Hame he has to his ladye gane, says, " Madam, on the morrow,
I've pledged mysel' to keep a tryste on the bonnie banks o' Yarrow."—
" O stay at hame, my lord !" she said, " O stay, my ain dear marrow !
My cruel brithers will you slay on the dowie dens o' Yarrow."—

" Now, haud your tongue, my ladye dear, for what needs a' this sorrow ?
For if I gae, I'll sune return frae the bonnie banks o' Yarrow."
She kissed his cheek, she kaimed his hair—her heart foreboded sorrow—
She belted him wi' his gude brand, and he's awa' to Yarrow.
As he gaed up the Tennies bank—I wot he gaed wi' sorrow—
It's there he spied nine armëd men, on the dowie dens o' Yarrow.

" Oh, come ye here to hunt or hawk the bonnie forest thorough ?
Or come ye here to part your land, upon the banks o' Yarrow ?"—

"I come not here to hunt or hawk the bonnie forest thorough;
  Nor come I here to part my land, but to fight wi' you on Yarrow.
  If you attack me nine to ane, then may God send you sorrow:
  Yet will I fight while lasts my brand, on the bonnie banks o' Yarrow."

Four has he hurt, and five has slain, on the bloody braes o' Yarrow,
  When a coward loon cam' him behind and ran his body thorough.
"Gae hame, gae hame, good-brother John, tak' to your sister sorrow;
  Gae hame, and tell my ladye dear that I sleep sound on Yarrow."
Her brother John oot ower the hill gaed wi' that word o' sorrow,
  And there he met his sister fair, was rinnin' fast to Yarrow.

"O gentle wind, that bloweth south, from where my love repaireth,
  Convey a kiss from his dear mouth, and tell me how he fareth!
  I dreamt a dreary dream yestreen—God keep us a' frae sorrow—
  I dreamt I pu'd the birk sae green wi' my true love on Yarrow."—
"I'll read your dream, my sister dear, I'll read it unto sorrow:
  You pu'd the birk wi' your true love?—he's killed! he's killed on Yarrow!"

She's torn the ribbons frae her hair, that were baith braid and narrow,
  And ower the hill she ran wi' speed, to the dowie dens o' Yarrow.

> She's ta'en him in her arms twa, and gi'en him kisses thorough;
> She sought to bind his mony wounds, but he lay deid on
>   Yarrow.
> She kissed his lips, she kaimed his hair, wi' mickle dule and
>   sorrow;
> Syne wi' a sigh her heart did break, on the dowie dens o'
>   Yarrow.   *Old Scottish Ballad.*

CHARLES EDWARD ON THE ANNIVERSARY OF CULLODEN.

Take away that Star and Garter—hide them from my aching
    sight!
Neither prince nor king shall tempt me from my lonely room
    this night.
Let the shadows gather round me while I sit in silence here,
Broken-hearted, as an orphan watching by his father's bier!
Let me hold my still communion far from every earthly sound,—
Day of penance! day of passion! ever as the year comes round!
Fatal day! wherein the latest die was cast for me and mine—
Cruel day! that quelled the fortunes of the hapless Stuart line!

Phantom-like, as in a mirror, rise the grisly scenes of death—
There before me, in its wildness, stretches bare Culloden's
    heath:
There the broken clans are scattered, gaunt as wolves, and
    famine-eyed,
Hunger gnawing at their vitals, hope abandoned, *all* but pride!
There they stand, the battered columns, underneath the murky
    sky,
In the hush of desperation, not to conquer, but to die!
Hark! the bagpipe's fitful wailing: not the pibroch loud and
    shrill
That, with hope of bloody banquet, lured the ravens from the
    hill;

But a dirge both low and solemn, fit for ears of dying men
Marshalled for their latest battle, never more to fight again.

Madness—madness! Why this shrinking? Were we less inured to war
When our reapers swept the harvest from the field of red Dunbar?
Bring my horse, and blow the trumpet! Call the riders of Fitz-James!
Let Lord Lewis head the column! Valiant chiefs of mighty names—
Trusty Keppoch! stout Glengarry! gallant Gordon! wise Lochiel!
Bid the clansmen hold together, fast and fell, and firm as steel!
Elcho! never look so gloomy—what avails a saddened brow?
Heart! man, heart!—we need it sorely, never half so much as now!
Had we but a thousand troopers, had we but a thousand more!
Noble Perth! I hear them coming! Hark! the English cannons roar!
Ah! how awful sounds that volley, bellowing through the mist and rain!
Was not that the Highland slogan? let me hear that shout again!
Oh, for prophet eyes to witness how the desperate battle goes!
Cumberland! I would not fear thee, could my Camerons see their foes!

Sound, I say, the charge at venture; 'tis not naked steel we fear!
Better perish in the *mêlée* than be shot like driven deer!
Hold! the mist begins to scatter! there, in front, 'tis rent asunder,
And the cloudy bastion crumbles underneath the deafening thunder.

Chief and vassal, lord and yeoman, there they lie in heaps
    together,
Smitten by the deadly volley, rolled in blood upon the heather!
And the Hanoverian horsemen, riding fiercely to and fro,
Deal their murderous strokes at random!......

Will that baleful vision never vanish from my aching sight?
Must those scenes and sounds of terror haunt me still by day
    and night?
Yes! the earth hath no oblivion for the noblest chance it gave—
None, save in its latest refuge: seek it only in the grave!
Love may die, and hatred slumber, and their memory will decay,
As the watered garden recks not of the drought of yesterday;
But the dream of power once broken, what can give repose
    again?
What can chain the serpent furies coiled around the maddening brain?
What kind draught can Nature offer strong enough to lull their
    sting?
Better to be born a peasant than to live an exiled king!

AYTOUN.

A PSALM OF LIFE.

    Tell me not, in mournful numbers, Life is but an empty dream! For the soul is dead that slumbers, and things are not what they seem. Life is real! life is earnest! and the grave is not its goal; "Dust thou art, to dust returnest," was not spoken of the soul. Not enjoyment, and not sorrow, is our destined end or way; but to act that each to-morrow finds us further than to-day. Art is long, and time is fleeting, and our hearts, though stout and brave, still, like muffled drums, are beating funeral marches to the grave. In the world's broad field of battle, in the bivouac of life, be not like dumb, driven cattle—be a hero in the strife! Trust no future, howe'er pleasant! Let the dead past bury its dead! Act—act in the living present! heart within, and God o'erhead! Lives of great men all remind us we can make our lives sublime, and, departing, leave behind us footprints on the sands of time; footprints that perhaps another, sailing o'er life's solemn main, a forlorn and shipwrecked brother, seeing, shall take heart again. Let us then be up and doing, with a heart for any fate; still achieving, still pursuing, learn to labour and to wait.

H. W. LONGFELLOW.

GIRLS THAT ARE IN DEMAND.

The girls that are wanted are good girls—
    Good from the heart to the lips;
Pure as the lily is white and pure
    From its heart to its sweet leaf-tips.

The girls that are wanted are home girls—
    Girls that are mother's right hand,
That fathers and brothers can trust to,
    And the little ones understand;

Girls that are fair on the hearthstone,
    And pleasant when nobody sees;
Kind and sweet to their own folks,
    Ready and anxious to please.

The girls that are wanted are wise girls,
    That know what to do and to say,
That drive with a smile and a soft word
    The wrath of the household away.

The girls that are wanted are girls of sense,
    Whom fashion can never deceive;
Who can follow whatever is pretty,
    And dare what is silly to leave.

> The girls that are wanted are careful girls,
>   Who count what a thing will cost,
> Who use with a prudent, generous hand,
>   But see that nothing is lost.
>
> The girls that are wanted are girls with hearts;
>   They are wanted for mothers and wives—
> Wanted to cradle in loving arms
>   The strongest and frailest lives.
>
> The clever, the witty, the brilliant girl,
>   There are few who can understand;
> But, oh! for the wise, loving, home girls
>   There's a constant, steady demand.

HOW HE SAVED ST. MICHAEL'S.

'Twas long ago—ere ever the signal-gun
That blazed above Fort Sumter had wakened the North as one;
Long ere the wondrous pillar of battle-cloud and fire
Had marked where the unchained millions marched on to their desire.

On roofs and glittering turrets, that night as the sun went down,
The mellow glow of the twilight shone like a jewelled crown.
And, bathed in the living glory, as the people lifted their eyes,
They saw the pride of the city, the spire of St. Michael's, rise,

High over the lesser steeples, tipped with a golden ball
That hung like a radiant planet caught in its earthward fall;
First glimpse of home to the sailor who made the harbour round,
And last slow-fading vision dear to the outward bound.

HOW HE SAVED ST. MICHAEL'S.

The gently-gathering shadows shut out the waning light;
The children prayed at their bedsides, as they were wont each
    night;
The noise from buyer and seller from the busy mart was gone;
And in dreams of a peaceful morrow the city slumbered on.

But another light than sunrise aroused the sleeping street;
For a cry was heard at midnight, and the rush of trampling feet.
Men stared in each other's faces, through mingled fire and
    smoke,
While the frantic bells went clashing, clamorous, stroke on
    stroke.

By the glare of her blazing rooftree the houseless mother fled,
With the babe she pressed to her bosom shrieking in nameless
    dread;
While the fire-king's wild battalions scaled wall and capstone
    high,
And planted their glaring banners against an inky sky.

From the death that raged behind them, and the crash of ruin
    loud,
To the great square of the city was driven the surging crowd,
Where, yet firm in all the tumult, unscathed by the fiery flood,
With its heavenward-pointing finger, the church of St.
    Michael's stood.

But e'en as they gazed upon it there rose a sudden wail,
A cry of horror blended with the roaring of the gale,
On whose scorching winds updriven a single flaming brand
Aloft on the towering steeple clung like a bloody hand.

"Will it fade?" The whisper trembled from a thousand
    whitening lips;
Far out on the lurid harbour they watched it from the ships—

A baleful gleam, that brighter and ever brighter shone,
Like a flickering, trembling will-o'-the-wisp to a steady beacon grown.

"Uncounted gold shall be given to the man whose brave right hand,
For the love of the perilled city, plucks down yon burning brand!"
So cried the Mayor of Charleston, that all the people heard;
But they looked each one at his fellow, and no man spoke a word.

Who is it leans from the belfry, with face upturned to the sky,
Clings to a column, and measures the dizzy spire with his eye?
Will he dare it, the hero undaunted, that terrible, sickening height?
Or will the hot blood of his courage freeze in his veins at the sight?

But, see! he has stepped on the railing, he climbs with his feet and his hands,
And firm on a narrow projection, with the belfry beneath him, he stands!
Now once, and once only, they cheer him—a single tempestuous breath;
And there falls on the multitude gazing a hush like the stillness of death.

Slow, steadily mounting, unheeding aught save the goal of the fire,
Still higher and higher, an atom, he moves on the face of the spire.
He stops! Will he fall? Lo! for answer a gleam like a meteor's track,
And, hurled on the stones of the pavement, the red brand lies shattered and black!

Once more the shouts of the people have rent the quivering air.
At the church door mayor and council wait with their feet on the stair;
And the eager throng behind them press for a touch of his hand—
The unknown saviour whose daring could compass a deed so grand.

But why does a sudden tremor seize on them as they gaze?
And what meaneth that stifled murmur of wonder and amaze?
He stood in the gate of the temple he had perilled his life to save,
And the face of the unknown hero was the sable face of a slave!

With folded arms he was speaking in tones that were clear, not loud,
And his eyes, ablaze in their sockets, burned into the eyes of the crowd:
" Ye may keep your gold—I scorn it!—but answer me, ye who can,
If the deed I have done before you be not the deed of a *man!*"

He stepped but a short space backward, and from all the women and men
There were only sobs for answers; and the mayor called for a pen,
And the great seal of the city, that he might read who ran:
And the slave who saved St. Michael's went out from its door
—a man!
MARY A. P. STANSBURY.

OUR FOLKS.

"Hi! Harry! halt a breath, and tell a comrade just a thing
  or two;
You've been on furlough—been to see how all the folks in
  Jersey do?
It's long ago since I was there,—I, and a bullet from Fair
  Oaks;—
When you were home, old comrade, say, did you see any of
  our folks?

"You did? Shake hands. That warms my heart; for, if I
  do look grim and rough,
I've got some feeling. People think a soldier's heart is
  naught but tough;
But, Harry, when the bullets fly, and hot saltpetre flames
  and smokes,
While whole battalions lie afield, one's apt to think about his
  folks.

"And so you saw them—when? and where? The old man—
  is he hearty yet?
And mother—does she fade at all? or does she seem to pine
  and fret
For me? And sis—has she grown tall? And did you see
  her friend—you know—that Annie Moss—How this pipe
  chokes!—
Where did you see her? Tell me, Hal, a lot of news about
  our folks.

"You saw them in the church, you say; 'tis likely, for they're
  always there.
Not Sunday? No?—A funeral? Who? Who, Harry?—
  How you shake and stare!

All well, you say, and all were out—What ails you, Hal?
  Is this a hoax?
Why don't you tell me, like a man, what is the matter with
  our folks?"

"I *said* all well, old comrade—true. I *say* all well; for He
  knows best
Who takes the young ones in His arms before the sun goes
  to the west.
Death deals at random, right and left, and flowers fall as well
  as oaks;
And so—fair Annie blooms no more!—and that's the matter
  with your folks.

" But see, this curl was kept for you, and this white blossom
  from her breast;
And look, your sister Bessie wrote this letter, telling all the
  rest.
Bear up, old friend!"—Nobody speaks; only the old camp-
  raven croaks,
And soldiers whisper: "Boys, be still; there's some bad
  news from Granger's folks."

He turns his back—the only foe that ever saw it—on this
  grief,
And, as men will, keeps down the tears kind Nature sends
  to woe's relief;
Then answers: "Thank you, Hal—I'll try; but in my throat
  there's something chokes,
Because, you see, I've thought so long to count her in among
  our folks.

" I daresay she is happier now; but still I can't help thinking,
  too,
I might have kept all trouble off by being tender, kind, and
  true.

But maybe not.—She's safe up there; and, when God's
    hand deals other strokes,
She'll stand by heaven's gate, I know, and wait to welcome
    in our folks."
                                                    ETHEL LYNN.

THE UNCLE.

I had an uncle once, a man
  Of threescore years and three,
And when my reason's dawn began
  He'd take me on his knee,
And often talk whole winter nights
  Things that seemed strange to me.

He was a man of gloomy mood,
  And few his converse sought;
But it was said, in solitude,
  His conscience with him wrought,
And there, before his mental eye,
  Some hideous vision brought.

There was not one in all the house
  Who did not fear his frown,
Save I, a little careless child,
  Who gambolled up and down,
And often peeped into his room,
  And plucked him by the gown.

I was an orphan, and alone;
  My father was his brother,
And all their lives I knew that they
  Had fondly loved each other;
And in my uncle's room there hung
  The picture of my mother.

There was a curtain over it,
　'Twas in a darkened place;
And few or none had ever looked
　Upon my mother's face,
Or seen her pale, expressive smile
　Of melancholy grace.

One night—I do remember well—
　The wind was howling high,
And through the ancient corridors
　It sounded drearily;
I sat and read in that old hall,
　My uncle sat close by.

I read, but little understood
　The words upon the book;
For, with a sidelong glance, I marked
　My uncle's fearful look,
And saw how all his quiv'ring frame
　In strong convulsions shook.

A silent terror o'er me stole,
　A strange unusual dread:
His lips were white as bone, his eyes
　Sunk far down in his head;
He gazed on me, but 'twas the gaze
　Of the unconscious dead.

Then, suddenly, he turned him round
　And drew aside the veil
That hung before my mother's face;—
　Perchance my eyes might fail,
But ne'er before that face to me
　Had seemed so ghastly pale.

THE UNCLE.

"Come hither, boy!" my uncle said.
   I started at the sound;
'Twas choked and stifled in his throat,
   And hardly utterance found.
"Come hither, boy!" then fearfully
   He cast his eyes around.

"That lady was thy mother once,
   Thou wert her only child,—
O God! I've seen her when she held
   Thee in her arms and smiled.
She smiled upon thy father, boy!
   'Twas that which drove me wild.

"He was my brother, but his form
   Was fairer far than mine.
I grudged not that; he was the prop
   Of our ancestral line,
And manly beauty was of him
   A token and a sign.

"Boy! I had loved her too—nay, more,
   'Twas I who loved her first;
For months, for years, the golden thought
   Within my soul was nursed.
He came—he conquered—they were wed!
   My air-blown bubble burst!

"Then on my mind a shadow fell,
   And evil hopes grew rife;
The madd'ning thought stuck in my heart
   And cut me like a knife,
That she, whom all my days I loved,
   Should be another's wife!

THE UNCLE.

"I left my home, I left the land,
　　I crossed the raging sea,—
In vain, in vain! where'er I went
　　My memory went with me;
My whole existence, night and day,
　　In memory seemed to be.

"I came again; I found them here,—
　　Thou'rt like thy father, boy,—
He doted on that pale face there;
　　I've seen them kiss and toy;
I've seen him locked in her fond arms,
　　Wrapped in delirious joy.

"By heaven! it was a fearful thing
　　To see my brother now,
And mark the placid calm that sat
　　For ever on his brow,
Which seemed in bitter scorn to say,
　　I am more loved than thou.

"He disappeared,—draw nearer, child,—
　　He died, no one knew how;
The murdered body ne'er was found;
　　The tale is hushed up now:
But there was one who rightly guessed
　　The hand that struck the blow.

"It drove her mad; yet not his death,
　　No, not his death alone,
For she had clung to hope when all
　　Knew well that there was none.
No, boy! it was a sight she saw
　　That froze her into stone.

THE UNCLE.

"I am thy uncle, child!—why star'st
　　So frightfully aghast?
The arras waves; but know'st thou not
　　'Tis nothing but the blast?
I too have had my fears like these;
　　But such vain fears are past.

"I'll show thee what thy mother saw;
　　I feel 'twill ease my breast,
And this wild, tempest-laden night
　　Suits with the purpose best.
Come hither, boy! thou'st often sought
　　To open this old chest.

"It has a secret spring; the touch
　　Is known to me alone."
Slowly the lid is raised.—" And now,
　　What see you that you groan
So heavily? That thing is nothing but
　　A bare-ribbed skeleton."

A sudden crash! the lid fell down;
　　Three strides he backward gave—
"O God! it is my brother's self
　　Returning from the grave!
His grasp of lead is on my throat!
　　Will no one help or save?"

That night they laid him on his bed,
　　In raving madness tossed;
He gnashed his teeth, and with wild oaths
　　Blasphemed the Holy Ghost;
And ere the light of morning broke,
　　A sinner's soul was lost!

H. G. BELL.

THE OLD MAN DREAMS.

O for one hour of youthful joy! give back my twentieth spring!
I'd rather laugh a bright-haired boy than reign a gray-beard king.
Off with the wrinkled spoils of age! away with learning's crown!
Tear out life's wisdom-written page, and dash its trophies down!

One moment let my life-blood stream from boyhood's fount of flame!
Give me one giddy, reeling dream of life all love and fame!
My listening angel heard the prayer, and, calmly smiling, said,
"If I but touch thy silvered hair, thy hasty wish hath sped.

"But is there nothing in thy track to bid thee fondly stay,
While the swift seasons hurry back to find the wished-for day?"
Ah, truest soul of womankind! without thee, what were life?—
One bliss I cannot leave behind: I'll take—my—precious wife!

The angel took a sapphire pen and wrote in rainbow dew,
"The man would be a boy again, and be a husband too!"—
"And is there nothing yet unsaid before the change appears?
Remember, all their gifts have fled with those dissolving years!"

Why, yes; for memory would recall my fond paternal joys;
I could not bear to leave them all: I'll take—my—girl—and —boys!
The smiling angel dropped his pen—"Why, this will never do;
The man would be a boy again, and be a father too!"

And so I laughed: my laughter woke the household with its noise—
And wrote my dream, when morning broke, to please the gray-haired boys.

C. W. HOLMES.

THE BOYS.

Has there any old fellow got mixed with the boys?
If there has, take him out, without making a noise!
Hang the Almanac's cheat and the Catalogue's spite!
Old Time is a liar! We're twenty to-night!

We're twenty! we're twenty! Who says we are more?
He's tipsy,—young jackanapes!—show him the door!—
"Gray temples at twenty?" Yes, white, if we please;
Where the snowflakes fall thickest there's nothing can freeze!

Was it snowing I spoke of? Excuse the mistake!
Look close,—you will see not a sign of a flake;
We want some new garlands for those we have shed,—
And these are white roses in place of the red!

We've a trick, we young fellows, you may have been told,
Of talking (in public) as if we were old.
That boy we call "Doctor," and this we call "Judge;"—
It's a neat little fiction,—of course it's all fudge.

That fellow's the "Speaker"—the one on the right;—
"Mr. Mayor," my young one, how are you to-night?
That's our "Member of Parliament," we say when we chaff;
There's the "Reverend" What's-his-name?—don't make me laugh.

That boy with the grave mathematical look
Made believe he had written a wonderful book;

And the Royal Society thought it was true!
So they chose him right in—a good joke it was too!

There's a boy—we pretend—with a three-decker brain,
That could harness a team with a logical chain;
When he spoke for our manhood in syllabled fire,
We called him "The Justice," but now he's "The Squire."

And there's a nice youngster of excellent pith—
Fate tried to conceal him by naming him Smith;
But he shouted a song for the brave and the free:
Just read on his medal—" My country—of thee!"

You hear that boy laughing? You think he's all fun;
But the angels laugh too at the good he has done;
The children laugh loud as they troop to his call;
And the poor man that knows him laughs loudest of all!

Yes, we're boys—always playing with tongue or with pen;
And I sometimes have asked, Shall we ever be men?
Shall we always be youthful, and laughing, and gay,
Till the last dear companion drops smiling away?

Then here's to our boyhood, its gold and its gray,
The stars of its winter, the dews of its May!
And when we have done with our life-lasting toys,
Dear Father, take care of Thy children, the Boys!

O. W. HOLMES.

LITTLE ORPHANT ANNIE.

Little Orphant Annie's come to our house to stay,
An' wash the cups and saucers up, and brush the crumbs away,
An' shoo the chickens off the porch, an' dust the hearth an' sweep,
An' make the fire, an' bake the bread, an' earn her board an' keep.

LITTLE ORPHANT ANNIE.

An' all us other children, when the supper things is done,
We set around the kitchen fire, an' has the mostest fun
A-lis'nin' to the witch-tales that Annie tells about,
An' the gobble-uns that gits you if you don't watch out!

Once't there was a little boy wouldn't say his prayers,
An' one night when he went to bed, away upstairs,
His mama heerd him holler, an' his papa heerd him bawl,
An' when they turned the kivers down, he wasn't there at all!
An' they seeked him in the rafter-room, an' cubby-hole, an' press,
An' seeked him up the chimbly-flue, an' ev'rywheres, I guess;
But all they ever found was jest his pants an' roundabout,—
An' the gobble-uns 'll git you if you don't watch out!

An' one time a little girl 'ud allas laugh an' grin,
An' make fun of ev'ry one, an' all her kith an' kin;
An' once't when there was company, an' old folks was there,
She mocked 'em, and shocked 'em, an' said she didn't care!
An' jest as she kicked her heels, an' turn'd to run an' hide,
There was two great black things a-standin' by her side!
An' they snatched her through the ceilin' afore she knowed what she's about!—
An' the gobble-uns 'll git you if you don't watch out!

An' little Orphant Annie says, when the blaze is blue,
An' the lamp-wick splutters, an' the wind goes *woo-oo*,
An' you hear the crickets quiet, an' the moon is gray,
An' the fire-flies in dew is all squenched away,
You'd better mind yer parents, an' yer teachers fond an' dear,
An' cherish 'em 'at loves you, an' dry the orphant's tear,
An' help the poor an' needy ones 'at clusters all about,
Or the gobble-uns 'll git you if you don't watch out!

J. W. RILEY.

THE KITCHEN CLOCK.

Knitting is the maid o' the kitchen, Milly ;
Doing nothing sits the boy in buttons, Billy :
  "Seconds reckoned
    Every minute,
    Sixty in it,
    Milly, Billy,
    Billy, Milly.
  Tick-tock, tock-tick,
  Nick-knock, knock-nick,
  Knockety-nick, nickety-knock,"
  Goes the kitchen clock.

Closer to the fire is rosy Milly ;
Every whit as close and cozy, Billy.
  "Time's a-flying,
    Worth your trying ;
    Pretty Milly—
    Kiss her, Billy !
    Milly, Billy,
    Billy, Milly.
  Tick-tock, tock-tick !
  Now, now,—quick, quick ;
  Knockety-nick, nickety-knock,"
  Goes the kitchen clock.

Something's happened : very red is Milly !
Billy boy is looking very silly !
  "Pretty missis, plenty kisses !
  Make it twenty, take a-plenty !
    Billy, Milly ! Milly, Billy !
    Right, left ; left, right ;
    That's right, all right,

Knockety-nick, nickety-knock,"
Goes the kitchen clock.

Weeks gone, still they're sitting, Milly, Billy!
Oh, the winter winds are wondrous chilly.
"Winter weather, close together;
Wouldn't tarry, better marry;
Milly, Billy! Billy, Milly!
Two, one—one, two;
Don't wait, 'twon't do;
Knockety-nick, nickety-knock,"
Goes the kitchen clock.

Winters two have gone, and where is Milly?
Spring has come again, and where is Billy?
"Give me credit, for *I* did it;
Treat me kindly, mind you mind me!
Mister Billy, Mistress Milly,
My—oh! oh—my!
Bye, bye! bye, bye!
Nickety-knock, cradle rock,"
Goes the kitchen clock.   J. V. CHENEY.

THE OWL CRITIC.

" Who stuffed that white owl?"   No one spoke in the shop;
The barber was busy, and *he* couldn't stop;
The customers, waiting their turns, were all reading
The Daily, *The Herald*, *The Post*, little heeding
The young man who blurted out such a blunt question;
Not one raised a head, or even made a suggestion;
            And the barber kept on shaving.

"Don't you see, Mister Brown,"
Cried the youth with a frown,

"How wrong the whole thing is,
   How preposterous each wing is,
How flattened the head is, how jammed down the neck is —
In short, the whole owl, what an ignorant wreck 'tis!
   I make no apology:
   I've learned owl-eology;
I've passed days and nights in a hundred collections,
And cannot be blinded to any defections
Arising from unskilful fingers that fail
To stuff a bird right from his beak to his tail.
   Mister Brown! Mister Brown!
   Do take that bird down,
Or you'll soon be the laughing-stock all over the town!"
               And the barber kept on shaving.

   "I've studied owls,
     And other night fowls,
     And I tell you
     What I know to be true:
     An owl cannot roost
     With his limbs so unloosed;
     No owl in this world
     Ever had his claws curled,
     Ever had his legs slanted,
     Ever had his bill canted,
     Ever had his neck screwed
     Into that attitude;
     He can't *do* it, because
     'Tis against all bird laws.
     Anatomy teaches,
     Ornithology preaches,
     An owl has a toe
     That *can't* turn out so!
I've made the white owl my study for years,
And to see such a job almost moves me to tears!

Mister Brown, I'm amazed
You should be so gone crazed
As to put up a bird
In that posture absurd!
To *look* at that owl really brings on a dizziness.
The man who stuffed him don't half know his business!"
And the barber kept on shaving.

"With some sawdust and bark,
I could stuff in the dark
An owl better than that.
I could make an old hat
Look more like an owl
Than that horrid fowl
Stuck up there so stiff, like a side of coarse leather—
In fact, about *him* there's not one natural feather."
Just then, with a wink and a sly normal lurch,
The owl, very gravely, got down from his perch,
Walked round, and regarded his fault-finding critic
(Who thought he was stuffed) with a glance analytic.
And then fairly hooted, as if he should say:
"Your learning's at fault this time, anyway;
Don't waste it again on a live bird, I pray.
I'm an owl; you're another. Sir Critic, good day!"
And the barber kept on shaving

From Harper's Magazine.

LITTLE "LORD FAUNTLEROY."

(Adapted by Mr. Harrower, *and inserted with the author's permission.)*

Captain Cecil was the second son of the Earl of Dorincourt; he had incurred his father's bitter anger by marrying a young American lady.

The old earl wrote his son, saying, "he might live where he pleased, and die where he pleased, for that he was done with him."

The result was that Captain Cecil left the army, and went to live in New York.

When their only child, Cedric, was between six and seven, Captain Cecil took fever; he became so ill that Cedric was sent away for a time.

When he was brought back, his mother looked pale and thin, and she was dressed in black.

"Dearest," he said—his father had always called his mother by that name—"Dearest, is my papa better? is he well?"

"Yes, darling, he is well, quite well; but we have no one left but each other now—no one at all."

Then, young though he was, he knew that his papa would not come back any more.

One day, Mr. Havisham, the Earl of Dorincourt's legal adviser, called on Mrs. Cecil; he had come to New York, to take Cedric back with him to England. The earl's eldest son having been killed by a fall from his horse, Cedric was heir to the title, and the earl, naturally enough, wished his grandson to stay with him in England.

"Must he be taken away from me? He is all I have! You don't know what he has been to me!"

"I am sorry to have to tell you, Mrs. Cecil, that the earl is not very friendly towards you: he proposes that his grandson shall stay with him at the Castle of Dorincourt. He offers to you Court Lodge, a very nice house, not far from the castle. He also proposes to settle upon you a suitable income. The only stipulation is that, while your boy may visit you at Court Lodge, the earl does not wish you to call at the castle. Not *very* hard terms, I think, Mrs. Cecil?"

"My husband was very fond of England. 'Twill be the best for my little boy; and since we may see each other, I ought not to suffer very much."

At that moment Cedric came into the room and ran up to his mother.

"And so," said Mr. Havisham—"and so this is little Lord Fauntleroy!"

Next morning his young lordship stepped in to see his old friend Mr. Hobbs the grocer.

"Helloh! Cedric! 'Mornin'."

"Good-morning, Mr. Hobbs! Do you remember what we were talking about yesterday?"

"Wal, Cedric, 'pears to me 'twas about England an' the aristocracy."

"Yes; and I think you said, Mr. Hobbs, you wouldn't have any Earls sitting around on your biscuit-boxes?"

"That's so, Cedric; and I meant it too. Let 'em try it, that's all!"

"Do you know, Mr. Hobbs, one is sitting on this box—now!"

"Eh! What's that?"

"Well, I *am* one—or going to be."

"Got any pain, Cedric? How d'ye feel? Thar is thunder in the atmosphere."

"I'm all right, thank you."

"*One* o' us has got a sunstroke!"

"Oh no, we haven't. You see, it's this: the lawyer came all the way from England to tell us. My grandpapa sent him."

"Yer grandfather, Cedric! An' who *is* yer grandfather?"

"Oh, he's the Earl of Dorincourt."

"Great Scott!"

"An' what may *your* name be, Cedric?"

"Well, the lawyer said I was Lord Fauntleroy."

"The lawyer said you was Lord Fauntleroy, Cedric?"

"Yes; he just said, 'And so this is little Lord Fauntleroy.'"

"Great Cæsar's ghost!"

That afternoon he said to the lawyer,—

"Do you know, Mr. Havisham, I don't know what an Earl *is?*"

"Don't you?"

"No. And when a boy is going to be an Earl, I think he ought to know; don't you?"

"Well, yes."

"Would you mind 'splaining it? What *made* my grandpapa an Earl?"

"Well, let me see. The *first* Earl of Dorincourt was made five hundred years ago."

"Well, well, that's a long time since. And what else do Earls do besides being made?"

"Well, some Earls have been very brave men, and have fought for their country."

"I'm glad of that! My papa was a soldier, and Dearest says he was a very brave man."

"Then, some Earls have a great deal of money."

"That's a good thing to have. I wish *I* had a great deal of money."

"Do you, and why?"

"Because Dearest says one can do so much with money. And if I were rich, I'd buy Dearest all sorts of beautiful things. And then there's Dick."

"And who is Dick?"

"Dick's a boot-black—one of the nicest boot-blacks you ever knew. I've known him for years."

"Oh, indeed! And if you were rich, now, what would you buy for him?"

"I'd buy Jake out."

"And who is Jake?"

"Jake's Dick's partner; but Jake isn't square—he cheats. And that makes Dick so wild, you know. If you were blacking boots all day, Mr. Havisham, and your partner wasn't square, 'twould make you wild, too, wouldn't it?"

"I daresay it would. But if you were rich now, what would you buy for yourself?"

"Oh, lots of things; but, first, I'd give Mary some money."

"And who is Mary?"

"A partic'lar friend of mine. She has twelve children and a husband, and he's got the fever, and they're very badly off."

[*Aside*] "This is the most singular boy I ever came across! Ah! Mrs. Cecil, I am very glad you've come in. Before I left England the Earl said, 'Let my grandson understand he can have anything he wants.'"

And thus it was that before little Lord Fauntleroy left New York for the home of his ancestors, he was able to give Mary and Dick enough money to help them out of all their difficulties.

He spent his first night in England with his mother at Court Lodge.

"Will you please tell the Earl, Mr. Havisham, that I would rather not take the money?"

"The money, Mrs. Cecil! You can't mean the income the Earl proposes to settle upon you?"

"Yes: if I took it, I should feel as if I were selling my boy to him. I am giving him up only because I love him enough to forget myself for his good, and because—because *his father* would have wished it to be so. And will you please ask the Earl not to tell my boy the reason I am not allowed to stay with him?"

"I shall deliver both messages, Mrs. Cecil."

"Thank you, Mr. Havisham."

On arriving at the castle, Mr. Havisham found the Earl of

Dorincourt recovering from an attack of his old complaint—the gout.

"Well, Havisham, got back? What sort of a lad is he?"

"Well, my lord, it's rather difficult to say."

"Ah! a fool is he, or a clumsy cub?"

"No, I don't think so. You will find him different, I daresay, from most English children."

"Haven't a doubt of it! Cheeky little beggars! These Americans call it smartness and precocity. I call it downright cheek and impudence."

"Mrs. Cecil has asked me to say, my lord, that she would rather not take the money."

"Ah! she wants to wheedle me into seeing her, does she? But I won't see her. I hate to think of her—a mercenary woman!"

"You can hardly call her mercenary, my lord; she has asked for nothing, and won't even accept the money you offer her."

"All done for effect, Havisham; all done for effect, I tell you."

"I have another message from Mrs. Cecil. She asks you not to tell her boy the reason she is not allowed to stay with him."

"Come, now, Havisham; you don't mean to tell me she hasn't told him the reason?"

"Not a syllable."

"So much the better, Havisham. He'll forget her in a week; he's only seven!"

"Yes, my lord, he is only seven; but he has spent those seven years by his mother's side, and I know she has all his affection."

"Nonsense, Havisham, nonsense! He'll forget her in a week; he's only seven."

It was the Earl's wish to see his grandson first alone.

As he stepped into the room in his black velvet suit, white lace collar, and flowing golden locks, the little fellow looked a perfect picture.

"Are you the Earl? I'm your grandson, you know. I hope you're quite well. I'm very glad to see you."

The old Earl could hardly believe his eyes or ears.

"Do you know, grandpapa, I've been wondering if you would look like my papa."

"Well, and do I—do I?"

"Well, I was very young when he died, you know, and I mayn't remember 'zactly *how* he looked; but I don't think you look like him."

"Ah, you're disappointed, I suppose!"

"Oh no; a person can't help his looks, you know. And, of course, a boy would love his grandpapa, even though he *wasn't* like his papa, 'specially one who had been so kind as you."

"Oh, I've been kind, have I?"

"Yes, grandpapa, very. I'm awfully obliged to you about Mary and Dick."

"Mary and Dick?"

"Yes: they're partic'lar friends of mine; and Michael had the fever."

"Michael! and who's Michael?"

"Michael's Mary's husband. When a man's got the fever and twelve children, *you* know how it is; but the money you sent me made them all right. And then there's Dick. You'd like Dick. Dick's so square, you know."

"Square! what do you mean by square?"

"It means Dick wouldn't cheat."

"Dick! and who's Dick?"

"Oh, Dick's a boot-black!"

"Oh, Dick's a boot-black!"

"Yes; and the money you sent me bought out Jake, Dick's partner, who wasn't square at all. So, you see, grandpapa, you've made Mary, and Michael, and their twelve children, and Dick very, very happy."

"Oh, have I?"

"Yes, grandpapa; and Dearest says that's the best kind of goodness, and when I grow up I hope I shall be just like you."

"Just like me?"

"If I can; I'm going to try."

Dinner was now announced.

"O grandpapa, you're lame! Would you like me to help you?"

"Do you think you could, Fauntleroy?"

"I think I could. Dick says I've a good deal of muscle for a boy that's only seven."

"Well, you may try, Fauntleroy—you may try."

"Lean on me, grandpapa. Don't be afraid. I'll walk very slowly. Lean on me; I'm all right if it isn't a very long way. —It's a hot night, grandpapa."

"Well, Fauntleroy, you've been doing some hard work."

"Oh, it wasn't 'zactly hard, grandpapa; but a person *will* get warm in summer. Grandpapa, this is a very big house for only just *two* people to live in."

"Do you find it too large, Fauntleroy?"

"Well, I was thinking, grandpapa, that if only just *two* people lived here, who weren't very fond of each other, they might feel a little lonely, sometimes. I wish Dearest was with us."

"Dearest! and who is Dearest?"

"My mamma! You know my papa always called her Dearest. But she isn't very far away; she told me to remember that. And I can always look at the picture she gave me. My papa used to wear it. She's in here. You touch this spring. Ah, there she is!"

"And that's your mamma, Fauntleroy?"

"Yes, that's Dearest!"

"And are you very fond of her, Fauntleroy?"

"Yes, grandpapa, very! You see, my papa left her to me to take care of, and when I'm a man I'm going to work, and earn money for Dearest."

"And do you think you'll miss her much, Fauntleroy?"

"Yes, grandpapa, I'll miss her all the time. She said she'd put a light in her window, and I might see it after dark. Ah, there it is, grandpapa! I see it shining through the leaves, and I know what it says."

"And what does it say, Fauntleroy?"

"It says, 'Good-night, darling! God keep you all the night.' And I know I am quite safe, grandpapa."

"Quite safe, Fauntleroy, my boy, quite safe."

The room was very still. A large St. Bernard dog was asleep on the rug; little Lord Fauntleroy was asleep also, his head resting on the dog's shoulder.

As the old man sat watching the child, many strange, new thoughts were passing through his mind.

By-and-by, Mr. Havisham was shown in.

"Ah, Havisham, I'm very glad to see you. You were right, Havisham, and I was wrong—utterly wrong. Call on Mrs. Cecil in the morning, ask her to forgive me, and bring her with you here, Havisham, as little Lord Fauntleroy's mother, and as my daughter.—Look at him, Havisham, look at him! That child has taught me more to-night than I have ever learned in all my past life, the dear, noble little fellow. God bless him!"

FRANCES HODGSON BURNETT.

EDITHA'S BURGLAR.

(*Adapted by* Mr. Harrower, *and inserted with the author's permission.*)

Mr. and Mrs. Hamilton lived in a suburb of London.

Their only child, Editha, was a bright little girl about eight years of age.

One morning she said, "Papa, what do you think of burglars as a class?"

"As a class, Edie?"

"Yes, papa, as a class."

"Well, I think they're a bad lot, Edie—a very bad lot."

"Are there no good burglars, papa?"

"Well, no, Edie; I rather think not. As a rule they are a class of gentlemen not distinguished for moral rectitude or blameless character."

"What ever has possessed the child? Why do you talk about burglars, Edie?"

"Well, mamma, I'm rather sorry for them. They must be often up all night."

"Sorry for them, the scoundrels! If I should waken and find a burglar in my room, I think I should die!"

One day Mr. Hamilton came home, saying, "I must go down to Glasgow by the 9.15 Pullman to-night."

"O Frank, what *shall* I do? You know the servants sleep in the attics. I shall be *so* frightened!"

"Nonsense, Polly! I'll leave Edie in charge of you."

That night Edie couldn't go to sleep. She thought of her father rushing through the dark night on his way to Scotland. At last she did doze off. About midnight something wakened her. Listening, she heard a stealthy filing of iron.

"It's a burglar! he'll frighten mamma!"

She slipped out of bed, out of the room, and down the stair. The filing had stopped, but she heard a step in the kitchen as she quietly opened the door. Imagine the astonishment of that burglar when he saw a little girl in white, on whom the light of his lantern shone—a little girl, whose large lustrous eyes looked at him in a by no means unfriendly manner.

"O Lor', wot a start!"

"Hush! don't be frightened, Mr. Burglar. I don't want to hurt you."

"She don't want to 'urt me!"

"Hush! I've come to ask a favour from you. Are you really a burglar?"

"Not at all! I'm a dear friend o' yer par's; an' not a-wishin' to disturb the servants by ringin' the bell, I stepped in by the winder. D'ye twig, little 'un?"

"Well, I'm very sorry! My papa's from home, and my mamma's so easily frightened; and if you are going to burgle, would you please to burgle as quiétly as you can?"

"Well, I'm blow'd!"

"Why don't you say you're blown? It isn't correct to say 'you're blow'd,' you know."

"Now, look 'ere, little 'un! I ain't got no time to waste, yer know."

"No, I s'pose you haven't. Well, what are you going to burgle first? If you don't mind, I'll show you some things you might burgle."

"Wot things?"

"Well, you can burgle *my* things."

"Wot kin' o' things?"

"Well, there's my gold watch, and my gold locket, and my pearl ear-rings, and necklace. They're worth a great deal of money. And then there's my books."

"I don't want no books!"

"Don't you? Thank you very much. Shall I step upstairs for my jewel-box?"

"No, not yet. I wants to 'ave a squint o' the knives an' forks first. Come into the pantry."

"It's very curious, Mr. Burglar, that you should know 'zactly where to look for things, and that your keys should fit our locks so nicely."

"Well, yes, it *is* kin' o' sing'lar. O' course, there's a good deal in bein' edercated, yer know."

"And are you educated, Mr. Burglar?"

"Did yer think as 'ow I weren't?"

"Well, you pronounce some words so strangely."

"Oh, it's all a matter o' taste. Hoxford an' Cambridge, Hedinburgh an' Glasgow 'as diff'rent vocabilleries, don't yer know?"

"And did you go to college, Mr. Burglar?"

"Did yer think as 'ow I didn't? Well, I *am* blowed!—blown!"

"Will you please leave a few silver knives and forks? We shan't have any to use at breakfast."

"Ain't yer got no steel 'uns?"

"Oh yes; but we don't use steel ones to fish. You can burgle *my* silver knife and fork, but, please, do leave one for my dear mamma!"

"Oh, wery well! It's agin' the rules o' the perfession, but there's a knife an' fork for yer precious mar."

"Thank you; you are very kind and considerate. Talking of professions, would you rather be a burglar than anything else?"

"Well, no; can't say as 'ow I would. Now I comes to think on't, I'd raither be the Lord Mayor, or a member o' the 'Ouse o' Lords, or even 'is R'yal 'Ighness Halbert Hed'ard, Prince o' Wales!"

"Oh, you could never be the Prince of Wales, you know."

"Well, no; I dessay you're about right, little 'un. There are a few hobstacles in the way."

"I meant some other *profession*. My papa's an editor; how would that suit you?"

"Fust-rate! Now I comes to think on't, I'm a born heditor!"

"I'm afraid my papa wouldn't change professions with you."

"Oh, d'ye think not?"

"No; but if you were to give me your name and address, he might speak to his friends about you."

"Well, now, honly to think! if I ain't went an' forgot my card-case! I left it on the pianner in the drorin'-room. I'm a-hallays a-leavin' my card-case!"

"Oh, never mind. If you tell me your name and address, I think I could remember them."

"No, I'm afeard yer couldn't."

"I think I could."

"Oh, yer think yer could, could yer? Well, 'ere goes. My name is Lord Halbert Hed'ard Halgernon de Pentonwille, 'Yde Park."

"And are you really a lord? How very strange!"

"Well, yes, it *is* kin' o' sing'lar. I've often thought so myself. An' now show us the libery; I wants to inspeck yer par's things."

"Very well, come this way. This is my papa's room; and now, dear Mr. Burglar, I want to ask *another* favour from you. I'll make you a present of all my jewels if you won't burgle any of my papa's things. He's very fond of them, and he is very good."

"Oh, wery well; go an' fetch yer jew'ls, as ye calls 'em.— She's the rummiest little kid I *ever* see'd."

In a few minutes she came back.

"My papa gave me this gold watch, my mamma gave me this gold locket, my grandmamma left me these pearl ear-rings and this necklace; and my dear grandmamma's in heaven."

"Oh, yer grandmamma's in 'eaven, is she? Then *she's* all right, little 'un! An' now I think I'll be movin'."

She followed him back to the kitchen.

"Are you going out by the window, my lord?"

"Well, yes. Yer see, it's a kin' o' a sort o' an 'abit o' mine.

I prefers 'em to doors, 'cause my medical hadwiser tells me the hexercise is good for my constitootion."

"Well, good-bye, my lord; and thank you very much for burgling so quietly."

* * * * * *

A few weeks after this a parcel was left at Mr. Hamilton's house by a very queer, shabby-looking man. It contained Edie's box of jewels and a very large, old-fashioned silver watch, on the lid of which were scratched these words,—

"To the little 'un, from 'er friend and well-wisher, Lord Halbert Hed'ard Halgernon de Pentonwille, 'Yde Park."

FRANCES HODGSON BURNETT.

ARTEMUS WARD'S LECTURE ON "THE MORMONS."

(*Adapted by* MR. HARROWER.)

Ladies and Gentlemen, I don't expect to do great things here to-night; but I thought if I could make enough money to take me to New Zealand, I should not have lived in vain. I don't want to live in Vain; I'd rather live in Margate or London. I really don't care for money. How often do large fortunes ruin young men! I should like to be ruined.

I'm not an artist, but I have always been mixed up with art. I have an uncle who takes photographs, and I have a servant who takes anything she can lay her hands on. I like art; I admire dramatic art, although I failed as an actor. The play was "The Ruins of Herculaneum." I played "The Ruins." "The Ruins" was not a success. A friend of mine played "The Burning Mountain." He was worse than "The Ruins"—he was a bad "Vesuvius."

The remembrance often makes me ask, Where are the boys of my youth? Some are with you here, some are abroad, some are in jail. Hence arises a most touching question—Where are the girls of my youth? Some are married, some would like to be. O my Maria! Alas! she married another—they frequently do. I hope she is happy, because I am.

I like music. I can't sing. As a singist I am not a success. I am saddest when I sing; so are those who hear me—they are sadder than I am. Some silver-voiced young men came under my window the other night and sang, "Come where my love lies dreaming." But I didn't go.

"The Great American Desert in Winter." This is a great work of art—an oil-painting, done in petroleum. It is by the old masters. This is the last thing they did before dying: they did this, and then they expired. Some of the greatest living artists come here every morning before daybreak with lanterns to look at it. They say they never saw anything like it before, and they hope they never shall again.

The overland mail-coach. In this den I was locked up for fourteen days and nights. Those of you who have been in jail, and stayed there any length of time as visitors, can realize how I felt.

I don't like to speak about it, but I once made the great speech of my life. I wish you could have heard it. I have a fine education. I speak six different languages—London, Chatham, and Dover, Margate, Brighton, and Hastings. I wish you could have heard that speech. If Cicero—he's dead now, he has gone from us—but if dear old Cis could have heard that effort, it would have given him the rinderpest. I spoke that speech to two battalions of soldiers, and I worked them up to such a pitch of enthusiasm that they came very near shooting me on the spot.

I remember being once surrounded by a band of Indians. They were armed with rifles, knives, and pistols. I'm a brave man. On the very day before the battle of Bull's Run, I was on the highway, when the bullets, those awful messengers of death, were passing all round me in waggons on their way to the battle-field. I *am* a brave man. But there were too many of those Indians—there were five thousand of them, and only one of me—so I said, "Great chief, I surrender." His name was "Wocky-Bocky." He approached me. I saw his tomahawk glisten in the morning sunlight. He mingled his swarthy fingers with my golden locks; he waved his dreadful Thomashawk before my lily-white face; he exclaimed, "Forsha, arrah, darrah, booksheesh!" Says I, "Mr. Wocky-Bocky," says I, "old Wocky, I've thought so for years, and so have all our family."

I regret to say that efforts were made to make a Mormon of me when I was in Utah. Seventeen young widows, wives of a deceased Mormon, offered me their hands and hearts. Taking their soft white hands in mine, which made eighteen hands altogether, I found them in tears. I said, "Why is this thus?" They hove a sigh, seventeen sighs, of different size. Then they said, "Doth not like us?" I said, "I doth, I doth!" I also remarked, "I hope your intentions are honourable, as I am a lone child, my parients being far, far away." Then they said, "Wilt not marry us?" I said, "Oh no, it cannot was." Then they said, "O cruel, cruel man! This is too much, too much!" "Yes," says I, "I think it is. It's on account of the muchness I beg to decline."

THE CELEBRATED JUMPING FROG.

(By kind permission of Messrs. CHATTO AND WINDUS.*)*

There was a feller here, once, by the name of Jim Smiley— in the winter o' '49, or maybe it was the spring o' '50; but anyway, he was the curiousest man about—always bettin' on anything that turned up. If there was a horse race, you'd find him flush, or you'd find him busted, at the end of it. If there was a dog fight, he'd bet on it; if there was a cat fight, he'd bet on it; if there was a chicken fight, he'd bet on it. Why, if there was two birds sittin' on a fence, he'd bet you which one would fly first. It never made no difference to him—he would bet on anything. The dangdest feller!

This yer Smiley had a mare, an' he used to win money on that horse for all she was so slow, and always had the asthma, or the distemper, or the consumption, or something o' that sort. They used to give her two or three hundred yards start, and then pass her on the way; but always at the fag-end o' the race she'd get excited, an' desperate like, an' come cavortin' an' straddlin' up—scatterin' her legs around—an' kickin' up more dust, an' raisin' more racket, wi' her coughin', an' sneezin', an' blowin' her nose—an' always fetch up at the stand, jest about a neck ahead, as near as you could cipher it down.

An' he had a little small bull-pup, that to look at you'd think he weren't worth a cent, but to set around an' look or'nery, an' lay for a chance to steal somethin'. But as soon as money was upon him, he was a different dog: his under-jaw began to stick out, like the fo'castle o' a steamboat; his teeth would uncover, an' shine savage, like the furnaces. An' a dog might tackle him, an' bully-rag him, an' bite him, an' throw him over his shoulder two or three times, an' Andrew Jackson —that was the name o' the pup—Andrew Jackson would never let on but what he was satisfied, an' hadn't looked for nothin' else. An' the bets bein' doubled an' doubled on the other side all the time, till the money was all up, an' then, all o' a sudden, he would grab that other dog, jest by the jint o' his hind-leg, and freeze to it; not chaw, you understand, but only jest grip, an' hang on, till they throwed up the sponge—if it was a year.

Wal, this yer Smiley had rat-terriers, an' chicken-cocks, an' tom-cats, an' all them kin' o' things, till you couldn't rest, an' you couldn't fetch nothin' for him to bet on, but he'd match you.

He ketched a frog one day, an' took him home with him, an' said he calc'lated to edercate him; an' so he never done nothin' for three months, but set in his back-yard an' learn that frog to jump. You bet, he did learn him too. He'd give him a little punch, an' the next minute you'd see that frog whirlin' in the air like an acrobat—see him turn one summerset, or maybe a couple, if he got a good start, and come down flat-footed, an' all right, like a cat, an' fall to scratchin' the side o' his head wi' his hind-foot, as indifferent as if he hadn't no idea he'd been doin' any more'n any frog might do. You never see such a frog so modest an' straightfor'ard as he was for all he was so gifted.

Wal, this yer Smiley kep' the frog in a little lattice-box, an' used to fetch him down town, an' lay for a bet. One day a feller, a stranger in the camp he was, comes up to Smiley, an' says, "What might it be you've got in the box?"

"Wal," says Smiley, sorter indifferent-like, "it might be a parrot, or it might be a canary, maybe; but it ain't—it's only jest a frog."

The feller took the box, an' looked at it careful, an' turned it round this way an' that, an' give it back to Smiley, an' says, "H'm! so 'tis. Wal, what's he good for?"

"Wal," Smiley says, easy an' careless, "he's good enough for one thing, I should jedge—he can out-jump any frog in Calaverous County."

The feller took the box again, an' took another long partic'lar look, an' give it back to Smiley, an' says, very deliberate, "Wal, I don't see no p'ints about that frog that's any better'n any other frog."

"Maybe you don't," says Smiley; "maybe you understand frogs, an' maybe you don't understand 'em. Maybe you've had experience, an' maybe you ha'n't—only a amateur, as it were. Anyways, I've got my opinion, an' I'll risk forty dollars that he can out-jump any frog in Calaverous County."

An' the feller studied a minute, an' then says, kinder sadlike, "Wal, I'm only a stranger here, an' I ain't got no frog; but if I had a frog, I'd bet you."

"That's all right," says Smiley, "if you'll hold my box a minute, I'll go an' get you a frog."

The feller took the box, put up his forty dollars, along with Smiley's, an' sat down to wait. He sat there a long while, thinkin' an' thinkin' to hisself. At last he took the frog out, forced his mouth open, took a teaspoon an' filled him full o' quail shot, filled him pretty nigh to the chin, an' set him on the floor. Smiley, he went to the swamp, an' slopped around in the mud for a long time. At last he ketched a frog, fetched him in, an' give him to the feller, an' says, "Now, if you're ready, set him alongside o' Dan'l"—Dan'l Webster was the name of the frog—"an' I'll give the word."

Then he says, "One, two, three—jump!"

An' him an' the other feller touched up the frogs behind. The new frog hopped off, but Dan'l gave a heave, an' h'isted up his shoulders—so—like a Frenchman; but it warn't no use, he couldn't budge. The feller took the money and started away. Goin' out at the door, he sorter jerked his thumb over his shoulder—this way—at Dan'l, an' says again, very deliberate—"Wal, I don't see no p'ints about that frog, that's any better'n any other frog."

Smiley, he stood scratchin' his head, an' lookin' down at Dan'l a long time, an' at last he says, "I do wonder what in thunder that frog throwed off for. He 'pears to look mighty baggy, somehow."

He ketched Dan'l by the nape o' the neck, an' says, "Why, blame my cats! if he don't weigh five pounds!" He turned him upside down, an' he belched out a double handful o' shot. An' then he sees how it was, an' he was the maddest man. He set the frog down, took out after that feller—but he never ketched him.

MARK TWAIN.

THE THREE PARSONS.

[FROM "QUEER FISH:" DEAN AND SON, LONDON.]

(*By kind permission of the Author.*)

I don't b'long to the 'Stablished Church myself, sir, as am a Independent, a-beggin' your pardon, as I knows for to be a 'Stablished Church parson. But yer see wot I says is this: you takes a lot o' us fisher-folks as works 'ard all the week, a-doin' wot the skipper tells us—a-haulin' in ropes, a-settin' sails, a-draggin' nets, an' one thing or t'other. Well, now, if we chaps goes in for the 'Stablished Church, we ain't nobody— we ain't got no woice, an' we ain't got no sort o' power or command like. But if so be as we goes in for the Baptists, or the Methodies, or any o' the sectises, why, bless you, sir, we get made a lot of—some bein' made stooards, some deacons, an' some ev'n a-takin' round the 'at. You should see me an' old Cockles in the westry o' a Sunday—an' our names, sir, our wery names called out from the pulpit, sometimes—" Brother Cockles, an' Brother Coleman." Then again, if we wants a change o' minister, we can tell our man to look out for a call to some place else; an' afore we elects a new 'un, we 'ave a lot down on trial, don't ye know? We pays our money, an' we takes our choice. Now, our usual way o' electin' a minister is this—We 'ave one man down one Sunday, 'nother on the follerin' Sunday, an' so on till we're satisfied. It so 'appened one time as 'ow we couldn't satisfy ourselves; we 'ad *six* down runnin', consecativ' like, but none o' 'em didn't suit. At last, by some little misunderstandin', we 'ad *three* come down to preach their trial sermons on the same Sunday. So we arranged that the Rev. Paul Duster should 'old forth in the mornin', the Rev. Halgernon Sydney Crackles in the arternoon, an' the Rev. John Brown in the evenin'. "You mark my words," says old Cockles to me in the westry that Sunday mornin'— "you mark my words: there'll be some close sailin' to-day. I'm rayther inclined to bet on the old gen'l'm as goes first, as is wery orthodox, an' seems to me to carry a deal o' canvas." An awful severe-lookin' man were the Rev. Paul Duster, wi' an immense 'ead an' face, both of 'em bald an' shinin', 'is 'ead all over bumps; 'e certainly were awful impressive—to look at! Old Duster's sermon caused a tremenjous sensation, the langidge bein' full o' Latin an' Greek, an' all sorts. In the arternoon we meets for to hear the second preacher, the Rev. Halgernon Sydney Crackles, as turned out so wery poetical, 'e seemed like takin' the wind out o' old Duster's sails. His woice had a bee-u-ti-ful shivery-shakery in it; an' 'e wept, bless you, sir, 'e wept that copious, I thought we'd 'ave to bail the pulpit out, an' ask him to kindly weep over the side. In the evenin' we meets for to hear the last preacher, the Rev. John Brown. The Rev. John Brown! Why, sir, his name alone were dead agin' 'im. Then 'e were only about five-an'-twenty, an' a trifle under-sized. I could see at once as 'ow 'e didn't go down like wi' the congregation. Well, 'e preached 'is sermon—a short, straight-away dociment, wich ev'rybody could understand. It weren't doctrinal; nor it weren't poetical. But it were just practical—a-tellin' us as 'ow ev'rybody in the world 'ad dooties to perform, an' 'ow we ought to stick to 'em, an' never-say-die-like; sort o' standin' by the ship, 'owever the wind might blow or the sea might rage. On the followin' Wensday night there was to be a church meetin' to eleck one o' 'em; but none o' us knowed, sir, none o' us knowed 'ow wery soon our choice was to be made.

That Sunday night will never be forgotten, sir, so long as this 'ere place has a boat on the water or a 'ouse on the shore—the night o' the great storm, we calls it, when the Spanish *San Perdro* went to pieces. Afore I turned in, I 'ad a look out, as usual, an' I sees a wessel in the offing. An old sailor like me, sir, al'ays sleeps wi' one eye open; so when the winds began to blow, an' the waves was a-tumblin' an' a-rollin' bang against the jetty there, I wakes up, an' I thought o' that ship wot I 'ad seen passin'. So I jumps into my clo's, clapped on a sou'-wester, an' made for the beach.

Wot a night! wot a night! The sky were as black as ink; the wind a-blowin' fit to wake the dead. By-an'-by blaze went the lightnin'; the thunder pealin' right above our 'eads, an' then rollin' away over that awful sea. Nigh ev'ry man an' 'ooman in the place was on the beach, an' even little uns had crep' away from 'ome, an' were a-clingin' to their mothers' gowns.

The first flash showed us an awful sight—a wessel, 'er riggin' all entangled on 'er deck, driftin' straight on for the rocks. Nought on earth could save her. There she was, a noble, 'an'some craft, drivin' right ashore—drivin' fast an' sure into the jaws o' death. The women were weepin'; an' many a brave man's heart, as we stood there grimly silent, was wild wi' sorrow at its own 'elplessness. Despairin' cries from the wreck were borne to the shore, as she struck wi' a great shiverin' shock on that black rock out there. The women shuddered an' fell on their knees, while from man to man went the question, "Can we do nothin', *nothin'* to 'elp 'em now?" But what *could* we do? None o' our boats could live in a sea like that; an' as for swimmin' off to the wreck—ah! little wonder our 'earts quailed a bit.

A lot o' lanterns 'ad been lit, so I could see things pretty plainly. Clingin' together in the background was the women an' little uns. Atween them an' us was two o' the parsons— the poetical chap on 'is knees; an' old Duster, 'is 'at blowed clean away, 'is bumps all wisible, a-'oldin' on tight to a jetty-post. I didn't see the young preacher chap, as I found out arterwards 'e 'ad gone to a farm-'ouse a few miles up-country; but as I were thinkin' about 'im, I sees 'im comin' wi' quick, 'asty strides towards the water. "Stand aside, women!" Calm and cool 'e orders 'em, an' to right an' left they scatter. Straight on 'e comes, to where we men was standin'. Off 'e flings 'is 'at an' coat an' boots, an' takes 'old of a rope. "Sir!" we cries, "you shall not go. Look at that sea; it's certain death. Wi' 'is own 'ands 'e ties the rope around 'is waist, a-wavin' us off as we press around 'im. An 'givin' one look towards the wreck, an' one look, bright an' quick, up to heaven, he takes one step back, and then—into the wild surf e' leaps!

Wi' bated breath an' strainin' eyes we watch the strugglin' swimmer—beaten an' buffeted—tossed 'ither an' thither. "Can 'e ever reach the ship?" To us on shore it seems impossible. But God Himself, sir, must 'ave filled that brave young 'eart wi' stren'th for the darin' deed. We can 'ear the poor fellows on the wreck a-wavin' 'im on wi' wild an' thankful cries. But we on shore are silent; our 'earts are too full for word or sound. At last, thank God, we sends up a shout as I can almost 'ear yet, for the swimmer 'as reached the wreck! Well, sir, by that there rope ev'ry soul on board the *San Perdro* was saved. An' now, pale an' bruised an' bleedin', last o' all there comes ashore young Parson Brown, ev'ry man an' 'ooman eager to see 'is face an' shake 'is 'and. "Mates," says old Cockles, "I can't say much, but wot I do say is" —an' 'e takes tight 'old o' young Brown's 'and—" wot I do say is, God bless our minister!"

An' then, sir, we all sends up a uniwersal shout—" God bless our minister!"

A-beggin' your pardon, as I knows for to be a 'Stablished Church parson, but that was the way as 'ow we elected our minister that time.   ROBERT OVERTON.

MR. PICKWICK AND THE WELLERS.

(*By kind permission of* Messrs. CHAPMAN AND HALL.)

Mr. Pickwick (*solus*). It is the fate of a lonely old man, that those about him should form new attachments and leave him. But I have no right to be selfish. No, no; I should rather be happy that I am able to provide for my faithful Sam; and I am happy—of course I am. [*Knock.*] Come in, Sam, come in.

Enter SAM WELLER *and his* FATHER.

Sam. My father, sir.

Mr. P. Glad to see you, Mr. Weller. How do you do?

Old W. Wery 'earty, thankee, sir. 'Ope I see you vell, sir?

Mr. P. Quite well, Mr. Weller, thank you, quite well.—Sam, give your father a chair.

Old W. No, thankee, sir; I'd rayther stand. Huncommon fine day, sir.

Mr. P. Uncommonly so, Mr. Weller; very fine weather indeed.

Old W. Wery much so, sir.—I never see sich a haggerawatin' boy as you, Samivel, never in all my born days.

Mr. P. What is Sam doing, Mr. Weller?

Old W. Vy, sir, 'e von't begin; that's wot 'e's a-doin' of.

Sam. You said you'd begin, guv'nor. 'Ow wos I to know you wos done up at the wery beginnin'?

Old W. You might ha' seen I warn't able to start, Samivel. I'm on the wrong side o' the road, an' a-backin' into the palin's, an' yet you von't put out a 'and to 'elp me. It ain't fillal conduck, Sammy; wery far from it.

Sam. All right, guv'nor.—Vell, you see, sir, the fact is the guv'nor's been a-drawin' out his money.

Old W. Wery good, Samivel; wery good, my boy. I didn't mean to speak 'arsh to you, Sammy. That's the vay to begin; come to the pint at vunce, as the young 'ooman remarked wen 'er sweet'eart wos a-courtin' o' her.

Sam. The guv'nor's drawed out eleven 'undred an' eighty pound.

Old W. Redooced *coun*cils, Sammy.

Sam. It don't signerfy vether it's redooced or hunredooced. Eleven 'undred an' eighty pound is the figger, ain't it?

Old W. Right you har, Sammy; eleven .'undred an' eighty pound.

Mr. P. Really, Mr. Weller, I am surprised. I had no idea—

Old W. Vait a minit, sir.—Get on, Samivel.

Sam. I'm a-gettin' on.—The guv'nor's wery anxious to put this 'ere money vere 'e knows it'll be safe. An' I'm wery anxious, too; for if 'e keeps it, 'e'll go an' inwest in 'osses, or deposit it in some bloomin' Australian bank.

Old W. Wery good, Sammy, my boy. Drive ahead.

Sam. For the aforesaid reasons, the guv'nor's come 'ere vith me to say—leastways to hoffer—or in other vords to—

Old W. To say this 'ere, sir, that this money ain't o' no use to me; an' if you'll take care of it, I shall be wery much obleeged. All I say is, you keep it till I ask you for it; an' I vishes you a wery good mornin'. [*Exit Old W.*

Mr. P. Bless my soul! Stop him, Sam! Overtake him—bring him back! [*Exit Sam.*

Enter SAM, *dragging* OLD WELLER.

Mr. P. Mr. Weller, my good friend, I assure you I have more money than I can ever use. Take this back, Mr. Weller. You must really take it back.

Old W. Oh wery well, sir, wery well! Mark my vords, Sammy; I'll go an' do somethin' desp'rate vith this 'ere property.

Mr. P. No, no, Mr. Weller, you must not do anything rash. I'll keep your money in trust for you.

Old W. You vill, sir?—Then, Sammy, I von't do nothin' desp'rate.

Mr. P. Ah! that's all right. And now, Mr. Weller, I wish to ask your advice on a very important subject.—Sam, will you wait outside for a few minutes? [*Exit Sam.*] And now, Mr. Weller, sit down. Oblige me—sit down. You are not, I think, Mr. Weller—you are not an advocate for matrimony?

Old W. No, sir, I ain't.

Mr. P. No, I thought not.—Did you see a young woman downstairs, Mr. Weller?

Old W. The old gent's a-goin' it.—Yes, I did see a young 'ooman downstairs.

Mr. P. Yes; and what did you think of her, Mr. Weller? Candidly now, what did you think of her?

Old W. Vell, I thought she wos rayther good-lookin', an' a wery tidy sort o' gell.

Mr. P. So she is, Mr. Weller, so she is. And what did you think of her manners, Mr. Weller?

Old W. Vell, I thought they wos wery pleasant and obligin' like.

Mr. P. So they are, Mr. Weller, so they are. Do you know, Mr. Weller, I take a very great interest in that young woman.

Old W. The old gent is a-goin' it.—Oh, ye do, sir?

Mr. P. Yes, I do, Mr. Weller, because that young woman is attached to your son.

Old W. Hattached to—hattached to Samivel!

Mr. P. Yes, Mr. Weller, attached to Sam.

Old W. Vell, I'm blowed. Oh, it's nat'ral, but alarmin'. Sammy must be wery careful. You ain't never safe vith 'em, sir, ven they vunce begins to 'ave designs on you.

Mr. P. But, Mr. Weller, she is not only attached to Sam—Sam is attached to her.

Old W. Samivel hattached! Vell, I *am* blowed. This 'ere's a pretty sort o' thing to come to a father's ears!

Mr. P. Suppose, now, Mr. Weller, suppose I wished to help Sam to marry this young woman. What would you say, Mr. Weller?

Old W. The young 'ooman not bein' a widder!

Mr. P. The young woman not being a widow, Mr. Weller.

Old W. Oh, vell, it ain't for me to hoppose your vishes, Mr. Pickwick.

Mr. P. Ah, that's all right.—Sam! Sam! [*Enter Sam.*

Sam. Yes, sir!

Mr. P. Your father and I have been talking about you, Sam.

Old W. About *you*, Samivel!

Mr. P. I am not so blind, Sam, as not to have seen that you entertain something more than a friendly feeling towards Mrs. Winkle's maid.

Sam. I 'ope there ain't no 'arm in that, sir?

Mr. P. Certainly not, Sam; certainly not.

Old W. Not by no manner o' means, Samivel; certainly not —oh no—not at all!

Mr. P. I am happy to find, Sam, your father is of my opinion.

Old W. The young 'ooman not bein' a widder!

Mr. P. The young woman not being a widow, Mr. Weller.— I wish to help you in this matter, Sam. I therefore free you from your situation as my servant. And I shall be proud, Sam, proud and happy to make your future prospects in life my grateful and peculiar care.

Sam. Wery much obliged to ye, sir; but it can't be done!

Mr. P. Can't be done, Sam!

Old W. Can't be done, Samivel!

Sam. I say it *can't* be done!

Mr. P. My good lad, I am growing old. My rambles, Sam, are over.

Sam. Wery good, sir. If you vant a more polishter servant, vell an' good—'ave 'im, 'ave 'im. But vages or *no* vages, board or *no* board, lodgin' or *no* lodgin', Sam Veller as you took from the old inn in the Borough sticks by you, come wot come may; an' let ev'rythin' and ev'rybody do their wery fiercest, nothin' nor nobody shall ever perwent it!

Old W. Wery good, Sammy; wery good, my boy!

Mr. P. But, Sam, you must think of the young woman.

Sam. I do think o' the young 'ooman. I 'ave thought o' the young 'ooman. I've told 'er 'ow I'm sitivated, an' she's willin' to vait till I'm ready, an' I believe she vill. If she don't, she's not the young 'ooman I takes 'er for, an' I gives 'er up vith pleasure. You've knowed me afore, sir. My mind's made up, an' nothin' can ever alter it.

Old W. Wery good, Sammy; wery good, my boy!

Mr. P. Sam, dear, faithful Sam! I assure you I feel more pleasure in your unselfish attachment than ten thousand protestations from the greatest men living could awaken in my breast......

Old W. Sammy, my boy, I'm proud o' ye!

CHARLES DICKENS.

HELEN AND MODUS.

[FROM "THE HUNCHBACK."]

Enter HELEN R—— *and* MODUS L——.

Helen. What's that you read?

Modus. Latin, sweet cousin.

Helen. 'Tis a naughty tongue, I fear, and teaches men to lie.

Modus. To lie!

Helen. You study it. You call your cousin sweet, and treat her as you would a crab.—Why, how the monster stares and looks about!—You construe Latin, and can't construe that.

Modus. I never studied women.

Helen. No, nor men; else would you better know their ways, nor read in presence of a lady.

[*Strikes book out of Modus's hand.*

Modus. Right you say, and well you served me, cousin. I own my fault. So please you, may I pick it up again? I'll put it in my pocket.

Helen. Pick it up.—He fears me as I were his grandmother.—What is the book?

Modus. 'Tis Ovid's "Art of Love."

Helen. That Ovid was a fool.

Modus. In what?

Helen. To call that thing an art which art is none.

Modus. And is not love an art?

Helen. Are you a fool as well as Ovid, cousin? Better stay at home and study homely English.

Modus. Nay; you know not the argument.

Helen. I don't? I know it better than ever Ovid did. The

face, the form, the heart, the mind—that's the argument. Cousin, you are no soldier. You'll never win a battle. You care too much for blows. [*Crosses to Modus.*

Modus. You wrong me there, sweet cousin. At school I was the champion of my form, and since I went to college—

Helen. *That* for college!

Modus. Nay, but hear me, cousin! [*Crosses to Helen.*

Helen. Well, what since you went to college? Was there not one Quentin Halworth there? You know there was, and that he was your master—

Modus. *He* my master! Thrice was he beaten by me.

Helen. Still was he your master. Confess it, cousin; 'tis the truth. A proctor's daughter you did both affect. Look at me and deny it! I've caught you now, bold cousin. Of the twain she more affected you, and yet *he* won her—won her, because he wooed her like a man. Now, sir, protest that you are valiant.

Modus. Cousin Helen!

Helen. Well, sir?

Modus. The tale is all a forgery.

Helen. A forgery?

Modus. From first to last ne'er spoke I to a proctor's daughter.

Helen. 'Twas a scrivener's then, or somebody's. Enough, you loved her, and, shame upon you! let another take her.

Modus. I tell you, cousin, if you'll only hear me, I loved no woman while I was at college save one, and her I fancied ere I went there.

Helen. Indeed!—Now I'll retreat if he's advancing. Comes he not on? Oh, what a stock's the man!—Well, cousin?

Modus. Well, sweet cousin, what more wouldst have me say? I think I've said enough.

Helen. And so think I. I did but jest with you. You're not angry? Well, shake hands. Why, cousin, do you squeeze me so?

Modus. I swear I squeezed you not.
Helen. You did not?
Modus. No. I'll die if I did.
Helen. Why, then, you did not, cousin. So let's shake hands again. Oh, go and now read Ovid. Cousin, will you tell me one thing?
Modus. What, sweet cousin?
Helen. Wore lovers ruffs in Master Ovid's time? Behoved him teach them then to put them on, and that you have to learn. Hold up your head. Why, cousin, how you blush! Plague on the ruff! I cannot give't a set. You're blushing still! Why do you blush, dear cousin? So—no! Oh, 'twill beat me. I'll give it up.
Modus. Nay, prithee, don't. Try on.
Helen. And if I do, I fear you'll think me bold.
Modus. For what?
Helen. To trust my face so near to thine!
Modus. I don't know what you mean.
Helen. I'm glad you don't. Cousin, I own right well behaved you are—most marvellously well behaved. They've bred you well at college. With another man, my lips would be in danger. Oh, hang the ruff!
Modus. Nay, give it up, nor plague thyself, dear cousin.
Helen. Dear fool! I swear the ruff is good for just as little as its master. There! 'tis spoiled. You'll have to get another. Hie for it, and wear't in fashion of a wisp ere I adjust it for thee. Farewell, *sweet* cousin! You'd *need* to study Ovid's "Art of Love." [*Exit Helen.*

Modus. Went she in anger? I will follow her. No, I will not. Heigh-ho! I love my cousin. Sees she I love her, and so laughs at me because I lack the front to woo her? I *will* woo her then! Her lips *shall* be in danger. A bold heart, master. 'Tis a saying, "Faint heart never won fair lady." I'll *woo* my cousin, come what will on't! Hang Ovid's "Art of Love"! I'll *woo* my cousin! [*Exit Modus.*

Enter HELEN.

Helen. Marry Master Wilford! never; I'll leap out of the window first. I'll hang myself ere I'd be forced to marry. [*Enter Modus.*] Why, cousin Modus! What! will you stand by and see me forced to marry? Cousin Modus, have you not a tongue? Have you not eyes? Do you not see I'm very, very ill, and not a chair in all the corridor?

Modus. I'll find one in the study.

Helen. Hang the study!

Modus. My room's at hand; I'll fetch one thence.

Helen. You shan't! I'd faint ere you came back.

Modus. What shall I do?

Helen. Why don't you offer to support me? Well, give me your arm. Be quick! Is that the way to help a lady when she's faint? I'll drop unless you hold me. *That* will do; I'm better now. Don't leave me. Is one well because one's better? Hold my hand. Keep so. I'll soon recover, so you move not. —Loves he? which I'll be sworn he does. He'll own it now. —Well, Cousin Modus?

Modus. Well, sweet cousin?

Helen. You heard what Master Walter said?

Modus. I did.

Helen. And would you have me marry Master Wilford? Can't you speak? Say yes or no.

Modus. No.

Helen. Bravely said; and why, my gallant cousin?

Modus. Why?

Helen. Ay, why? Women, you know, are fond of reasons. Why would you not have me marry? How stupid you are, cousin! Let me go.

Modus. You are not well yet.

Helen. Yes.

Modus. I'm sure you're not.

Helen. I'm sure I am.

Modus. Nay, let me hold you, cousin. I like it

Helen. Do you? I would wager you could not tell me why you like it. Why, how you stare! What see you in my face to wonder at?

Modus. A pair of eyes.

Helen. At last he'll find his tongue.—-And saw you ne'er a pair of eyes before?

Modus. Not such a pair; they are so bright! You have a Grecian nose.

Helen. Indeed!

Modus. Indeed!

Helen. What kind of mouth have I?

Modus. A handsome one. I never saw so sweet a pair of lips; I ne'er saw lips at all till now!

Helen. Cousin, I'm well! Do you not hear? I tell you I am well! I need your arm no longer—take it away. So tight it locks me, 'tis with pain I breathe. Let me go, cousin. Wherefore do you hold your face so close to mine? What do you mean?

Modus. You've questioned me, and now I'll question you.

Helen. What would you learn?

Modus. The use of lips.

Helen. To speak.

Modus. Naught else?

Helen. How bold my *modest* cousin grows! Other use know you?

Modus. I do.

Helen. Indeed! You're wondrous wise! And pray what is it?

Modus. This—

Helen. Soft. My hand thanks you, cousin; for my lips, I keep them for a husband. Nay, stand off! I'll not be held in manacles again. Why do you follow me?

Modus. I—I love you, cousin.

Helen. O cousin! say you so? That's passing strange—falls out most crossly—is a dire mishap—a thing to sigh for—weep for—languish for, and die for—

Modus. Die for!

Helen. Yes, with laughter, cousin; for, cousin, I love you.

Modus. And you'll be mine?

Helen. I will.

Modus. Your hand upon't.

Helen. Hand and heart. Hie thee to thy dressing-room—I'll to mine. Attire thee for the altar; so will I. But hark you, ere you go—ne'er brag of reading Ovid's "Art of Love."

Modus. And, cousin, stop! One little word with you.

[*Exeunt Helen and Modus.*
SHERIDAN KNOWLES.

DIALOGUE FROM "SHE STOOPS TO CONQUER."
KATE HARDCASTLE *and* YOUNG MARLOW.

Scene.—Mr. Hardcastle's House.

Enter MARLOW.

Mar. I'm in such a flurry. I've just heard that Miss Hardcastle, whom I've never seen, is in this confounded inn. To me the most terrible thing in the world is to be left alone with a young—

Enter MISS HARDCASTLE.

Miss H. I'm glad of your safe arrival, Mr. Marlow. I'm told you had some accidents by the way.

Mar. Only a few, madam. Yes, we had some—a good many. But I'm sorry, madam—I mean happy, madam—of any accidents which are so agreeably concluded!

Miss H. I'm afraid you flatter, sir. You, who have seen so much of the finest company, can find little entertainment in an obscure corner of the country.

Mar. I have lived, indeed, in the world, madam, but have kept very little company. I have been only an observer of life, madam, while others were enjoying it.

DIALOGUE FROM "SHE STOOPS TO CONQUER."

Miss H. An observer of life, like you, Mr. Marlow, must, I fear, have been disagreeably employed, since you must have seen much more to censure than to approve.

Mar. Pardon me, madam. I was always willing to be amused.

Miss H. But you have not been wholly an observer, I presume, sir? The ladies, I should hope, have formed some part of your addresses?

Mar. Pardon me, madam; I—I as yet have studied—only to —deserve them.

Miss H. And that, some say, is the very worst way to obtain them.

Mar. Perhaps so, madam; but I love to converse only with the more grave and sensible part of your charming sex. But, madam, I fear I grow tiresome.

Miss H. Not at all, sir. There is nothing I like so well myself as grave conversation; I could listen to it for ever. Indeed, I have often been surprised how a man of sentiment could ever admire those light, airy pleasures where nothing reaches the heart.

Mar. It's a disease of the mind, madam. In the great variety of tastes there must be some who, wanting a relish for —ah—um—ah—

Miss H. I understand you, sir. There must be some who, wanting a relish for refined pleasures, pretend to despise what they are incapable of tasting.

Mar. My meaning exactly, madam. And I can't help observing, madam, that in this age of hypocrisy—ah—um—ah—

Miss H. You were going to observe, sir—

Mar. I was going to observe, madam, that—ah—I protest, madam, I forget what I was going to observe.

Miss H. You were observing, sir, that in this age of hypocrisy—

Mar. Yes, madam. In this age of hypocrisy there are few— I will say there are very few—who do not—ah—um—ah—

Miss H. I understand you perfectly, sir.

Mar. [*Aside*] It's more than I do.—[*Rising*] Madam, shall I—

Miss H. I protest, sir, I never was more agreeably entertained in all my life. Pray go on.

Mar. Yes, madam. I was—Madam, shall I have the honour?

Miss H. Oh, very well; I'll follow.

Mar. Yes, madam; I can assure you.—[*Aside*] Confound it! this pretty mincing dialogue has done for me. [*Exit.*

Miss H. [*Laughing*] Was there ever such a sober, sentimental interview? I'm certain he scarce looked me in the face the whole time. And yet the fellow, but for his unaccountable bashfulness, is well enough. If I could only teach him a little confidence, it would be doing somebody that I know a little service. I have it. He thinks our house an INN; I'll act the part of a housemaid, and stoop to conquer. [*Exit.*

Enter MARLOW.

Mar. A nice fool I made of myself; what will Miss Hardcastle think of me? I can't account for my bashfulness. You may talk of an earthquake or a burning mountain, but to me a young lady is the most tremendous object in the whole world.

Enter MISS HARDCASTLE (*apron, servant's cap, keys at side.*)

Miss H. Did you call, sir? [*Curtsies.*

Mar. As for Miss Hardcastle, she's too sentimental for me.

Miss H. Did your honour call?

Mar. No, child.—From the glimpse I had of her, I think she squints.

Miss H. I'm sure, sir, I heard the bell ring.

Mar. Go away, child. I've pleased my father by coming here, and now I'll please myself by going home.

Miss H. Are you sure, sir, you didn't call?

Mar. I tell you no.—Yes, child, yes; I think I did call. I wanted—I vow, child, you are very handsome.

Miss H. O sir, you make one ashamed.

Mar. Yes, child, yes; I *did* call. Have you got any—what d'ye call it in the house?

Miss H. No, sir; we've been out of that these ten days.

Mar. Suppose, then, I should call for a taste, by way of sample, of the nectar of your lips.

Miss H. Nectar! nectar! That's a liquor there's no call for in these parts. French, I suppose?

Mar. No, child; English, I assure you.

Miss H. It's odd I shouldn't know it. We keep all sorts of wines in this house, and I've been here these eighteen years.

Mar. Eighteen years! How old are you, child?

Miss H. O sir! I mustn't tell my age.

Mar. To guess at this distance, you can't be much over forty. Yet nearer, I don't think quite so much. By coming close, you look younger still; and closer—

Miss H. Pray, sir, keep your distance. One would think you wanted to know one's age as they do horses, by mark of mouth. I'm sure you didn't treat Miss Hardcastle in this obstropolous manner. I'll warrant, now, before her you looked bashful enough, and talked as if you were before a Justice of the Peace.

Mar. [*Aside*] She's hit me, sure enough!—In awe of her, child? Ha! ha! ha! A mere awkward, squinting thing! No, no, child; you don't know me. I laughed and joked with her.

Miss H. I suppose, sir, you'll be a great favourite with the ladies?

Mar. Oh yes, child; a great favourite. In London, at the ladies' club, my friends call me their lively rattle. Rattle's not my real name, child. My name is Solomons; Mr. Isaac Solomons, at your service.

Miss H. The ladies' club 'll be a very merry place, sir?

Mar. Rather; we keep up the fun till three in the morning.

Miss H. And you are their lively rattle. Ha! ha! ha!

Mar. [*Laughs with her*] I don't quite understand this chit. She looks too knowing.—What are you, child?

Miss H. A relation of the family, sir.

Mar. A poor relation?

Miss H. [*Nods*] I keep the keys, and see that the guests want for nothing.

Mar. In plain English, you are the barmaid of this inn.

Miss H. Inn! what brought that into your head? One of the best families in the county keep an inn! Ha! ha! ha! Mr. *Hard*castle's house an inn!

Mar. Mr. *Hard*castle's house! Is this Mr. Hardcastle's house?

Miss H. Ay, sir; whose else should it be?

Mar. Confound my stupidity! To mistake this house for an inn, and you for the barmaid!

Miss H. I'm sure, sir, there's nothing in my behaviour to—

Mar. Nothing, child, nothing; quite the reverse. I was in for a list of blunders, and made you a subscriber. But this house I no more show my face in!

Miss H. I hope, sir, I've done nothing to offend you. I'm sure I should be sorry to offend any gentleman who has been so polite, and who has said so many civil things to me. I'm sure I should be sorry if he left the family on my account; and I'm sure my family's as good as Miss Hardcastle's, and though I'm poor, that's no great misfortune to a contented mind.

Mar. Madam, you are the only member of the family I am sorry to part with.

Miss H. As our acquaintance began, sir, so let it end, in indifference—because *I* am Miss Hardcastle—

Mar. W—w—what!

Miss H. Yes, sir, that very identical "awkward, squinting thing" you were pleased to call me—she whom you addressed as the mild, modest, sentimental man of gravity; and when you thought I was a barmaid, spoke to me as the bold, rollicking, "lively rattle" of the ladies' club. In which of these characters, sir, will you give me leave to address you—as the faltering, bashful gentleman, with looks downcast, and who hates hypocrisy? or as the loud, confident man of fashion who keeps up the fun till three in the morning?

Mar. Madam, I am dumb! Can you forgive me?

Miss H. I only stooped to conquer. GOLDSMITH.

CARDINAL RICHELIEU.

[EXTRACTS.]

(*By kind permission of* Messrs. GEO. ROUTLEDGE AND SONS.)

CHARACTERS.

JULIE DE MORTIMAR (*Ward to Richelieu*); CARDINAL RICHELIEU; ADRIEN DE MAUPRAT; JOSEPH (*a Monk, Richelieu's Confidant*); HUGUET (*an Officer of Richelieu's Household Guard*).

RICHELIEU *and* JOSEPH.

Rich. And so you think this new conspiracy the craftiest trap yet laid for the old fox. Fox! Well, I like the nickname.

Jos. Orleans heads the traitors.

Rich. A very wooden head, then—well?

Jos. The favourite, Count Baradas—

Rich. A weed of hasty growth : it cost me six long winters to mount as high as in six little moons this painted lizard. But I hold the ladder, and when I shake, he falls. What more?

Jos. A scheme to make your orphan ward an instrument to aid your foes. Your ward has charmed the king.

Rich. Out on you! Have I not, one by one, from such fair shoots plucked the insidious ivy of his love? The king must have no goddess but the state—the state—that's Richelieu.

Jos. This is not the worst. Baradas—

Rich. I have another bride for Baradas.

Jos. You, my lord?

Rich. Ay, more faithful than the love of fickle woman—when the head lies lowliest, clasping him fondest.

Enter HUGUET.

Hug. Mademoiselle de Mortimar.

Rich. Most opportune; admit her. [*Exit Huguet.*]—In my closet you'll find a rosary, Joseph. Ere you tell three hundred beads I'll summon you. Stay, Joseph! I did omit an *Ave* in my matins—a grievous fault—atone it for me, Joseph. There is a scourge within. I am weak, you strong; it were but charity to take my sin on such broad shoulders.

Jos. I guilty of such criminal presumption as to mistake myself for you! No, never think it.—[*Aside*] I' faith, a pleasant invitation. [*Exit Joseph.*

Enter JULIE DE MORTIMAR.

Jul. Cardinal! are you gracious? May I say father?

Rich. Now, and ever.

Jul. Father! a sweet word to an orphan.

Rich. No! not orphan while Richelieu lives. Thy father loved me well, my friend, ere I had flatterers. He died young in years, not service, and bequeathed thee to me; and thou shalt have a dowry, girl, to buy thy mate amidst the mightiest. Drooping! Sighs! Art thou not happy at the court?

Jul. Not often.

Rich. Thou art admired, art young; does not the king commend thy beauty? ask thee to sing to him?

Jul. He's very tiresome, our worthy king.

Rich. Fie! kings are never tiresome—save to their ministers.

Enter HUGUET.

Hug. The Chevalier de Mauprat waits below.

Jul. De Mauprat!

Rich. H'm! he has been tiresome too—anon!

[*Exit Huguet.*

Jul. What doth he? I mean—does your eminence—that is—know you Monsieur de Mauprat?

Rich. Well! And you? has he addressed you often?

Jul. Often? No, nine times—nay, ten—the last time by the lattice of the great staircase. The court sees him but rarely.

Rich. A bold and forward roisterer!

Jul. He! Nay! modest, gentle, and sad, methinks.

Rich. Wears gold and azure?

Jul. No! sable.

Rich. So you note his colours, Julie? Shame on you, child! Look loftier. By the mass! I have business with this modest gentleman.

Jul. You are angry with poor Julie. There's no cause.

Rich. No cause! You hate my foes?

Jul. I do.

Rich. Hate Mauprat.

Jul. Not Mauprat! no, not Adrien, father.

Rich. Adrien! familiar—go, child—not that way—wait in the tapestry chamber—I will join you—go!

Jul. His brows are knit. I dare not call him father—but I must speak.—Your eminence!

Rich. Well?

Jul. Do not rank De Mauprat with your foes. He is not—I know he is not; he loves France too well.

Rich. Not rank De Mauprat with my foes? so be it. I'll blot him from that list.

Jul. That's my own father. [*Exit Julie.*

Rich. Huguet! [*Enter Huguet.*] De Mauprat struggled not nor murmured?

Hug. No; proud and passive.

Rich. Bid him enter. Hold! Look he hide no weapon. When he has entered, place thyself yonder, and watch him. If he show violence—[Let me see thy carbine—so—a good weapon]—If he play the lion, why—the dog's death.

Hug. I never miss my mark. [*Exit Huguet.*

RICHELIEU *sits at table and arranges papers. Enter* HUGUET *and* DE MAUPRAT. HUGUET *retires behind screen.*

Rich. Approach, sir! Can you call to mind the hour, now three years since, when in this room, methinks, your presence honoured me?

Mau. It is, my lord, one of my most—

Rich. Delightful recollections.

Mau. [*Aside*] Doth he make a jest of axe and headsman?

Rich. I did then accord you a mercy ill requited; you still live.

Mau. To meet death face to face at last.

Rich. Your words are bold, Adrien de Mauprat, doomed to sure death. How hast thou since consumed the time allotted thee for serious thought and solemn penitence?

Mau. The time, my lord?

Rich. Is not the question plain? I'll answer for thee. Thou hast sought nor priest nor shrine; no sackcloth chafed thy delicate flesh; the rosary and the death's-head have not, with pious meditation, purged earth from thy carnal gaze. What thou hast *not* done, brief told; what *done*, a volume. Wild debauch, turbulent riot; for the morn, the dice-box, noon claimed the duel, and the night the wassail. Do I wrong you, sir?

Mau. My lord, I was not always thus. If changed my nature, blame that which changed my fate. Were you accursed with that which you inflicted, night and day, by bed and board, dogged by one ghastly spectre; the while within you youth beat high, and life grew lovelier from the neighbouring frown of death,—were this *your* fate, perchance you would have erred like *me*.

Rich. I might, like you, have been a brawler and a reveller; not, like you, a trickster and a thief.

Mau. Lord Cardinal, unsay these words!

[*Huguet steps out and slowly takes aim.*

Rich. Not quite so quick, friend Huguet; Monsieur de

Mauprat is a patient man, and he can wait. [*Huguet retires.*]
—You have outrun your fortune; I blame you not that you would be a beggar—each to his taste. But I do charge you, sir, that, being beggared, you would coin false moneys out of that crucible called debt. To live on means not yours, be brave in silks and laces, gallant in steeds, magnificent in banquets,—all *not yours*—ungiven, unmerited, unpaid for,—this is to be a trickster; and to filch men's art and labour, which to them is wealth, life, daily bread—quitting all scores with, " Friend, you're troublesome ! "—why this—forgive me—is what, when done with a less dainty grace, plain folks call theft. [*Reads paper.*] You owe eight thousand pistoles, minus one crown, two liards.

Mau. [*Aside*] The old conjurer !

Rich. This is scandalous !—shaming your birth and blood ! I tell you, sir, that you must pay your debts.

Mau. With all my heart, my lord. Where shall I borrow then the money ?

Rich. [*Aside*] A humorous dare-devil ; the very man to suit my purpose—ready, frank, and bold.—Adrien de Mauprat ! men have called me cruel. I am not ; I am just. I found France rent asunder ; the rich men, despots, and the poor, banditti ; sloth in the mart and schism in the temple ; brawls festering to rebellion, and weak laws rotting away with rust in antique sheaths. I have re-created France, and, from the ashes of the old feudal and effete carcass, Civilization, on her luminous wings, soars phœnix-like to Jove. What was my art? Genius, some say ; some, fortune ; witchcraft, some. Not so ; my art was justice. Force and fraud misname it cruelty. You shall confute them, my champion, you. You met me as my foe—depart my friend ; you shall not die. France needs you. You shall wipe off all stains—be rich, be honoured, be great. I ask, sir, in return, this hand, to gift it with a bride, whose dower shall match yet not exceed her beauty.

Mau. My lord, I—I have no wish to marry.

Rich. Surely, sir, to die were worse!

Mau. The poorest *coward* must die; but knowingly to march to marriage, my lord, it asks the courage of a *lion.*

Rich. Adrien de Mauprat, I know all. Thou hast dared to love my ward, my charge!

Mau. As rivers may love the sunlight—basking in the beams, and hurrying on.

Rich. Renounce her! take life and fortune with another! Silent?

Mau. Your fate has been one triumph. You know not how blest a thing it was in my dark hour to nurse the one sweet thought you bid me banish. Base knight, false lover he who bartered all that brightened grief and sanctified despair for life and gold. Revoke your mercy! I prefer the fate I looked for.

Rich. Huguet! [*Huguet comes down.*] To the tapestry chamber conduct your prisoner.—[*To De Mauprat.*] You will there behold the executioner. Your doom be private, and Heaven have mercy on you!

Mau. When I'm dead, tell her I loved her.

Rich. Keep such follies, sir, for fitter ears. Go!

[*Exit De Mauprat, followed by Huguet.*

Rich. Joseph! [*Enter Joseph.*] Methinks your cheek hath lost its rubies, Joseph. I fear you have been too lavish of the flesh; the scourge is heavy.

Jos. I pray you, change the subject.

Rich. You good men are so modest. Well, to business. Bid my stewards arrange my house by the Luxembourg—a bridal present to my ward, who weds to-morrow.

Jos. Weds! With whom?

Rich. De Mauprat.

Jos. H'm! A penniless husband.

Rich. Bah! The mate for beauty should be a man, not a money-chest. When her brave sire lay on his bed of death, I vowed to be a father to his Julie. And so he died, the smile upon his lips; and when I spared the life of her young lover, methought I saw that smile again. He has honour and courage; besides, he has taste, this Mauprat. When my play was acted to dull tiers of lifeless gapers, who had no soul for poetry, I saw *him* applaud at the proper places. Trust me, Joseph, he is a man of most uncommon promise.

Jos. And yet your foe.

Rich. Have I not foes enow? Great men gain doubly when they make foes friends. Remember my grand maxims: first, employ all methods to conciliate.

Jos. Failing these?

Rich. All means to crush. As with the opening and the clenching of this little hand, I will crush the small venom of these stinging courtiers.

Jos. And when check the conspiracy?

Rich. Check! check! Full way to it! Let it bud, ripen, flaunt i' the day, and burst to fruit!—the Dead Sea's fruit of ashes!—ashes which I will scatter to the wind. Go, Joseph; when you return, I have a feast for you—the last great act of my great play. [*Exit Joseph.*

Enter JULIE *and* MAUPRAT.

Mau. O speak, my lord! I dare not think you mock me— and yet—

Rich. Eh! how now?—O sir! you live?

Julie. My father, from my heart for ever now I'll blot the name of orphan.

Rich. My children! ye are mine—mine both; and in your sweet and young delight, your love, my own lost youth breathes musical. Go, my children; be lovers while ye may. —How is't with *you*, sir? You bear it bravely. You know "it asks the courage of a lion." [*Exeunt Julie and Mauprat.*] O God-like power! woe, rapture; penury, wealth; marriage and death, for one infirm old man through a great empire to dispense, withhold, as the will whispers. And shall things like motes that live in my daylight, lackeys of court wages, dwarfed starvelings, mannikins, upon whose shoulders the burden of a province were a load more heavy than the globe of Atlas, cast lots for my robes and sceptre? France! I love thee! All earth shall never pluck thee from my heart. My wedded wife! sweet France! who shall proclaim divorce for thee and me?

LORD LYTTON.

SCENES FROM "KING LOUIS THE ELEVENTH."

CHARACTERS.

KING LOUIS, DUKE DE NEMOURS, DR. COITIER (*the King's Physician*), FRANÇOIS (*a Monk*), TRISTAN (*a Member of the King's Bodyguard*).

Enter COITIER *and* NEMOURS.

Coit. Let me look well upon you, dear Nemours, son of my benefactor!

Nem. Whose fate I shall share.

Coit. By heaven, thou shalt not die!

Nem. How can I escape?

Coit. Thou art in the king's chamber.

Nem. This Louis's room?

Coit. He would speak with you, and bade me bring you here.

Nem. See me, and here! What would he with me?

Coit. You may yet obtain a pardon.

Nem. How?

Coit. Be useful.

Nem. To *him!* the butcher of my father!

Coit. Nemours, save your life.

Nem. No, Coitier; I'd sooner die than do thy will.

Coit. You are resolved?

Nem. Yes, Coitier; a thousand times, yes!

Coit. And so am I. All the gold the king could give me would have failed to have secured my services, had he not granted me freedom. I alone have power to come and go, to pass the sentinels unquestioned. Here is the talisman—this master-key. Take it, Nemours; it gave *me* liberty, it now gives liberty to *thee*.

Nem. But, Coitier, his rage will fall on you.

Coit. Perhaps.

Nem. Your life will answer for it.

Coit. No; he's ill, and cannot do without me. Take this dagger; descend the vaulted stair; at the foot you'll find a door; use that key, and then—liberty! Away! I fear the king's arrival. I'll haste below and stop him if I can. Farewell!

Nem. Farewell, good Coitier! [*Exit Coitier.*] O Fate! this is thy work. He's in my power; his weapon in my hand! Assemble here, ye spectres of his victims!—my father first: gather round his bed, his bed of torture; the altar of revenge and justice. Hark! he comes!

[*Nemours goes behind curtain.*

Enter LOUIS, COITIER, *and* TRISTAN.

Louis. How dark the night is, and how cold! I tremble.

Coit. Warm yourself.

Louis. The sun is not so sweet. Fire—'tis life! But Nemours? what said Nemours?

Coit. Follow my advice: to bed, sire.

Louis. No, Coitier, not till I have seen Nemours.—Go fetch him, Tristan.

Trist. He's not in my charge, sire.

Louis. True; I had forgot.—I bade *you* bring him here, Coitier.

Coit. I could not persuade him to come.

Louis. *I* could.

Coit. I think not.

Louis. No?

Coit. No; he'd have defied you, and you'd have slain him.

Louis. Well?

Coit. So I saved him.

Louis. Saved! saved! And hast thou dared to brave me, wretch?—And has he, too, escaped thy vigilance? Where is he?—quick, Tristan!

Coit. Save yourself the trouble; he's beyond your reach.

Louis. Dead or alive, I'll have him!—Away, Tristan. [*Exit Tristan.*]—For you, traitor, death to-morrow!

Coit. Strike to-day; but of your after-sufferings have a care. I give you but a week to live!

Louis. Well, then, I'll die—I will! Think not to escape! I'll crush you!

Coit. So you have said.

Louis. Ay, ay. Your learning may deceive the vulgar crowd—not me; your art, your medicines—I laugh at them. I'll do without you, and live just as long—I will, I will! The saint whom I expect to-night can, with a single word, give me health.

Coit. Indeed! then speed him here quickly.

Louis. Whilst thou, deprived of light and air, shalt from between thy prison bars look out and see my new youth laugh at thy rage.

Coit. Agreed!

Louis. Ay, ay.

Coit. It may be so.

Louis. False friend! Ah, Coitier, ungrateful!

Coit. It was to avoid that charge I saved Nemours.

Louis. But my kindness—mine—*that* you have betrayed! Gold I o'erload you with: what more did Nemours to be so loved?

Coit. What did he? Why, he gave me all his heart. You! what claim have you to love? Let's understand each other. You give from fear; I take from interest. I sell; you purchase. 'Tis a contract; and where the heart is not, there can be no ingratitude. Kings think that gold can purchase everything. You pay a courtier or a servant: friends, sire, we love; and though their salary be but one kind look, one pressure of the hand, they feel they're paid with love ten thousandfold.

Louis. O Coitier! I'm a wretched man. Good Coitier! you know I love you.

Coit. Yes, for yourself.

Louis. No, no; not from selfishness. My sufferings are extreme; but Father François will this night give me strength. Still, as a simple friend, there's my hand! [*François, a monk, enters.*]—See, my father, he has braved his king, yet I pardon him.—Good night, good Coitier; good night. [*Exit Coitier.*] Ah, traitor, I'll watch ye!—Father, I tremble at thy feet with hope and fear.

Fran. What would you?

Louis. Restore my health—efface the lines of age—extend thine hand and bid me live again. Ten years, my father!—grant but ten years, and I'll heap on thee honours twentyfold. In thy name great cathedrals will I found. I'll—

Fran. King! Heaven permits not this feeble worm even to know, much less to change, the laws of nature; and to assume such power were blasphemy.

Louis. I'm growing tired of this. Come, do thy duty, monk! Exert for me thy supernatural power—or, if need be, I'll resort to force. I'm king!—

Fran. I fear, king, that in your heart remorse is like a burning wound, kept fresh by crime, and dragging your body slowly to the grave.

Louis. Priests have absolved me.

Fran. Vain hope! True penitence alone can wash your sins away.

Louis. Shall I find mercy?

Fran. Heaven grant you may.

Louis. You promise, if I confess? Listen, then, and to thee I'll tell that which hath never reached the ears of man.

Fran. What hast thou done?

Louis. It was rumoured that the fear the dauphin caused the late king hastened him to heaven.

Fran. A son abridge his aged father's life!

Louis. I was that dauphin.

Fran. You!

Louis. But his weak rule would have ruined France. State interests—

Fran. Confess; do not excuse thy faults.

Louis. I had a brother who by poison died.

Fran. By your orders?

Louis. Some suspected so. But he deserved it.

Fran. Fratricide! repent!

Louis. I do. See, my father, I confess another sin: the old Nemours he had conspired, and at his death, beneath the scaffold, I placed his two weeping sons.

Fran. Barbarian!

Louis. Others I have put to death. Prisoners even now in dungeons deep groan out forgotten lives.

Fran. Since these are wrongs thou canst still repair, come!

Louis. Whither?

Fran. To release them.

Louis. No; 'tis enough that I repent. The church has pardons which a king can buy.

Fran. God sells not pardon. Miserable man, appease the torture of thy guilty soul: an act of mercy may give back thy sleep, and some, at least, will bless thy waking hours.

Louis. Well, I'll see about it.

Fran. Heaven will not wait.

Louis. To-morrow.

Fran. Ere to-morrow death may—

Louis. Death! no—I have Coitier, and am well defended.

Fran. Adieu then!

Louis. Father, stay!

Fran. Pray.

Louis. I will—I will.

Fran. Not with vain words. Pray with deeds, and thus alone atone the past. Farewell! [*Exit François.*

Louis. Father, stay! I repent!—He's gone. No, I don't!—

What's that I hear? Their merry dancing o'er, the village peasants wander home. Happy souls! gentle sleep is theirs. They slumber on—but I—I— [*Enter Nemours.*

Louis. Nemours!
Nem. Silence!
Louis. Yes.
Nem. Not a cry!
Louis. No.
Nem. Thy guards defend thee well.
Louis. Nemours, what wouldst thou?
Nem. Vengeance!
Louis. Judge not in passion.
Nem. I am not thy judge.
Louis. Who is, then?
Nem. My father.
Louis. Thou, Nemours!
Nem. My father.
Louis. Thou alone!
Nem. My father!
Louis. He would kill me.
Nem. Thou hast judged thyself.
Louis. Nemours, be merciful!
Nem. Wert thou?
Louis. Hear my prayer!
Nem. Dost recollect his prayer to thee—his last appeal? 'Tis here!
Louis. I ne'er received—
Nem. Thou liest! 'Twas by thee rejected, and which, when dead, I found upon his breast—my only heritage!
Louis. Nemours, forgive!
Nem. Beneath this dagger read.
Louis. I cannot.
Nem. Beneath the axe he well could write; read what he wrote.
Louis. I cannot. This dagger blinds me. No, I cannot.

Nem. Then, listen :—" My Sovereign Liege, I humbly recommend me to your mercy. I will serve thee well and loyally. Have mercy on my poor children. Let me not die, that they may survive me in disgrace and beggary. For God's sake, sire, have pity on my poor children !"—Look, murderer, read—

Louis. Where?

Nem. There !

Louis. [*Reads*] "Your poor friend, NEMOURS."

Nem. And there, see, his blood ! his blood ! Oh what punishment can meet thy crimes? how make it equal with thy matchless guilt? There is but one torture can suffice !

Louis. It is my death.

[*Louis falls at Nemours' feet insensible.*

Nem. No, it is thy life ! What ! I free thee? No; live on—or, rather, *living*, die. Die slowly too ! that all thy cruel schemes may add accumulated woe, and foretaste give of thine eternity. Ay, wait till death, both just and pitiless, shall seize that soul that never mercy felt—laden with crimes so deep that even Heaven's mercy hath no measure for thee ! Live on. It is thy prayer—thy wish. Heaven grant it, then. Prolong his damnèd life, until his crimes reach Babel-like to heaven to bring its righteous judgment down !—Father, now art thou avenged ! DELAVIGNE.

DOGBERRY, VERGES, AND THE WATCH.

[*From "Much Ado About Nothing."*]

Characters—DOGBERRY, VERGES ; SEACOAL *and* OATCAKE (*Watchmen*).

Scene I.—A Street in Messina.

Dog. Are you good men and true?

Verg. Yea, or else it were pity but they should suffer salvation, body and soul.

Dog. Nay, that were a punishment too good for them.

Verg. Well, give them their charge, neighbour Dogberry.

Dog. First, who think you the most desartless man to be constable?

Verg. Hugh Oatcake, or George Seacoal; for they can write and read.

Dog. Come hither, neighbour Seacoal. God hath blessed you with a good name: to be a well-favoured man is the gift of fortune; but to write and read comes by nature.

Sea. Both which, master constable,—

Dog. You have; I knew it would be your answer. Well, for your favour, sir, give God thanks, and make no boast of it; and for your writing and reading, let that appear when there is no need of such vanity. Neighbour Seacoal, you are thought here to be the most senseless and fit man for the constable of the watch; therefore bear you the lantern. This is your charge:— you shall comprehend all vagrom men; you are to make any man stand, in the prince's name.

Sea. How if he will not stand?

Dog. Why, then, take no note of him, but let him go; and presently call the rest of the watch together, and thank God you are rid of a knave.

Verg. If he will not stand when he is bidden [*Coughs*], he is none of the prince's subjects.

Dog. True, Master Verges; and they are to meddle with none but the prince's subjects. You shall also make no noise in the streets; for—for the watch to babble and to talk is most tolerable and not to be endured.

Oat. We will rather sleep than talk: we know what belongs to a watch.

Dog. Why, Master Oatcake, you speak like an ancient and most quiet watchman; for I cannot see how sleeping should offend: only, have a care that your bills be not stolen. Well, you are also to call at all the ale-houses, and bid them that are the worse of liquor get them to bed.

Sea. How if they will not?

Dog. Why, then, let them alone till they are sober : if they make you not then the better answer, you may say they are not the men you took them for.

Sea. and Oat. Well, sir.

Dog. If you meet a thief, you may suspect him, by virtue of your office, to be no true man ; and, for such kind of men, the less you meddle or make with them, why, the more is for your honesty.

Sea. If we know him to be a thief—

Oat. Shall we not lay hands on him ?

Dog. Truly, by your office, you may ; but I think they that touch pitch will be defiled : the most peaceable way for you, if you do take a thief, is to let him show himself what he is, and steal out of your company.

Verg. You have always [*Coughs*] been called [*Coughs*] a merciful man, Master Dogberry.

Dog. Truly, I would not hang a dog by my will, much less a man.

Verg. If you hear a [*Coughs*] child cry in the night [*Coughs*], you must call to the nurse and [*Coughs*] bid her still it.

Sea. How if the nurse be asleep—

Oat. And will not hear us ?

Dog. Why, then, depart in peace, and let the child wake her with crying; for the ewe that will not hear her lamb when it bleats will never answer a calf when it "bâs."

Verg. 'Tis very true.

Dog. This is the end of the charge :—you, neighbour Seacoal, are to present the prince's own person. If you meet the prince in the night, you may stay him.

Verg. Nay, by'r lady, that I think he cannot.

Dog. Five shillings to one on't, with any man that knows the statues, he may stay him. Marry, not without the prince be willing ; for, indeed, the watch ought to offend no man ; and it is an offence to stay a man against his will.

Verg. Yea, by'r lady, I think it be so.

Dog. Ha! ha! ha! Well, neighbours Seacoal and Oatcake, give you good-night. [*Going.*] Ah, if there be any matter of weight chances, call up me. Keep your fellows' counsels and your own. Good-night. Come, neighbour Verges.

Verg. Good-night. [*Exit with Dogberry.*

Sea. Well, Master Oatcake, we hear our charge. Let us go sit upon the church-bench till two, and then to bed. [*Exeunt.*

Scene II.—*A Prison.*

Characters—DOGBERRY, VERGES, SEXTON, SEACOAL, OATCAKE, CONRADE, *and* BORACHIO.

Dog. Is our whole dissembly appeared?

Sex. [*Very old, at table with writing materials*] Which be the malefactors?

Dog. Marry, that am I and my partner, Master Verges!

Verg. Nay, that's certain; we have the exhibition to examine.

Sex. But which are the offenders that are to be examined? let them come before master constable!

Dog. Yea, marry, let them come before me.

Enter SEACOAL *and* OATCAKE, *with* CONRADE *and* BORACHIO.

Dog. What is your name, friend?

Bora. Borachio.

Dog. Write down,—Borachio.—Yours, sirrah?

Conrade. I am a gentleman, sir, and my name is Conrade.

Dog. Write down,—master gentleman Conrade.—Masters, do you serve God?

Bora. and Con. Yea, sir, we hope.

Dog. Write down, that they hope they serve God.—Masters, it is proved already that you are little better than false knaves; and it will go near to be thought so shortly. How answer you for yourselves?

Con. Marry, sir, we say we are none.

Dog. H'm! a marvellous witty fellow, I assure you; but I

will go about with him.—Come you hither, sir [*to Bora.*]; a word in your ear: sir, I say to you, it is thought you are false knaves.

Bora. Sir, I say to you we are none.

Dog. H'm! well, stand aside!—Ah, have you writ down, that they are none?

Sex. Master constable, you go not the way to examine: you must call forth the watch that are their accusers.

Dog. Yea, marry, that's the eftest way.—Masters Seacoal and Oatcake, I charge you, in the prince's name, accuse these men.

Sea. [*Points to Bora.*] This man said, sir, that Don John, the prince's brother, was a villain.

Dog. Write down,—Prince John a villain.—Why, this is flat perjury, to call a prince's brother villain!

Bora. Master constable,—

Dog. Prithee, fellow, peace: I do not like thy look, I promise thee.

Sex. What heard you him say else?

Oat. Marry, that he had received a thousand ducats of Don John for accusing the Lady Hero wrongfully.

Dog. Flat burglary as ever was committed!

Sex. What else?

Sea. And that Count Claudio did mean to disgrace the Lady Hero before the whole assembly, and not marry her.

Dog. O villain! thou shalt be condemned into everlasting redemption for this.

Sex. What else?

Sea. and Oat. This is all.

Sex. And this [*Points with quill to book*] is more, masters, than you can deny. Prince John is this morning stolen away; the Lady Hero was in this manner accused, and upon the grief of this suddenly died.—Master constable [*To Dog.*], let these men be bound, and brought to Signior Leonâto's: I will go before and show him their examination.   [*Exit Sexton.*

Dog. Come, let them be opinioned.

Con. Off, coxcomb!

Dog. Where's the sexton? let him write down the prince's officer coxcomb.—Thou naughty varlet!

Con. Away! you are an ass!

Dog. Dost thou not suspect my place? dost thou not suspect my years?

Con. You are an ass!

Dog. Oh, that he were here to write me down an ass!—But, masters, remember that I am an ass; though it be not written down, yet forget not that I am an ass.—O thou villain, thou art full of piety. I am a wise fellow; and, which is more, a householder; and, which is more, one that knows the law, go to; and, which is more, a rich fellow; and one that hath two gowns, and everything handsome about him.—Bring him away.—Oh, that I had been writ down an ass!

[*Exeunt omnes.*
SHAKESPEARE.

SCENES FROM "LOVE'S LABOUR'S LOST."

CHARACTERS.

KING OF NAVARRE; BIRON, LONGAVILLE, DUMAIN (*Lords attending on the King*); COSTARD (*a Clown*); JAQUENETTA (*a Country Wench*).

Scene I.—A Park.

Discovered, KING, BIRON, LONGAVILLE, *and* DUMAIN.

King. Let fame, that all hunt after in their lives,
Live registered upon our brazen tombs,
And make us heirs of all eternity.
Therefore, brave conquerors,—for so you are,
That war against your own affections,
And the huge army of the world's desires,—
Our late edict shall strongly stand in force:
Navarre shall be the wonder of the world;
Our court shall be a little Academe,

Still and contemplative in living art.
You three, Biron, Dumain, and Longaville,
Have sworn for three years' term to live with me,
My fellow-scholars, and to keep those statutes
That are recorded in this schedule here;
Your oaths are passed, and now subscribe your names,
That his own hand may strike his honour down
That violates the smallest branch herein:
If you are armed to do, as sworn to do,
Subscribe to your deep oath, and keep it too.

   Long. I am resolved; 'tis but a three years' fast:
The mind shall banquet, though the body pine:
Fat paunches have lean pates, and dainty bits
Make rich the ribs, but bankrupt quite the wits.

   Dum. My loving lord, Dumain is mortified:
To love, to wealth, to pomp, I pine and die;
With all these living in philosophy.

   Biron. I can but say their protestation over;
So much, dear liege, I have already sworn,
That is, to live and study here three years.
But there are other strict observances;
As, not to see a woman in that term,
Which, I hope well, is not enrollèd there;
And one day in a week to touch no food,
And but one meal on every day beside,—
The which I hope is not enrollèd there;
And then, to sleep but three hours in the night,
And not be seen to wink of all the day,—
Which I hope well is not enrollèd there:
Oh, these are barren tasks, too hard to keep;
Not to see ladies, study, fast, not sleep!

   King. Your oath is passed to pass away from these.

   Biron. Let me say no, my liege, an if you please:
I only swore to study with your grace,
And stay here in your court for three years' space.

Long. You swore to that, Biron, and to the rest.
Biron. By yea and nay, sir, then I swore in jest.
What is the end of study? let me know.
King. Why, that to know, which else we should not know.
Biron. Things hid and barred, you mean, from common sense?
King. Ay, that is study's god-like recompense.
Biron. Come on, then; I will swear to study so,
To know the thing I am forbid to know.
If study's gain be thus, and this be so,
Swear me to this, and I will ne'er say no.
King. Biron is like an envious nipping frost
That bites the first-born infants of the spring.
Biron. Well, say I am; why should proud summer boast,
Before the birds have any cause to sing?
At Christmas I no more desire a rose
Than wish a snow in May's new-fangled shows:
But like of each thing that in season grows.
So you, to study now it is too late,
Climb o'er the house to unlock the little gate.
King. Well, sit you out: go home, Biron: adieu!
Biron. No, my good lord; I have sworn to stay with you,
And confident I'll keep to what I swore.
Give me the paper; let me read the same;
And to the strict'st decrees I'll write my name.
King. How well this yielding rescues you from shame!
Biron. [*Reads*] "Item, That no woman shall come within a mile of my court:"—Hath this been proclaimed?
King. [*Nods*] Four days ago.
Biron. Let's see the penalty. [*Reads*] "On pain of losing her tongue."—Who devised this penalty?
Long. Marry, that did I.

Biron. Sweet lord, and why?
Long. To fright them hence with that dread penalty.
Biron. A dangerous law against gentility!
[*Reads*] "If any man be seen to talk with a woman within the term of three years, he shall endure such public shame as the rest of the court can possibly devise."—
This article, my liege, yourself must break;
For well you know here comes in embassy
The French king's daughter with yourself to speak,—
A maid of grace and complete majesty,—
Therefore this article is made in vain,
Or vainly comes the admired princess hither.
King. What say you, lords? why, this was quite forgot.
We must of force dispense with this decree;
She must stay here on mere necessity.
Biron. Necessity will make us all forsworn
Three thousand times within this three years' space;
If I break faith, this word shall speak for me,
I am forsworn "on mere necessity."—
So to the laws at large I write my name:
And he that breaks them in the least degree,
Stands in attainder of eternal shame:
But I believe, although I seem so loth,
I am the last that will last keep his oath.
[*Subscribes.*
King. Now go we, lords, to put in practice that
Which each to other hath so strongly sworn.
Biron. I'll lay my head to any good man's hat,
These oaths and laws will prove an idle scorn.
[*Exeunt or Curtain.*

Scene II.—*A Forest.*
Enter BIRON, *with a paper.*
Biron. The king he is hunting the deer; I am coursing myself: they have pitched a toil; I am toiling in a pitch,—pitch

that defiles: defile? a foul word. Well, set thee down sorrow! for so, they say, the fool said, and so say I, and I the fool. Well proved, wit! By the Lord, this love is as mad as Ajax: it kills sheep; it kills me, I a sheep. Well proved again on my side! I will not love: if I do, hang me: i'faith, I will not. Oh, but her eye,—by this light, but for her eye, I would not love her; yes, for her two eyes. Well, I do nothing but lie, and lie in my throat. By heaven, I *do* love: and it hath taught me to rhyme, and to be melancholy; and here is part of my rhyme, and here my melancholy. Well, she hath one o' my sonnets already; the clown bore it, the fool sent it, and the lady hath it: sweet clown, sweeter fool, [*Sighs*] sweetest lady! By the world, I would not care a pin if the other three were in. Here comes one with a paper: Heaven give him grace to groan!
[*Retires.*

Enter KING, *with a paper.*
King. Ah me!
Biron. Shot, by Venus!—Proceed, sweet Cupid: thou hast thumped him with thy bird-bolt under the left breast. I'faith, secrets.— [*Retires.*
King [*reads*].
" So sweet a kiss the golden sun gives not
    To those fresh morning drops upon the rose,
As thine eye-beams, when their fresh rays have smote
    The dew of night that on my cheeks down flows:
O queen of queens, how far thou dost excel
No thought can think, nor tongue of mortal tell!"
How shall she know my griefs? I'll drop the paper.
Sweet leaves, shade folly!—Who is he comes here? [*Retires*
What, Longaville! and reading! listen, ear.
Biron. Now, in my likeness, one more fool appear.

Enter LONGAVILLE, *with a paper.*
Long. Ah me! I am forsworn.
King. In love, I hope: Sweet fellowship in shame!

Biron. One drunkard loves another of the name.
Long. Am I the first that have been perjured so?
Biron. I could put thee in comfort: not by two, that I know.
Long. O sweet Maria, empress of my love! [*Reads.*
  "Did not the heavenly rhetoric of thine eye
    'Gainst whom the world cannot hold argument,
  Persuade my heart to this false perjury?
  Vows for thee broke deserve not punishment.
  A woman I forswore; but I will prove,
    Thou being a goddess, I forswore not thee:
  My vow was earthly, thou a heavenly love;
    If by me broke, what fool is not so wise,
    To lose an oath to win a paradise?"
Biron. This is the liver-vein, which makes flesh a deity:
A green goose, a goddess: pure, pure idolatry.
Heaven amend us, Heaven amend! we are much out o' the way.
Long. By whom shall I send this?—Company! stay.
                                                  [*Retires.*
Biron. All hid, all hid, an old infant play.
More sacks to the mill! By Venus, I have my wish!

        Enter DUMAIN, *with a paper.*

Biron. Dumain transformed: four woodcocks in a dish!
Dum. O most divine Kate!
Biron. O most profane coxcomb!
Dum. By heaven, the wonder of a mortal eye!
Biron. By earth, she is not, corporal; there you lie.
Dum. As upright as the cedar.
Biron.   Stoops, I say.
Dum. As fair as day.
Biron. Ay, as some days; but then no sun must shine.
Dum. Oh that I had my wish!
Long.   And I had mine!
King. And I mine, too, good lord!

Biron. Amen, so I had mine!
Dum. Once more I'll read the ode that I have writ.
Biron. Once more I'll mark how love can vary wit.
Dum. [*reads*].
　　　　"On a day—alack the day!—
　　　　Love, whose month is ever May,
　　　　Spied a blossom, passing fair,
　　　　Playing in the wanton air!
　　　　But, alack, my hand is sworn
　　　　Ne'er to pluck thee from thy thorn.
　　　　Do not call it sin in me,
　　　　That I am forsworn for thee;
　　　　Thou, for whom Jove would swear
　　　　Juno but an Ethiope were."
Oh, would the king, Biron, and Longaville,
Were lovers too!
　Long. [*Advancing*] Dumain, thy love is far from charity,
That in love's grief desir'st society:
You may look pale, but I should blush, I know,
To be o'erheard, and taken napping so.
　King. [*Advancing to Longaville*] Come, sir, you blush; as
　　　his, your case is such:
You chide at him, offending twice as much;
You do not love Maria; Longaville
Did never sonnet for her sake compile;
Nor never lay his wreathèd arms athwart
His loving bosom to keep down his heart!
I have been closely shrouded in this bush,
And marked you both, and for you both did blush.
What will Biron say, when he shall hear?
How will he scorn! how will he spend his wit!
How will he triumph, leap, and laugh at it!
For all the wealth that ever I did see,
I would not have him know so much by me.
　Biron. Now step I forth to whip hypocrisy.—

Ah, good my liege, I pray thee pardon me:
Good heart, what grace hast thou, thus to reprove
These worms for loving that are most in love?
You'll not be perjured, 'tis a hateful thing:
Tush, none but minstrels dream of sonneting.
But are you not ashamed? nay, are you not,
All three of you, to be thus much o'ershot?
You [*To Longaville*] found his [*To Dumain*] mote; the king
    [*To Longaville*] your mote did see;
But I a beam do find in each of three.
Oh, what a scene of foolery have I seen,
Of sighs, of groans, of sorrow, and of teen!
Where lies thy grief, O tell me, good Dumain?
And, gentle Longaville, where lies thy pain?
And where my liege's? all about the breast.

  King. Too bitter is thy jest.
Are we betrayed thus to thy over-view?

  Biron. Not you by me, but I betrayed by you;
I, that am honest; I, that hold it sin
To break the vow I am engagèd in.
When shall you see me make a thing in rhyme?
When shall you hear that I
Will praise a hand, a foot, a face, an eye?

Enter JAQUENETTA *and* COSTARD.

  Jaq. God bless the king!
  King.   What paper hast thou there?
  Cost. Some certain treason.
  King.   What makes treason here?
  Cost. Nay, it makes nothing, sir.
  King.   If it mar nothing neither,
The treason and you go in peace away together.
  Jaq. I beseech your grace, let this letter be read:
Our parson misdoubts it; 'twas treason, he said.
  King. Biron. read it over.   [*Biron takes letter from Jaq.*

King. Where hadst thou it?
Jaq. From Costard.
[*Biron tears letter, and throws it down.*
King. How now! what is in you? why dost thou tear it?
Biron. A toy, my liege, a toy; your grace needs not fear it.
Long. It did move him to passion, and therefore let's hear it.
[*Dumain picks up paper.*
Dum. It is Biron's writing, and here is his name.
Biron. [*To Costard*] Ah, you loggerhead!
You were born to do me shame.—
Guilty, my lord, guilty; I confess, I confess.
King. What?
Biron. That you three fools lacked me fool to make up the mess;
He, he, and you, and you, my liege, and I,
Are pick-purses in love, and we deserve to die.
Will these turtles be gone?
King. Hence, sirs; away!
Cost. Walk aside the true folks, and let the traitors stay.
[*Takes Jaq.'s arm.*
Jaq. The gods give us joy! the gods give us joy!
[*Exeunt Cost. and Jaq.*
Biron. Sweet lords, sweet lovers, oh, let us embrace!
As true we are as flesh and blood can be!
The sea will ebb and flow, heaven show his face;
We cannot cross the cause why we were born;
Therefore, on all hands must we be forsworn.
It is religion to be thus forsworn,
For charity itself fulfils the law,
And who can sever love from charity? SHAKESPEARE.

SLEEP-WALKING SCENE.
[*From* "*Macbeth.*"]

Lady Macbeth. Yet here's a spot. Out, damnëd spot! out, 1 say!—One: two: why, then 'tis time to do't.—Fie, my lord, fie! a soldier, and afeard? What need we fear who knows it, when none can call our power to account?—Yet who would have thought the old man to have had so much blood in him.— What! will these hands ne'er be clean?—No more o' that, my lord, no more o' that: you mar all with this starting.—Here's the smell of blood still: all the perfumes of Arabia will not sweeten this little hand. Oh, oh, oh!—Wash your hands; look not so pale.—I tell you, Banquo's buried; he cannot come out on's grave.—There's knocking at the gate.—To bed, to bed! Give me your hand. What's done cannot be undone! To bed, to bed, to bed! SHAKESPEARE.

HAMLET'S ADVICE TO THE PLAYERS.

Speak the speech, I pray you, as I pronounced it to you, trippingly on the tongue; but if you mouth it, as many of your players do, I had as lief the town-crier spoke my lines. Nor do not saw the air too much with your hand, thus, but use all gently; for in the very torrent, tempest, and (as I may say) the whirlwind of your passion, you must acquire and beget a temperance that may give it smoothness. Oh, it offends me to the soul to hear a robustious periwig-pated fellow tear a passion to tatters, to very rags, to split the ears of the groundlings, who, for the most part, are capable of nothing but inexplicable dumb-show and noise. I would have such a fellow whipped for o'erdoing Termagant; it out-herods Herod: pray you, avoid it. Be not too tame neither, but let your own discretion be your tutor: suit the action to the word, the word to the action; with this special observance, that you o'erstep not the modesty of nature; for anything so overdone is from the purpose of playing, whose end, both at the first and now, was and is to hold, as 'twere, the mirror up to nature; to show virtue her own feature, scorn her own image, and the very age and body of the time his form and pressure. Now this overdone, or come tardy off, though it make the unskilful laugh, cannot but make the judicious grieve; the censure of the which one must, in your allowance, o'erweigh a whole theatre of others. Oh, there be players that I have seen play,—and heard others praise, and that highly, not to speak it profanely, —that, neither having the accent of Christians nor the gait of Christian, pagan, nor man, have so strutted and bellowed, that I have thought some of nature's journeymen had made men, and not made them well, they imitated humanity so abominably.

SHAKESPEARE.

POLONIUS'S ADVICE TO LAERTES.

Yet here, Laertes! aboard, aboard,—for shame! The wind sits in the shoulder of your sail, and you are stayed for. There, —my blessing with thee! And these few precepts in thy memory see thou character:—Give thy thoughts no tongue, nor any unproportioned thought his act. Be thou familiar, but by no means vulgar. The friends thou hast, and their adoption tried, grapple them to thy soul with hooks of steel; but do not dull thy palm with entertainment of each new-hatched, unfledged comrade. Beware of entrance to a quarrel; but, being in, bear it that the opposèd may beware of thee. Give every man thine ear, but few thy voice; take each man's censure, but reserve thy judgment. Costly thy habit as thy purse can buy, but not expressed in fancy; rich, not gaudy, for the apparel oft proclaims the man. Neither a borrower nor a lender be; for loan oft loses both itself and friend, and borrowing dulls the edge of husbandry. This above all—to thine own self be true; and it must follow, as the night the day, thou canst not then be false to any man. SHAKESPEARE.

HAMLET ON A FUTURE STATE.

To be, or not to be : that is the question :
Whether 'tis nobler in the mind to suffer
The slings and arrows of outrageous fortune,
Or to take arms against a sea of troubles,
And by opposing end them ! To die :—to sleep ;—
No more ; and, by a sleep, to say we end
The heart-ache and the thousand natural shocks
That flesh is heir to,—'tis a consummation
Devoutly to be wished ! To die,—to sleep ;
To sleep : perchance to dream ;—ay, there's the rub ;
For in that sleep of death what dreams may come
When we have shuffled off this mortal coil,
Must give us pause : there's the respect
That makes calamity of so long life ;
For who would bear the whips and scorns of time,
The oppressor's wrong, the proud man's contumely,
The pangs of despised love, the law's delay,
The insolence of office and the spurns
That patient merit of the unworthy takes,
When he himself might his quietus make
With a bare bodkin ? who would fardels bear,
To groan and sweat under a weary life,
But that the dread of something after death,
That undiscovered country from whose bourn
No traveller returns, puzzles the will,
And makes us rather bear those ills we have
Than fly to others that we know not of ?
Thus conscience does make cowards of us all ;
And thus the native hue of resolution
Is sicklied o'er with the pale cast of thought,
And enterprises of great pith and moment
With this regard their currents turn awry,
And lose the name of action. SHAKESPEARE.

CASSIUS INSTIGATING BRUTUS.

Well, honour is the subject of my story. I cannot tell what you and other men think of this life; but, for my single self, I had as lief not be as live to be in awe of such a thing as I myself. I was born free as Cæsar; so were you: we both have fed as well, and we can both endure the winter's cold as well as he: for once, upon a raw and gusty day, the troubled Tiber chafing with her shores, Cæsar said to me, "Darest thou, Cassius, now leap in with me into this angry flood, and swim to yonder point?" Upon the word, accoutred as I was, I plungëd in, and bade him follow; so indeed he did. The torrent roared, and we did buffet it with lusty sinews, throwing it aside and stemming it with hearts of controversy; but ere we could arrive the point proposed, Cæsar cried, "Help me, Cassius, or I sink!" I, as Æneas, our great ancestor, did from the flames of Troy upon his shoulder the old Anchises bear, so from the waves of Tiber did I the tired Cæsar. And this man is now become a god, and Cassius is a wretched creature, and must bend his body, if Cæsar carelessly but nod on him.

He had a fever when he was in Spain, and when the fit was on him, I did mark how he did shake: 'tis true,—this god did shake: his coward lips did from their colour fly, and that same eye whose bend doth awe the world did lose its lustre: I did hear him groan: ay, and that tongue of his that bade the Romans mark him, and write his speeches in their books, alas, it cried, "Give me some drink, Titinius," as a sick girl.

Ye gods, it doth amaze me a man of such a feeble temper should so get the start of the majestic world, and bear the palm alone. Why, man, he doth bestride this narrow world like a Colossus, and we petty men walk under his huge legs, and peep about to find ourselves dishonourable graves. Men at some time are masters of their fates: the fault, dear Brutus, is not in our stars, but in ourselves, that we are underlings. Brutus and Cæsar: what should be in that "Cæsar"? Why should that name be sounded more than yours? Write them together, yours is as fair a name; sound them, it doth become the mouth as well; weigh them, it is as heavy; conjure with them, Brutus will start a spirit as soon as Cæsar.

Now, in the names of all the gods at once, upon what meats doth this our Cæsar feed, that he is grown so great? Age, thou art shamed! Rome, thou hast lost the breed of noble bloods! When went there by an age, since the great flood, but it was famed with more than with one man? When could they say till now, that talked of Rome, that her wide walls encompassed but one man? Oh, you and I have heard our fathers say, there was a Brutus once that would have brooked the eternal devil to keep his state in Rome, as easily as a king!

SHAKESPEARE.

BRUTUS ON THE DEATH OF CÆSAR.

Romans, countrymen, and lovers! hear me for my cause, and be silent, that you may hear: believe me for mine honour, and have respect to mine honour, that you may believe: censure me in your wisdom, and awake your senses, that you may the better judge. If there be any in this assembly, any dear friend of Cæsar's, to him I say, that Brutus' love to Cæsar was no less than his. If then that friend demand why Brutus rose against Cæsar, this is my answer:—Not that I loved Cæsar less, but that I loved Rome more. Had you rather Cæsar were living, and die all slaves, than that Cæsar were dead, to live all free men? As Cæsar loved me, I weep for him; as he was fortunate, I rejoice at it; as he was valiant, I honour him: but, as he was ambitious, I slew him. There are tears for his love; joy for his fortune; honour for his valour; and death for his ambition. Who is here so base that would be a bondman? If any, speak; for him have I offended. Who is here so rude that would not be a Roman? If any, speak; for him have I offended. Who is here so vile that will not love his country? If any, speak; for him have I offended. I pause for a reply.

None? Then none have I offended. I have done no more to Cæsar than you shall do to Brutus. The question of his death is enrolled in the Capitol; his glory not extenuated, wherein he was worthy; nor his offences enforced, for which he suffered death.

Here comes his body, mourned by Mark Antony; who, though he had no hand in his death, shall receive the benefit of his dying, a place in the commonwealth; as which of you shall not?

With this I depart,—that, as I slew my best lover for the good of Rome, I have the same dagger for myself, when it shall please my country to need my death. SHAKESPEARE.

EXTRACTS FROM "ETERNAL HOPE."

(*By kind permission of the Author.*)

FROM SERMON I.

It is perfectly easy for a man to say, if he will, "I do not believe in God."......We can pluck the meanest flower of the hedgerow, and point to the exquisite perfection of its structure, the tender delicacy of its loveliness; we may pick up the tiniest shell upon the shore, so delicate that a touch would crush it, and yet a miracle of rose and pearl, of lustrous iridescence and fairy arabesque, and ask the atheist if he feels seriously certain that these things are but the accidental outcome of self-evolving laws. We can take him under the canopy of night, and show him the stars of heaven, and ask him whether he holds them to be nothing more than "shining illusions of the night; golden lies in dark-blue nothingness." Or we may appeal to the inner voices of his being, and ask whether *they* have no message to tell him. But if he deny or reject such arguments as these;

if he demand a kind of proof which is impossible, and which God has withheld, seeing that it is a law that spiritual things can only be spiritually discerned, and that we walk by faith and not by sight; if, in short, a man will not see God because clouds and darkness are round about Him, then we can do no more. He must believe or not believe as seems him best. We cannot argue about colour to the blind; we cannot prove the glory of music to the deaf.

That the blush of morning is fair, that the quietude of grief is sacred, that the heroism of conscience is noble, who will undertake to prove to one who does not see it? So wisdom, beauty, holiness are immeasurable things, appreciable by pure perception, but which no rule can gauge, no argument demonstrate.

Let us get near to God by faith and prayer, and we shall break with one of our fingers through the brain-spun meshes of these impotent negations. And when we believe in Him whom we have not seen, all else follows. We believe that He did not befool with irresistible longings, that He did not deceive with imaginary hopes, the man whom He had made. We believe that the breath of life which came from Him shall not pass away. We believe that He sent His Son to die for us and to save us. We believe that because He lives we shall live also. We believe; we are content.

In this belief, which we believe that He inspireth, we shall console ourselves amid all the emptiness and sorrow of life; we shall advance, calm and happy, to the very grave and gate of death.
Archdeacon Farrar.

From Sermon II.

Life is not all darkness: it has its crimson dawns, its rosy sunsets. It is not all clouds: it has its silvery embroideries, its radiant glimpses of heaven's blue. It is not all winter: it has its summer days, on which "it is a luxury to breathe the breath of life."

EXTRACTS FROM "ETERNAL HOPE."

'Life has its May, and all is joyous then;
The woods are vocal, and the winds breathe music,
The very breeze has mirth in it."

Ask the happy little child, with its round cheeks, and bright eyes, and flaxen curls, and pure, sweet face; ask the happy boy, tingling with life to the finger-tips, making the fields ring with his glad voice on summer holidays, when "the boy's will is the wind's will, and the thoughts of youth are long;" ask soldiers in the hour of victory; ask great thinkers when some immortal truth bursts upon them; ask the happy band who gather in the yet unbroken circle round the Christmas hearth—at such times, perhaps, all these will be inclined to tell you life *is* worth living......

But when, swiftly, imperceptibly, boyhood and youth are over, and manhood with all its cares is upon us, and we step forth into the thorny wilderness; when the splendid vision fades into the light of common day; when the brilliant ideals, and innocent enthusiasms of early years have been smirched, and vulgarized, and dimmed; when not one single ray of illusion or of enchantment rests, were it but for one instant, over the bleak hills and barren wilderness of life;—worn men and weary women—ye who must work, and ye who must weep—how is it with us then?

Is there one of us who has not known the throbbing head, the aching nerve, the sleepless night? Is there no household whose graves have been scattered far and wide? No father who has seen the dust sprinkled over the golden head of his dear little child? No mother whose heart has not ceased to ache since death plucked her "wee white rose"? No lonely man whose circle has ever narrowed and narrowed, and whose path in life has been marked by the gravestones of his early friends?

"Alas for man, if this were all,
And naught beyond, O earth!"......

If you ask me whether life without God in the world, and

no hope beyond, is worth living, I answer, No! Nor is it I only who say it, but all the best, and greatest, and wisest of mankind......

I am well aware that they who would rob us of all our hopes; who would change our God into a struggle of careless forces or a complexity of impersonal laws; who would turn all creation for us into a mask with no living face behind it, or a hollow eye-socket in which no eye of love or mercy ever shone,—I know that they tell us that all this makes no difference, and offer us for God I know not what goddess of humanity, and I know not what "posthumous activity" for a life beyond the grave. We do not need these sham gods and mock eternities; and as for the world, if religion fail to save it from wickedness, God only knows what atheism will do.

But when it is touched by one ray out of God's eternity, how does this blank materialism—this grotto of icicles in the Valley of the Shadow of Death—melt into mud and nothingness! How does this glaring metal colossus, with its golden head of intellectualism, tumble into impotency when the rock of faith smites it on its feet of miry clay!

But let but one whisper of God's voice thrill the deafened sense; let but one gleam of God's countenance flash on the blinded eyes; let His hand hold forth to us but one green leaf from the tree of life, and how is all changed!

Is life worth living, then? Ay, indeed, life is infinitely worth living, and death is infinitely worth dying; for to live is Christ, and to die is gain—to live is to have faith in God, and to die is to be with Him for evermore. ARCHDEACON FARRAR.

THE LONELINESS OF CHRIST.

(*By kind permission of* Messrs. KEGAN PAUL, TRENCH, AND Co.)

There are two kinds of solitude—the one, insulation in space; the other, isolation of the spirit. The first is simply separation by distance. When we are seen, touched, heard by none, we are said to be alone. But this is not solitude; for sympathy can people our solitude with a crowd. The fisherman on the ocean alone at night is not alone when he remembers the earnest longings which are rising up to Heaven at home for his safety. The traveller is not alone when the faces that will greet him on his arrival seem to beam upon him as he trudges on. The solitary student is not alone when he feels that human hearts will respond to the truths he is preparing to address to them.

The other is loneliness of soul. There are times when hands touch ours, but only send an icy chill of unsympathizing indifference to the heart; when eyes gaze into ours, but with a glazed look which cannot read into the depths of our souls; when words pass from our lips, but only come back as an echo reverberated without reply through a dreary solitude; when the multitude throng and press us, and we cannot say, as Christ said, "Somebody hath *touched me*," for the contact has been, not between soul and soul, but only between form and form......

To the superficial observer, Christ's life was a mass of inconsistencies and contradictions. The Pharisees could not comprehend how a holy teacher could eat with publicans and sinners. His own brethren could not reconcile His assumption of a public office with the privacy which he aimed at keeping. And hence it was that He lived to see all that acceptance which had marked the earlier stage of His career melt away. First the Pharisees took the alarm, then the Sadducees, then the people. *That* was the most terrible of all, for the enmity of the upper classes is impotent; but when the cry of brute force is stirred from the deeps of society, as deaf to the voice of reason as the ocean in its strength churned into raving foam by the winds, the heart of mere earthly oak quails before that— the apostles, at all events, did quail. One denied; another betrayed; all deserted. They "were scattered, each to his own," and the Truth Himself was left alone in Pilate's judgment hall......

There is a moment in every true life—to some it comes very early—when the old routine of duty is not large enough ; when the parental roof seems too low, because the Infinite above is arching over the soul ; when the old formulas seem to be too narrow, and they must either be thrown aside or else transformed into living, breathing realities. That is a lonely, lonely moment when the young soul first feels God ; when this earth is recognized as an "awful place, yea, the very gate of heaven;" when the dream-ladder is seen planted against the skies, and we wake, and the dream haunts us as a sublime reality......

The Redeemer's soul was alone in dying. The hour had come. They were all gone, and He was, as He predicted, left alone. All that is human drops from us in that hour. Human faces flit and fade, and the sounds of the world become confused. "I shall die alone." There is a feeble and sentimental way in which we speak of the Man of sorrows. We turn to the cross, the agony, the loneliness, to touch the softer feelings, to arouse compassion. You degrade that loneliness by your compassion. Compassion! compassion for Him! Respect, reverence, adore if you will, but no pity. In that single human bosom dwelt the thought which was to be the germ of the world's life. Can you not feel the grandeur of those words when the Man, reposing on His solitary strength, felt the last shadow of perfect isolation pass across His soul : "My God, my God, why hast thou forsaken me?"

Even in human things, the strength that is in a man can be only learned when he is thrown upon his own resources and left alone. What a man can do in conjunction with others does not test the man. Tell us what he can do *alone*. It is one thing to defend the truth when you know that your hearers are already prepossessed, and that every argument will meet a willing response ; it is another thing to hold the truth, when truth must be supported, if at all, alone—met by cold looks and unsympathizing suspicion. It is one thing to rush on to danger with the shouts and the sympathy of numbers ; it is another thing when the lonely captain of the sinking ship sees the last boatful disengage itself, and folds his arms to go down into the majesty of darkness, crushed but not subdued.

This is self-reliance : to repose calmly on the thought which is deepest in our bosoms, and be unmoved if the world will not accept it. To live on your own convictions against the world is to overcome the world—*that* is independence. It is not difficult to get away into retirement, and there live upon your own convictions ; it is not difficult to mix with men and follow their convictions ; but to enter into the world, and there live out firmly and fearlessly according to your own conscience—*that* is Christian greatness.

There is a cowardice in this age which is not Christian. We shrink from the consequences of truth. We ask what men will think, what others will say—whether they will not stare in astonishment. Perhaps they will ; but he who is calculating that will accomplish nothing in this life. The Father—the Father who is with us and in us—what does *He* think ? A man is got some way in the Christian life when he has learned to say humbly and yet majestically, " I dare to be alone."

F. W. ROBERTSON.

ADDITIONAL STUDIES.

THIRD SERIES.

DEATH OF GENERAL WAUCHOPE.

On that fatal Monday, December 12, our brave Highlanders reeled before the shock. General Wauchope was down, riddled with bullets. Yet, though dying, bleeding from every vein, the Highland chieftain raised himself on his hands and knees and cheered his men forward.

The Black Watch charged, and the Gordons and Seaforths, with a yell that stirred the camp below, rushed onward to death or disaster.

The accursèd barbed wires caught them round the legs, until they floundered like trapped wolves; and all the time the bullets of the foe sang the song of death in their ears. Then they fell back, broken and beaten, leaving nearly thirteen hundred dead and wounded.

An hour afterwards morning dawned on the dreariest day Scotland has known for a generation past. Of her officers— the flower of her chivalry—but few remained to tell the tale. A sad tale indeed! but a tale unstained by dishonour or smirched with disgrace; for up those heights a brigade of devils could scarce hope to pass! All that mortal men could do, the Scots did. They fought—they failed—they fell.

* * * * * *

Three hundred yards to the rear of Modder River, as the sun was sinking in a blaze of African splendour, on the evening of Tuesday, December 13, a long, shallow grave lay exposed in the breast of the veldt.

DEATH OF GENERAL WAUCHOPE. 521

A few paces from that grave fifty dead Highlanders lay. "They had followed their chief to the field;" they were now to follow him to the grave. How grim and stern those dead men looked as they lay face upward to the sky, with great hands clenched in the last death-agony. His plaid—dear to every Highlander—was wrapped round each man. And as I looked, awe-struck, out of the distance came the sound of the pipes. It was the dead general coming to join his men.

There, right under the eyes of the enemy, moved with slow and solemn tread all that remained of the Highland Brigade. In front of them walked the chaplain; then came the pipers, sixteen in all. Behind them, with arms reversed, marched the Highlanders in all the regalia of their regiments; and in the midst the dead general, borne by four of his comrades. Out swelled the pipes to the strains of "The Flowers of the Forest," now ringing proud and high, until each soldier's head went back in haughty defiance, and eyes flashed through tears like sunlight on steel; now sinking to a moaning wail, like a mother mourning for her first-born, until the proud heads drooped, resting on heaving breasts, and choking sobs broke through the solemn rhythm of the march of death. Right up to the grave they marched, then broke away in companies, until the general was laid in his grave, with a square of Scottish armed men around him.

Then once again the pipes pealed out, and "Lochaber no More" cut through the stillness like a cry of pain. One could almost hear the widow, in her Highland home, moaning for the soldier she would welcome back no more.

Then, as if touched by the magic of one thought, every man turned his tear-stained eyes from that still form up to the heights where Cronje and his soldiers stood. Then, every cheek flushed crimson, the strong jaws set like steel, and that look from those silent armed men spoke more eloquently than ever spoke the tongues of orators.

At the head of the grave the general was laid to sleep. His

officers were laid around him. Behind him, his brave soldiers were laid in a double line, each wrapped in his Highland plaid. No shots were fired over the dead men, resting there so peacefully. Only a royal salute was given, and then the men marched campwards as the darkness rolled over the far-stretching breadth of the veldt.

From a War Correspondent's Letter, January 1900.

JAMIE DOUGLAS.

'Twas in the days when Claverhouse was scouring moor and glen,
To shake with fire and bloody sword the faith of Scottish men;
They had made a covenant with the Lord, firm in their faith to bide,
Nor break with Him their plighted troth, whatever might betide.

The sun was nearly setting, when o'er the heather wild,
And up a narrow mountain-path, alone there walked a child.
He was a bonnie, blithesome lad, lithe, and strong of limb;
A father's pride, a mother's love, were fast bound up in him.

His bright blue eyes glanced fearless round, his step was firm and light;
What was it underneath his plaid his little hands grasped tight?
'Twas the bannocks which that morn his mother made with care
From out her scanty store of meal, and now, with many a prayer,
Had sent by Jamie, her ain boy, a trusty lad and brave,
To good old Pastor Tammas Roy, now hiding in yon cave;

For whom the bloody Claverhouse had hunted long in vain,
And swore he would not leave that glen till old Tam Roy
was slain.

So Jamie Douglas went his way, with heart that knew no
fear,
He turned a great curve in the rock, nor dreamed that
death was near;
But lurking there were Claver's men, who laughed aloud
with glee.
He turns to flee, but all in vain; they drag him back a pace,
To where their cruel leader stands, and set them face to face.

The cakes concealed beneath his plaid soon tell the story
plain.
" 'Tis old Tam Roy the cakes are for," exclaims the angry
man.
" Boy, guide me to his hiding-place, and I will let you go."
But Jamie shook his yellow curls, and stoutly answered,
" No."

" I'll drop you down the mountain-side, and there among the
stones
The old gaunt wolf and carrion crow shall battle for your
bones."
And in his brawny, strong right hand he lifted up the child,
And held him o'er the clefted rock, a chasm deep and wild.

So deep it was, the trees below like willow wands did seem;
The poor boy looked in frightened maze—it seemed some
horrid dream.
He looked up to the sky above, then at the men near by;
Had they no little ones at home, and could they let him die?

But no one spoke, and no one moved, or lifted hand to save
From such a fearful, awful death the little lad so brave.

"It's waefu' deep," he shuddering cried; but no, I canna
   tell:
Sae drap me doon—then, if you will, it's no sae deep as hell."

A childish scream, a faint dull sound. Oh, Jamie Douglas
   true!
Long, long within that lonely cave shall Tam Roy wait
   for you;
And long for your welcome coming waits the mother on the
   moor,
And watches and calls, "Come, Jamie lad," through the
   half-open door.

No more adown the rocky path you come with fearless tread,
Or on the moor and mountain take the good man's daily
   bread.
But up in heaven the shining ones a wondrous story tell,
Of a child snatched up from a rocky gulf, that's no sae deep
   as hell.

And there before the great white throne, for ever blest and
   glad,
His mother dear and old Tam Roy shall meet their bonnie
   lad. *Scotch Ballad.*

ME AND HIM.

[DIALECT READING.]

I wuz out in the medder pickin' danderli'ne roots,
When I heerd the chumpin' o' Jim's big boots.
Ma heart mos' stopped beatin', but I tossed ma bunnet
   brim—
We wuz thar by ourselves, jes' me an' him.
Sez I, "How do, Jim? How's yer par an' mar?"
He didn't do nothin' 'cep' grin an' run his fingers
   through his har;

Then he comes up close, an' I says, "Jim!"
An' blushed, though thar wuz jes' me an' him.
Terreckly he put his arm roun' my waist—sassy like—
Turn't me roun' till we faced. Then he kissed me,
    did Jim;
But nobuddy wuz thar—jes' me an' him.

ANON.

THE MINUET.

Grandma told me all about it—
Told me so I couldn't doubt it—
How she danced—my grandmamma—long ago;

How she held her pretty head,
How her dainty skirts she spread,
As she danced the minuet, long ago.

Grandma's hair was bright and shining;
Dimpled cheeks, too—oh, *so* funny!
Bless me! *now* she wears a cap—
My grandma does—and takes a nap
Every single day; yet she danced the minuet, long ago.

Now she sits there, rocking, rocking,
Always knitting grandpa's stocking.
All the girls were taught to *knit*, long ago.

But her figure is so neat,
And her ways so staid and sweet,
I can almost see her now
Bending to her partner's bow,
As she danced the minuet, long ago.

Grandma says, "Our modern jumping,
Rushing, dashing, whirling, bumping,
Would have *shocked* the *gentle* people, long ago.

"Ah, they moved with *stately* grace—
Everything in *proper* place;
Gliding gently forward, slowly curtsying back again,
As they danced the minuet, long ago.

"*Modern* ways are quite alarming,"
Grandma says; but boys were *charming*—
Girls and boys I mean, of course—long ago.

Sweetly modest, bravely shy,
What if each of us should try
To feel like those who met
In the stately minuet, long ago?

With the minuet in fashion,
Who could fly into a passion?
All would wear the calm *it* wore, long ago.

And if in years to come, perchance,
I should tell *my* grandchild of our dance,
I should really like to say
We did it in some *such* way, long ago.

ANON.

A FEAST OF ALL NATIONS.

A feast, I have read,
There was recently spread,
Where this novel arrangement existed:
Each fortunate guest,
When his choice he expressed,
To his favourite dish was assisted.

Said Mickey M'Guire,
As he sat by the fire,

A FEAST OF ALL NATIONS.

Faith, thin, but it's warmin' the heat is;
  An', sure, for a party
  Of appitite hearty,
There's nothing quite aqual to praties."

"Ach! donner and blitz!"
  Cried fat little Fritz,
Regarding his neighbour so bony,
  "Dot poy vas so droll.
  I vould gif der whole bowl
For vun leetle bite of *bologna.*"

The fair Yum Yan
  Waved her beautiful fan
As she smiles his enjoyment to see.
  She would taste of no dish
  Save an *entrée* of fish,
But she never once stopped drinking tea.

"Me velly hunglee,"
  Said the guileless Chung See,
With an evident yearning for rice.
  He smiled and he sighed,
  And his chopsticks applied,
And was ready for more in a trice.

"*Carissima mia!*"
  Said little Maria,
"Der is nosing so lofely as dese."
  And she fondly surveyed,
  On the table displayed,
Her beloved macaroni and cheese.

"Non, non!" said Helene,
  With a shrug of disdain,

"I vish but un morsel petite.
　　Nosing hot, *s'il vous plaît*,
　　But some vater *sucré*,
And von bon-bon *je vous remercie.*"

Quoth brave John Bull,
　　With his mouth rather full,
And his waist with a napkin begirt,
　　"Of dainties the chief
　　Is our noble roast beef,
With plum-pudding, of course, for dessert."

Mustapha the bland,
　　With a wave of his hand,
Declined to partake of the feast
　　Till the coffee was served,
　　When he visibly swerved,
And drank twenty cups at the least.

"Jest hab your own way,"
　　Said George Washington Clay,
'And go 'long with those fibs you's a-tellin'.
　　Der's nothin' like dis,"
　　And chuckling with bliss,
He extinguished himself in a melon.

"Wal, mebbe you're right,"
　　Said young Jonathan Bright,
With a wink of his merry young eye;
　　"But for all yer so knowin',
　　The dish ain't a-goin'
That can come up, I reckon, to pie."

"Aweel an' aweel,"
　　Said Jimmy M'Neil,

"O' maggots and freaks there's a mony;
  But there's naething I know
  Like the parritch I lo'e,
To mak' a braw lad and a bonny."

IF I COULD KEEP HER SO.

Just a little baby, lying in my arms:
Would that I could keep you with your baby charms—
Helpless, clinging fingers, downy golden hair,
Where the sunshine lingers, caught from otherwhere;
Blue eyes asking questions, lips that cannot speak,
Roly-poly shoulders, dimple in your cheek.
Dainty little blossom in a world of woe!
Thus I fain would keep you, for I love you so.

Roguish little maiden, scarcely six years old,
Feet that never weary, hair of deeper gold;
Restless, busy fingers, all the time at play;
Tongue that never ceases talking all the day;
Blue eyes learning wonders of the world about.
Here you come to tell them: what an eager shout!
Winsome little damsel, all the neighbours know;
Thus I long to keep you, for I love you so.

Sober little school-girl, with your bag of books,
And such grave importance in your puzzled looks;
Solving weary problems, poring over sums,
Yet with mouth for sponge-cake and tooth for sugar-plums.
Reading books of fiction in your bed at night,
Waking up to study with the morning light;
Anxious as to ribbons, deft to tie a bow;
Full of contradictions—I would keep you so.

Sweet and thoughtful maiden, sitting by my side,
All the world's before you, and the world is wide.
Hearts are there for winning, hearts are there to break;
Has your own, shy maiden, just begun to wake?
Is that rose of dawning, glowing on your cheek,
Telling us in blushes what you will not speak?
Shy and tender maiden, I would fain forego
All my golden fortune just to keep you so.

Ah! the listening angels saw that she was fair,
Ripe for rare unfolding in the upper air.
Now the rose of dawning turns to lily white,
And the close-shut eyelids veil the eyes from sight.
All the past I summon as I kiss her brow;
Babe, and child, and maiden—all are with me now.
Though my heart is breaking, yet God's love I know—
Safe among the angels, I would keep her so.

ANON.

THE STORY OF A FAITHFUL SOUL.

The fettered spirits linger in purgatorial pain,
With penal fires effacing their last faint earthly stain
Which life's imperfect sorrow had tried to cleanse in vain.
Yet on each "Feast of Mary" their sorrow finds release,
For the great archangel Michael comes down and bids it cease,
And the name of these brief respites is called "Our Lady's Peace."

Yet once, so runs the legend, when the archangel came,
And all these holy spirits rejoiced at Mary's name,
One voice alone was wailing, still wailing on the same;
And though a great "Te Deum" the happy echoes woke,
This one discordant wailing through the sweet voices broke.
So when St. Michael questioned, thus the poor spirit spoke:

"I am not cold or thankless, although I still complain;
I prize 'Our Lady's' blessing—although it comes in vain
To still my bitter anguish, or quench my ceaseless pain.
On earth a heart that loves me still lives and mourns me there,
And the shadow of his anguish is more than I can bear;
All the torment that I suffer is the thought of his despair.
The evening of my bridal death took my life away,
Not all love's passionate pleading could gain an hour's delay,
And he I left has suffered a whole year from this day.
If I could only see him, if I could only go
And speak one word of comfort and of solace, then I know
He would endure with patience, and strive against his woe."

Then the archangel answered, "Your time of pain is brief,
And soon the peace of heaven will give you full relief;
Yet if this earthly comfort so much outweighs your grief,
Then, through a special mercy, I offer you this grace:
You may seek him who mourns you, and look upon his face,
And speak to him of comfort for one short minute's space;
But when that time is ended, return here and remain
A thousand years in torments, a thousand years in pain—
Thus dearly must you purchase the comfort he will gain."

The lime trees' shade at evening is spreading broad and wide,
Beneath their fragrant arches pace slowly side by side,
In low and tender converse, a bridegroom and his bride.
      The night is calm and stilly,
No other sound is there, except their happy voices—
      What is that cold, bleak air
That quivers through the lime trees, and stirs the bridegroom's hair?
One low, lone cry of anguish, like the last dying wail
Of some dumb, hunted creature, is borne upon the gale!
Why does the bridegroom shudder, and turn so deathly pale?

Near purgatory's entrance the radiant angels wait,
It was the great St. Michael who closed that gloomy gate
When the poor, wandering spirit came back to meet her fate.
"Pass on!" thus spoke the angel; "heaven's joy is deep and vast.
Pass on, pass on, poor spirit, for heaven is yours at last!
In that one minute's anguish your thousand years have passed!"
         ADELAIDE PROCTER.

THE DOG AND THE TRAMP.

A tramp went up to a cottage door,
To beg for a couple of pence or more;
The cottage door was open wide,
So he took a cautious look inside.
Then over his features there spread a grin,
As he saw a lovely maid within—
A lonely maid within the gloom
Of the shadiest part of a roomy room.
Into the room the tramper went;
Over a dog the maiden bent,
His eyes were red and full of fire,
And he viewed the tramp with ardent ire.
"Run for your life!" the maiden cried;
"I have forgotten to have him tied!
Run for your life through yonder door;
I cannot hold him a minute more!"
Without a word he turned his face,
And leaped the fence with careless grace;
Then lightly along the road he ran,
A very much-put-out young man.
The maiden loosed her bulldog's neck,
And gazed at the tramp—a vanishing speck;
And peal after peal of laughter rent
The air with the maiden's merriment.

The dog was of terra-cotta ware;
She had won him that week at a "fancy fair."

EVA BEST.

ABOU BEN ADHEM AND THE ANGEL.

Abou Ben Adhem—may his tribe increase!—
Awoke one night from a deep dream of peace,
And saw, within the moonlight in his room,
Making it rich, and like a lily in bloom,
An angel writing in a book of gold.
Exceeding peace had made Ben Adhem bold,
And to the presence in the room he said,
"What writest thou?" The vision raised its head,
And, with a look made of all sweet accord,
Answered, "The names of those who love the Lord.
"And is mine one?" said Abou. "Nay, not so,"
Replied the angel. Abou spoke more low,
But cheerily still, and said, "I pray thee, then,
Write me as one that loves his fellow-men."
The angel wrote, and vanished. The next night
It came again with a great wakening light,
And showed the names whom love of God had blest,
And, lo, Ben Adhem's name led all the rest!

LEIGH HUNT.

DAINTY LITTLE LADY.

A DIALOGUE FOR CHILDREN.

"Dainty little lady, listen, pray, to me,
  Canst thou ever love me? canst thou? say to me."

"Ere I tell you that, sir, you must prove to me
  That my heart with you, sir, safely kept will be."

"Prudent little lady, thou hast stolen mine;
  Surely, while thou hast it, I must value thine."

"That is proof enough, sir. Further would I know
  What about me 'tis, sir, makes you love me so?"

"Simple little lady, hast thou not been told
  That thy silken tresses shine like burnished gold?"

"Answer that is none, sir. I need scarcely say,
  Even golden hair, sir, quickly turns to gray."

"Modest little lady, clearest summer skies—
  Blue, and calm, and cloudless—pale beside thine eyes."

"Ah! but you must own, sir, though that may be true,
  Age will never spare, sir, eyes of deepest blue."

"Cruel little lady, shall I praise thy lips,
  Or thy fairy fingers, with their rosy tips?"

"There will come a day, sir, when these hands shall lie
  Quiet, and these lips, sir, never frame reply."

"Then, my little lady, I can only say
  That it was thy goodness stole my heart away."

"Goodness, not my own, sir, given each day anew;
  Lov'st thou me for that, sir?—then I love thee too."

CAN I GO HOME?

Madge went to church one sultry day;
She kept awake, I'm glad to say,
Till "Fourthly" started on its way,
Then moments into long hours grew.
 "I'se tired an' sleepy; what will I do?"
Unseen she glided from the pew,

And up the aisle demurely went,
On some absorbing mission bent,
Her eyes filled with look intent;
She stopped, and said in plaintive tone,
"Please, preacher man, can I go home?"
The clear young voice, bell-like in sound,
Disturbed a sermon most profound,
And caused a titter all around.
A smile the pastor's face o'erspread,
He paused, and bent his stately head;
"Yes, little dear," he gently said.

BABY IN CHURCH.

Aunt Nelly has fashioned a beautiful thing
Of swan's-down, and ribbon, and lace;
And mamma said, as she settled it round
Our beautiful baby's face,
Where the dimples play, and the laughter lies
Like sunbeams hid in her violet eyes,—
"If the day is pleasant, and baby is good,
She may go to church and wear her new hood."

Then Ben, agèd six, began to say, in elder-brotherly way,
How very, very good baby must be
If she went to church next day.
He spoke of the church, and the choir, and the crowd,
And the man in the pulpit who spoke so loud;
But she mustn't talk, nor laugh, nor sing,
But just sit as quiet as anything.

And so, on a beautiful Sabbath in May,
When the fruit-buds had burst into flowers—
There wasn't a blossom on bush or on tree
So fair as this blossom of ours—

BABY IN CHURCH.

All in her white dress, dainty and new,
Our baby sat in the family pew.

The grand, sweet music, the reverent air,
The solemn hush, the voice of prayer,
Filled all her baby-soul with awe.
And now the grand organ pealed forth again,
The collection-bag came round,
And baby dropped her penny in,
And smiled at the chinking sound.

Alone in the choir Aunt Nelly stood,
Waiting the close of the soft prelude,
    Her solo to begin.
High and strong she struck the first note,
Clear and long she held it; and all were charmed
But one, who, with all the might she had,
Sprang to her feet and cried,—
"Aunt Nelly, you'se very, *very* bad!"

The audience smiled, the minister coughed,
The little boys in the corner laughed;
The tenor-man shook like an aspen leaf,
And hid his face in his handkerchief.
But poor Aunt Nelly never could tell
How she *finished* that terrible strain;
And says that nothing on earth would tempt her
    To go through the same again.
And so we've decided, perhaps 'tis best for *her* sake,
    Ours, and all the rest,
That we'll allow to elapse a year or two
Ere our baby re-enters the family pew

A PERFECT FAITH.

My darling kneeled down for her evening prayer,
And out from her gown peeped her little feet bare,
And a halo of light touched her golden hair,
And I thought of the dear Christ-child!
The moonbeams fell soft on my dear little girl,
And lovingly lingered on dimple and curl;
And peace mocked the presence of tumult and whirl,
And a holiness seemed to pervade!
Then the sweet words arose, "Dear God, everywhere,
Please listen to-night to a little girl's prayer.
Bless papa and mamma, and keep in Thy care
All the friends that I love and know,
And make them all happy, dear Father, I pray,
And help me to be a good girl every day.
And one thing more I'd like to say,
But it may not be right if I do—
I wish that to-morrow You would let
The blue sky with beautiful clouds covered get,
And You'd cause them to rain a little bit wet
For one who'd be glad if they would.
My papa has brought me only to-night
A gossamer cloak, and it fits me all right,
And I just want to see if it's leaky or tight
From the foot right up to the hood."
And with heart full of faith she slipped into bed,
And soon into dreamland her happy thoughts sped.
    And soon came a splash on the pane,
And all through the night and far into the day
The hot, burning earth drank its fever away.
And becloaked and behooded, I heard my little girl say,
  "I *knew* God would let the clouds rain."

THE AUCTIONEER'S GIFT.

The auctioneer leaped on a chair, and bold, and loud, and clear
He poured his cataract of words—just like an auctioneer.
A humorist of wide renown was this auctioneer;
He knocked down sideboards, beds, and stoves, and clocks, and chandeliers,
And a grand piano, which he swore would last a thousand years;
He rattled out the crockery, and sold the silver ware;
At last they passed him up to sell a little baby's chair.
"How much? how much? Come, make a bid! Is all your money spent?"
And then a would-be-clever wag called out and bid "One cent!"
Just then a sad-faced woman, who stood in silence there,
Broke down and cried, "My baby's chair! my poor dead baby's chair!"
"Here, mistress, take your baby's chair," said the kind-hearted auctioneer;
"I know its value all too well—my baby died last year.
And if the owner of the chair, our friend the mortgagee,
Objects to this proceeding, let him send the bill to me."
Gone was the tone of raillery—the lately humorous auctioneer
Turned shamefaced from his audience to brush away a tear.
The laughing crowd was awed and still, no tearless eye was there,
When the weeping woman reached and took her little baby's chair.

THE CHILD'S MIRROR.

"Where is the baby, grandmamma?"
The fair young mother calls
From her work in the cozy kitchen,
With its dainty whitewashed walls.
And grandma leaves her knitting,
And looks for her all around,
But not a trace of the baby can anywhere be found.
No sound of merry prattle, no gleam of sunny hair,
No patter of little footsteps—no sign of it anywhere!
All through the house and garden, far out into the field,
They search each nook and corner, but nothing is revealed,
And the mother's face grew pallid, grandma's eyes grew dim.
"Baby's lost! Where's Rover?"
The mother chanced to think of the old well in the orchard
Where the cattle used to drink.
"Where's Rover? I know he'd find her.—
Rover! Rover!" In vain they call.
They hurry away to the orchard,
And there, by the moss-grown wall,
Close to the well lies Rover,
Holding on to baby's dress;
She was leaning over the well's edge
In perfect fearlessness!
She was stretching her little arms down,
But Rover held her fast,
And never seemed to mind the kicks
The tiny bare feet cast
So spitefully upon him,
But joyfully wagged his tail
To greet the frightened searchers, while naughty baby said:
"Dere's a little girl in the water—
She's just as big as me—

Mamma, I want to help her out, and take her home to tea.
And bad Rover he won't let me, and I don't love him!—
Go away, you naughty Rover!—Mamma, why are you
   crying so?"
The mother kissed her, saying, "My darling, you don't
   understand :
Good Rover saved your life, my dear,
And see, he licks your hand. Kiss Rover."
Baby struck the dog—" Bad Rover."
But grandma understood. "It's hard," she said,
" To thank the friend who thwarts us for our good."

THE CHILD CHRIST.

I had fed the fire and stirred it, till the sparkles in delight
Snapped their saucy little fingers at the chill December night;
Like a fragrant incense rising, curled the smoke of my cigar,
With the lamp-light gleaming through it like a mist-enfolded
   star.
And as I gazed I marvelled, as I saw a mimic stage
Alive with little actors of a very tender age ;
And they each had little burdens, and a little tale to tell
Of fairy-lore, and giants, and delights delectable.
And they mixed and intermingled, weaving melody with joy,
Till the magic circle clustered round a blooming baby-boy.
He was a wondrous little fellow, with a dainty double chin,
And chubby cheeks and dimples for the smiles to blossom in.
And I saw the happy mother, and a group surrounding her,
That knelt with costly presents of frankincense and myrrh.
And I thrilled with awe and wonder as a murmur filled
   the air,
And came drifting on my hearing in a melody of prayer.
By the splendour in the heavens, and the hush upon the sea,
And the majesty of silence reigning over Galilee,

We feel Thy kingly presence, and we humbly bow the knee,
And lift our hearts and voices in gratefulness to Thee.
Thou hast given us a Shepherd, Thou hast given us a Guide,
And the light of heaven grew dimmer when Thou sent Him from Thy side ;
But He comes to lead Thy children where the gates will open wide,
To welcome His returning when His works are glorified.
By the splendour in the heavens, and the hush upon the sea,
And the majesty of silence reigning over Galilee,
We feel Thy kingly presence, and we humbly bow the knee,
And lift our hearts and voices in adoration unto Thee.
Then the vision slowly fading with the words of the refrain,
I saw nothing but the moonlight through the frosty window-pane,
And I heard the chimes proclaiming, like an eager sentinel,
Who brings the world good tidings, " It is Christmas ; all is well ! "

JAS. WHITCOMB RILEY.

TWO SURPRISES.

A workman plied his heavy spade, as the sun was going down ;
The German king, with a cavalcade, on his way to Berlin town,
Reined up his steed at the old man's side. " My toiling friend," said he,
" Why not cease work at eventide, when the labourer should be free ? "
" I do not slave," the old man said, " and I am always free,
Though I work from the time I leave my bed till I can hardly see."
" How much," said the king, " is thy gain in a day ? " " Eight groschen," the man replied.
" And thou canst live on this meagre pay ? " " Like a king," he said with pride.

"Two groschen for me and my wife, good friend, and two for
 a debt I owe,
   Two groschen to lend, and two to spend for those who can't
   labour, you know."
"Thy debt?" said the king. Said the toiler, "Yea, to my
 mother, with age oppressed,
   Who cared for me, toiled for me, many a day, and now
   hath need of rest."
"To whom dost lend of thy daily store?" "To my boys—for
 their schooling, you see;
   When I'm too feeble to toil any more, they will care for their
   mother and me."
"And thy *last* two groschen?" the monarch said. "My sisters
 are old and lame;
   I give them two groschen for raiment and bread, all in the
   Father's name."
Tears welled up in the good king's eyes. "Thou knowest
 me not," said he;
"As thou hast given me one surprise, here is another for
 thee :
   I am thy king, give me thy hand," and he heaped it high
   with gold—
"When more thou needest, I command that I at once be told;
   For I would bless with *rich reward* the man who can
   proudly say,
   That eight souls doth he keep and guard on eight poor
   groschen a day." R. W. M'ALPINE.

THE THREE KINGDOMS.

King Frederick William of Prussia walked in the green
 fields one day,
   When the trees and flowers were fresh with the life that
   wakes in the month of May;

THE THREE KINGDOMS.

Well pleased was he to leave a while Berlin's crowded streets,
And forget for a time his kingly cares, 'mid the blossoming hedgerows sweet.
Spring sunshine flickered across his path as he strolled through the leafy glade,
Till he came to a glen where a joyous group of village children played.
He called them all around him there, in the mossy flower-strewn dell;
And soon they came clustering about him, for they knew his kind face well.
Then smiling, he held up an orange that chanced in his hand to be:
"To which of the three kingdoms does this belong, my little folks?" said he.
There was silence awhile to the question, till a bright little fellow said,
"To the vegetable kingdom, Your Majesty." The king he nodded his head.
"Well said; quite right. The orange is *yours*, my brave little man;"
So saying, he tossed it to him. "There, catch my cowslip-ball, if you can!"
Then the good king took out a crown piece and held it up to view:
"To which of the kingdoms does this belong? Who guesses shall have it too."
"To the *mineral* kingdom, Your Highness," a little lad quick replies;
As the silver coin in the sunlight shone, so sparkled his eager eyes.
"*Well* answered, so here's your crown," and the king placed the prize in his hand,
While around him the *other* children delighted and wondering stand.

"One question more I will ask, and 'tis neither hard nor long:
Now tell me, my little friends, to which kingdom do *I* belong?"

In the group of little ones gathered there was a tiny, blue-eyed child;
Full of thoughtful grace was her childish face, like a starry primrose mild.
Wistfully gazing into his face, with an earnestness sweet to see,
Simply she answered the king, "To the kingdom of heaven, I think," said she.
King Frederick stooped down, and in his arms took the little maiden then,
And kissing her brow, he softly said, "Amen, dear child, amen!"

J. E. BENDALL.

AN ORDER FOR A PICTURE.

O good painter, tell me true—
Has your hand the cunning to draw
Shapes of things you never saw?
Ay? Well, here's an order for you.
Woods and cornfields, a little brown—
The picture must not be over-bright—
Yet all with the golden and gracious light
Of a cloud when the summer sun is down.
Woods upon woods, with fields of corn
Lying between them, some cattle grazing near,
With bright birds twittering all around—
Ah, good painter, you can't paint sound!
When you have done
With woods, and cornfields, and grazing herds,
A lady, the loveliest ever the sun
Looked down upon, you must paint for me.

AN ORDER FOR A PICTURE.

Oh! if I only could make you see
The clear blue eyes, the tender smile
That are beaming on me all the while,
I need not speak these foolish words;
Yet one word tells you all I would say. She
Was my mother. Two little urchins at her knee
You must paint, sir: one like me,
The other with a clearer brow,
And the light of his adventurous eyes
Flashing with boldest enterprise.
At twelve years old he went to sea,
God knoweth if he be living now!
He sailed in the good ship *Commodore;*
Nobody ever passed her track
To bring us news—she never came back.
It's twenty long years and more
Since that old ship went out of the bay
With my brave young brother on her deck;
I watched him till he shrunk to a speck,
And his face was toward me all the way.
Bright his hair was, a golden brown,
The time we stood at our mother's knee;
That golden head, if the ship went down,
Carried the sunshine into the sea.
Out in the fields, one summer night,
We were together—
Afraid to go home, sir: for one of us bore
A nest full of speckled and thin-shelled eggs;
The other, a bird held fast by the legs.
At last we stood at our mother's knee—
Do you think, sir, that if you try,
You can paint the look of a lie?
If you can, sir, pray have the grace
To put it only on the face
Of the urchin that is likest me.

I think it was solely mine, indeed ;
But that's no matter, paint it so—
The eyes of our mother, take good heed,
Looking not on the nestful of eggs,
Nor the fluttering bird held fast by the legs,
But straight through our faces down to our lies,
And oh! with such sad, reproachful surprise,
I felt my heart bleed where her look went, as though
A sharp blade had struck it. You, sir, know
That you on your canvas must repeat
Things that are fairest, things most sweet:
Woods and cornfields—one mulberry tree—
The mother—the lads, with their bird, at her knee.
But oh! that look of reproachful woe—
High as the heavens your name I'll shout,
If you'll paint me the picture, and leave that out.

A. M. CAREY.

HER HERO.

Ah! did you see him riding down,
And riding down, while all the town
Came out to see, came out to see,
And all the bells rang mad with glee?

Ah! did you hear those bells ring out,
The bells ring out, the people shout?
And did you hear that cheer on cheer
That over all the bells rang clear?

And did you see the waving flags,
The fluttering flags, the tattered flags—
Red, white, and blue—shot through and through,
Baptized in battle's deadly dew?

And did you hear the drums' gay beat,
The drums' gay beat, the bugles sweet,

HER HERO.

The cymbals' clash, the cannons' crash
That rent the sky with seam and gash?

And did you see me waiting there,
Just waiting there and watching there—
One little lass, amid the mass
That pressed to see the hero pass?

And did you see him riding down,
As riding down and smiling down,
With slowest pace and stately grace,
He caught the vision of a face—

My face uplifted, red and white,
Turned red and white with sheer delight
To meet his eyes, his smiling eyes,
Outflashing in their swift surprise?

Oh! did you see how swift it came,
How swift it came, like sudden flame,
That smile to me, to only me,
The little lass who blushed to see?

And at the windows all along
A lovely throng of faces fair
Beyond compare beamed down upon him riding
    there;
Each face was like a radiant gem,
A sparkling gem, and yet to them

No swift smile came,
No sudden glance took certain aim.
He turned away from all their grace,
From all their grace of perfect face;
He turned to me, to only me,
The little lass who blushed to see.

                      ANON.

BRITANNIA AND HER COLONIES.

BRITANNIA *in mourning: Attendant with cushion and crown.*

Brit. Weep with me, daughter, for our diadem shines dim through the mist of a nation's tears. The sceptre hath fallen from the kindliest hand that e'er swayed empire. A star hath set whose guiding ray shed light o'er the world's tempestuous sea; a voice is hushed that counselled "peace and good will" toward all the sons of men. Victoria, whose throne was every loyal heart, hath passed for ever from our yearning eyes, from war and weeping, to "heaven's perfect peace." Yet, ere she passed, she saw, athwart the cloud of war, the dawning of a glorious day, when all her children, ocean-severed, would muster to her aid, "and stand a wall of fire around their much-loved isle."

SCOTLAND, IRELAND, and WALES come forward and exhort Britannia to hold up her head again and think of the future.

Enter CANADA.

Can. O great sea-mother! from my prairies vast,
    From lonely forests ermined with the snow,
I come to do thee homage, who, though last,
    Shall mightier grow.   [*Take position.*

INDIA.

I who have read the wisdom of the seers,
    Where Himalayan ridges pierce the blue,
From plains and cities of two thousand years
    Bring greeting true.   [*Take position.*

SOUTH AFRICA.

My veldt late reeked with blood and bitterness;
    Now am I come to speak the heartfelt word
Of praise to her who heard my deep distress,
    And drew the sword.   [*Take position.*

New Zealand.

From island realms in fern and heather hid,
  From storm-scarred summits, frowning to the skies,
I come to greet my sister, and to bid
  Her star arise.   [*Take position.*

Britannia.

Let her approach, a virgin robed in white,
And let her handmaids gathered round her be,
That all to do her honour may delight,
And she be crowned supreme in all men's sight—
O'er the wide south—a queen, but not less free.

Enter Australia, *with one of her colonies on either side.*

Witness, my people, who are gathered round,
By love alone our mighty realms are bound;
Free-born was she, and before nations free
Shall she be crowned.

Australia *advances to throne.*

Brit. We come to crown thee, beautiful and brave
Child of the dawn on Southern seas that break
    On golden sands.
Alas! the shadow from that royal grave,
Where one who loved thee well her last rest takes.
Sister, thy sword flashed forth to guard her throne,
Thy tears are mingling with our own—
    Thy Queen's and ours!
It should have been her hand the golden circlet
    On thy brow to bind,
And send thee forth the youngest of her band,
Free and unfettered as the chainless wind,
Save but the tie which round thy heart she wove—
That one imperishable bond of love.

Sister, no mortal forecast can divine
What glories may await thee in God's plan,
What heights in future ages may be thine,
What bugle-note may call thee to the van;
O'er what wild skies the Southern Cross may ride
To unknown issues borne on time and tide.
But as the child remembers, so shalt thou
The empress-mother of these realms vast—
No duty left undone, no unkept vow,
Her hand upon the helm to the last!
Oh! many a star shall set, but hers
    Shall shine for aye;
Thy children's children rise and call her blessed.
    We crown thee now.

AUSTRALIA, after being crowned, goes in centre of her provinces, who kneel around her.

AUSTRALIA (*to her states*).

My states, by whose free will and toil-spent days
I stand a queen before you, hear my vow,
To wear this crown our great sea-mother lays
Upon my brow not vainly; nor with pride to overbear
    The weak, nor hold with careless hand the helm,
But to rule justly, without let or fear,
    This mighty realm.
The dawn is overpast—we stand upon
    The threshold of the morning and the year;
Down the white century where no feet have gone
    The path lies clear.
The scroll is blank before us; let us write
    Our words thereon in deeds of living fame:
Australia—freedom—in the whole world's sight
    Shall mean the same.
    Brit. Thou sayest well, my sister!

May all my children live in pulses stirred
    To generosity,
In deeds of daring rectitude, in scorn
For miserable aims that end with self ;
In thoughts sublime that pierce the night like stars,
And with their mild persistence urge man's search
    To vaster issues.
    [*Exeunt omnes, while choir sings* "*Rule Britannia.*"

THE LITTLE SCOTTISH MARTYRS.

A bonnie wee Scotch lassie, with rosy cheeks, sunny hair, laughing eyes, and bare brown feet, stood beside a brawling mountain stream. Poised on one foot, she touched the water lightly with the other.

"Eh, but it's cauld, an' it's deep. Will ye no lift me across, Sandy ?"

"No. If ye canna come yersel', ye maun jist gang hame."

"Weel, if I maun, I maun," and with a splash she bravely crossed the stream, and stood by her brother's side. "Eh, Sandy—look !"

"Wheest, Myzie, it's the sogers !"

Up the mountain pass came the glittering bayonets, and before the boy and girl could gain shelter they were surrounded by armed men.

"Dinna tell them onything. Be a brave lassie, Myzie."

"Here, boy ! has any one passed this way this morning ?"

"No mony folk pass this wiy."

"Perhaps not; but one has passed—not an hour ago. Do you know the man I speak of ?"

"What like was he ?"

"Do you know Robert Brock ?"

"I ken him for a guid man wha never did onybody herm."

"You saw him, then ?"

"Ay."

"Which road did he take?"

"What d'ye want him for?"

"To send a bullet through his head—as I'll send one through yours if you don't answer!"

"Ye can send a bullet through my heid gin ye like, but I'll no tell which wiy Robert Brock went."

"Ask the girl, captain; she'll tell fast enough."

"Dinna tell them, Myzie."

"Curse you, be quiet!" and a heavy hand fell with cruel force on his mouth.

"Now, girl, which way went this saintly man of God?"

"I canna tell."

"You will not, you mean. Did he take the right or the left road?"

"I canna tell."

"Then I must find some way to make you tell," and he caught her by the wrist, twisting it till she screamed with pain.

"Now, will you tell?"

"Let her be, ye black-herted cooard!"

"I'll let her be when she has answered my question.—Which way went Robert Brock?"

"I canna tell."

"Set her against that boulder. Present arms!—Now, for the last time, girl—which way went the godly Robert Brock?"

"I canna tell."

"Fire!"

A wreath of smoke curling upwards to the blue heaven, a mass of bright hair dabbled in blood, a wee white face on the green grass.

"Throw her into the stream!"

In a moment the pure water blushed in God's sunlight with the blood of one of His martyrs.

"Now, boy, which way went Robert Brock?"

"Ye hae killed my brave wee sister, an' noo ye can kill me."

"It's easy to talk of dying, boy."

"I wad raither dee wi' clean hauns than stain them wi' the bluid o' God's servant and leeve."

"We'll see.—Present arms!—For the first time—which way went Robert Brock?"

Steadfast and calm was the brave young face, silent the firm young lips.

"For the second time—which way went Robert Brock?"

He looked at the sunny sky, the smiling earth, the silvery stream murmuring o'er its rocky bed.

"For the last time—which way went Robert Brock?"

He heard the singing of the birds, and the approving voice of God in his brave young soul.

"Fire!"

Again the curling smoke, the bloodstained turf, the crimsoned water.

Down the mountain side pressed the soldiers on a bootless errand.

And God watched over the lonely resting-place of "The Little Scottish Martyrs."

ALPHABETICAL INDEX.

PROSE.

Babies, The	Mark Twain	365
Boat Race, The	O. W. Holmes	37
Caleb Plummer and his Blind Daughter	C. Dickens	43
Celebrated Jumping Frog, The	Mark Twain	459
Christmas Eve in a Belfry	L. Mosley	82
City by Night, A	T. Carlyle	71
Editha's Burglar	F. H. Burnett	453
Escape of Sir Arthur and Miss Wardour	Sir Walter Scott	56
European Guides	Mark Twain	370
General Wauchope, Death of	Letter	520
Houp-La	J. S. Winter	86
Irishman's Love for his Children, An	Anon	68
Jud. Brownin' on Rubenstein's Playing	M. Adams	362
Le Fevre, The Story of	L. Sterne	51
Little Lord Fauntleroy	F. H. Burnett	445
Marley's Ghost	C. Dickens	65
Mormons, The	Artemus Ward	457
Mother and her Dead Child, The	Hans Andersen	96
Noble Revenge, A	T. de Quincey	102
Old Parson Rayne	Geo. R. Sims	72
Old Scrooge	C. Dickens	62
One Niche the Highest	E. Burritt	93
Paul Dombey, The Death of	C. Dickens	39
President Garfield, The Death of	J. G. Blaine	49
Rapids, The	J. B. Gough	368
Reading, The Art of	Mrs. Ellis	21
Reading Aloud	R. Chambers	22
St. George, The	Scottish Annual	34
Scottish Martyrs, The Little	Anon	551
Three Cherry Stones, The	Anon	29
Three Parsons, The	Robert Overton	463
Vision of Mirza, The	Joseph Addison	24
Voyage, The	W. Irving	31
Wild Night at Sea, A	C. Dickens	60

ALPHABETICAL INDEX.

POETRY.

Abou Ben Adhem and the Angel	Leigh Hunt	533
Auctioneer's Gift, The	Anon	538
Baby in Church	Anon	535
Barbara Frietchie	J. G. Whittier	136
Battle of Blenheim, The	R. Southey	124
Becalmed	S. K. Cowan	160
Bells, The	E. A. Poe	207
Boys, The	O. W. Holmes	438
Bridge of Sighs, The	Hood	342
Can I Go Home?	Anon	534
Captain's Child, The	Mrs. Leeson	127
Catastrophe, A	P. Arkwright	118
Cato on the Immortality of the Soul	Joseph Addison	199
Charcoal Man, The	J. T. Trowbridge	113
Charles Edward on the Anniversary of Culloden	Aytoun	422
Child Christ, The	J. W. Riley	540
Child's Mirror, The	Anon	539
Coming	B. M	208
Cotter's Saturday Night, The	Robert Burns	414
Curfew must not ring to-night	Rose H. Thorpe	153
Dainty Little Lady	Anon	533
Dead Doll, The	American Magazine	323
Dimes and Dollars	Henry Mills	142
Dog and the Tramp, The	Eva Best	532
Dowie Dens o' Yarrow, The	Old Scottish Ballad	420
Drum, The	D. Jerrold's Magazine	129
Elegy written in a Country Churchyard	T. Gray	204
Elkano and the Widow	J. T. Trowbridge	143
Excelsior	H. W. Longfellow	134
Execution of Montrose, The	Aytoun	344
Falcon of Ser Federigo, The	H. W. Longfellow	183
Feast of all Nations, A	Anon	526
Field of Waterloo, The	Byron	347
Fireman's Wedding, The	W. E. Eaton	334
Fitz-James and Roderick Dhu	Sir Walter Scott	164
Gain of Giving, The	The Young Pilgrim	104
Gift of Tritemius, The	J. G. Whittier	107
Girls that are in Demand	Anon	425
Glove and the Lions, The	Leigh Hunt	119
Guilty, or not Guilty?	Anon	326
Her Hero	Anon	546
Horatius	Lord Macaulay	349
How he saved St. Michael's	M. A. P. Stansbury	426
If I could keep her so	Anon	529
Jack Chiddy	Alex. Anderson	332
Jamie Douglas	Scotch Ballad	522

ALPHABETICAL INDEX.

Jane Conquest	J. Milne	156
Karl the Martyr	Anon	338
King John and the Abbot of Canterbury	Old Ballad	109
King Robert of Sicily	H. W. Longfellow	188
King's Temple, The	Anon	105
Kitchen Clock, The	J. V. Cheney	441
Lady of Provence, The	Mrs. Hemans	162
Lapsus Linguæ, A	Anon	133
Leper, The	N. P. Willis	180
Little Help worth a Great Deal of Pity, A	A. H. Miles	108
Little Orphant Annie	J. W. Riley	439
Lochinvar	Sir Walter Scott	120
Maister and the Bairns, The	W. Thomson	413
Marjorie's Almanac	J. B. Aldrich	116
Marmion, The Death of	Sir Walter Scott	192
Mary, Queen of Scots	H. G. Bell	174
Maud Müller	J. G. Whittier	151
Me and Him	Anon	524
Measuring the Baby	E. A. Brown	135
Minute, The	Anon	525
Modest Wit, A	Anon	118
Moses, The Burial of	Mrs. Alexander	179
Mother's Answer, A	L. E. Barr	137
Mouse, The	Anon	322
"Nay; I'll stay with the Lad"	L. E. Barr	327
News-Boy's Debt, The	Harper's Magazine	131
Night before Christmas, The	C. S. Moore	114
Nottman	Alex. Anderson	329
Old Clock on the Stairs, The	H. W. Longfellow	203
Old Man Dreams, The	O. W. Holmes	437
Order for a Picture, An	A. M. Carey	544
Our Folks	Ethel Lynn	430
Owl Critic, The	Harper's Magazine	442
Papa's Letter	Anon	125
Perfect Faith, A	Anon	537
Pied Piper of Hamelin, The	Robert Browning	138
Psalm of Life, A	H. W. Longfellow	424
Raven, The	E. A. Poe	357
Ride of Jennie Macneal, The	Will Carleton	122
Robert of Lincoln	W. C. Bryant	112
Ruined Cottage, The	Mrs. Maclean	172
Scots wha hae	Robert Burns	419
Seven Ages, The	Shakespeare	198
Somebody's Mother	Anon	324
Story of a Faithful Soul, The	Adelaide Procter	530
Three Kingdoms, The	J. E. Bendall	542
To-morrow	N. Cotton	202

ALPHABETICAL INDEX.

Two Surprises.. *R. W. M'Alpine*..........541
Uncle, The... *H. G. Bell*..............432
Virginia.. *Lord Macaulay*..........353
Water-mill, The... *D. C. M'Callum*.........200
William Tell to his Native Mountains.............. *S. Knowles*..............196

DIALOGUES AND SCENES.

FROM

As You Like It.. *Shakespeare*...............277
Britannia and her Colonies.............................. *Anon*......................548
Canute and his Courtiers................................. *Barbauld*..................213
Cardinal Richelieu....................................... *Lord Lytton*...............481
Examination of Mr. Winkle and Sam Weller..... *C. Dickens*................372
Fortunes of Nigel, The.................................. *Sir Walter Scott*..........226
  (*King James and George Heriot.*)
Gaol Mouse, A.. *John Cox*.................219
Hamlet... *Shakespeare*...............261
  (*Hamlet and Horatio.*)
Hamlet... *Shakespeare*...............379
  (*Hamlet, Guildenstern, and Queen.*)
Hamlet... *Shakespeare*...............393
  (*The two Grave-diggers.*)
Hamlet... *Shakespeare*...............508
  (*Hamlet's Advice to the Players.*)
Hamlet... *Shakespeare*...............509
  (*Polonius's Advice to Laertes.*)
Hamlet... *Shakespeare*...............510
  (*Hamlet on a Future State.*)
Heart of Midlothian, The............................... *Sir Walter Scott*..........221
  (*1. Jeanie Deans and the Laird of Dumbiedykes; 2. Jeanie Deans and the Duke of Argyll; 3. Jeanie Deans and Queen Caroline.*)
Henry V.. *Shakespeare*...............253
  (*Henry and Katherine.*)
Henry VIII.. *Shakespeare*...............257
  (*Wolsey and his Secretary.*)
Hunchback, The... *Sheridan Knowles*.........471
  (*Helen and Modus.*)
Julius Cæsar.. *Shakespeare*...............387
  (*Brutus and Cassius.*)
Julius Cæsar.. *Shakespeare*...............511
  (*Cassius instigating Brutus.*)
Julius Cæsar.. *Shakespeare*...............512
  (*Brutus on the Death of Cæsar.*)

King John..Shakespeare.................246
                (*Arthur and Hubert.*)
King Louis the Eleventh ....*Delavigne*...................488
Love's Labour's Lost ....*Shakespeare*...............499
Macbeth ....*Shakespeare*...............384
                (*Murder of Duncan.*)
Macbeth ....*Shakespeare*...............506
                (*Sleep-walking Scene.*)
Merchant of Venice, The..............................*Shakespeare*...............265
                (*The Bond Scene.*)
Merchant of Venice, The..............................*Shakespeare*...............269
                (*The Trial Scene.*)
Merchant of Venice, The..............................*Shakespeare*...............391
                (*Shylock on Revenge.*)
Much Ado about Nothing..............................*Shakespeare*...............494
                (*Dogberry, Verges, and the Watch.*)
Old Lieutenant and his Son, The...................*Dr. Norman Macleod*....230
Pickwick Papers..*C. Dickens*...................466
                (*Mr. Pickwick and the Wellers.*)
Pygmalion and Galatea..................................*W. S. Gilbert*...............305
Richard III..*Shakespeare*...............255
                (*Clarence's Dream.*)
Rivals, The..*Sheridan*.....................243
                (*Mrs. Malaprop and Sir Anthony Absolute.*)
Rivals, The..*Sheridan*.....................396
                (*1. The Challenge; 2. The Duel.*)
Rob Roy...*Scott*..........................402
                (*The Tolbooth Scene.*)
Romeo and Juliet..*Shakespeare*...............250
                (*The Balcony Scene.*)
Sam Weller's Valentine.................................*C. Dickens*...................376
School for Scandal, The................................*Sheridan*.....................234
                (*Sir Peter and Lady Teazle.*)
School for Scandal, The................................*Sheridan*.....................239
                (*Charles Surface, Careless, "Mr. Premium," and Moses.*)
She Stoops to Conquer ....*Goldsmith*...................476
                (*Kate Hardcastle and Young Marlow.*)
Two Robbers, The ....*Barbauld*.....................214
William Tell ....*Sheridan Knowles*.........216
                (*Tell and Gesler.*)

SACRED.

All people that on earth do dwell ....*Psalm c.*.....................313
Comfort ye, comfort ye my people.................*Isaiah xl.*...................315
Extracts from "Eternal Hope"......................*Farrar*.......................513

Lead, kindly Light	*J. H. Newman*	319
Love one Another	*F. W. Robertson*	410
O God of Bethel	*Paraphrase ii*	312
Remember now thy Creator in the days of thy youth	*Eccles. xii.*	314
The Comforter	*H. Auber*	320
The Loneliness of Christ	*F. W. Robertson*	516
The Lord is my Shepherd	*Psalm xxiii*	314
The Parable of the Prodigal Son	*Luke xv.*	317
Though I speak with the tongues of men and of angels	*1 Cor. xiii.*	318

www.ingramcontent.com/pod-product-compliance
Lightning Source LLC
Chambersburg PA
CBHW031322230426
43670CB00006B/209